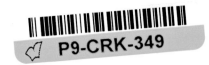
The Healthy Gluten-Free Life

Tammy Credicott

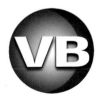

VICTORY BELT PUBLISHING INC.

Las Vegas

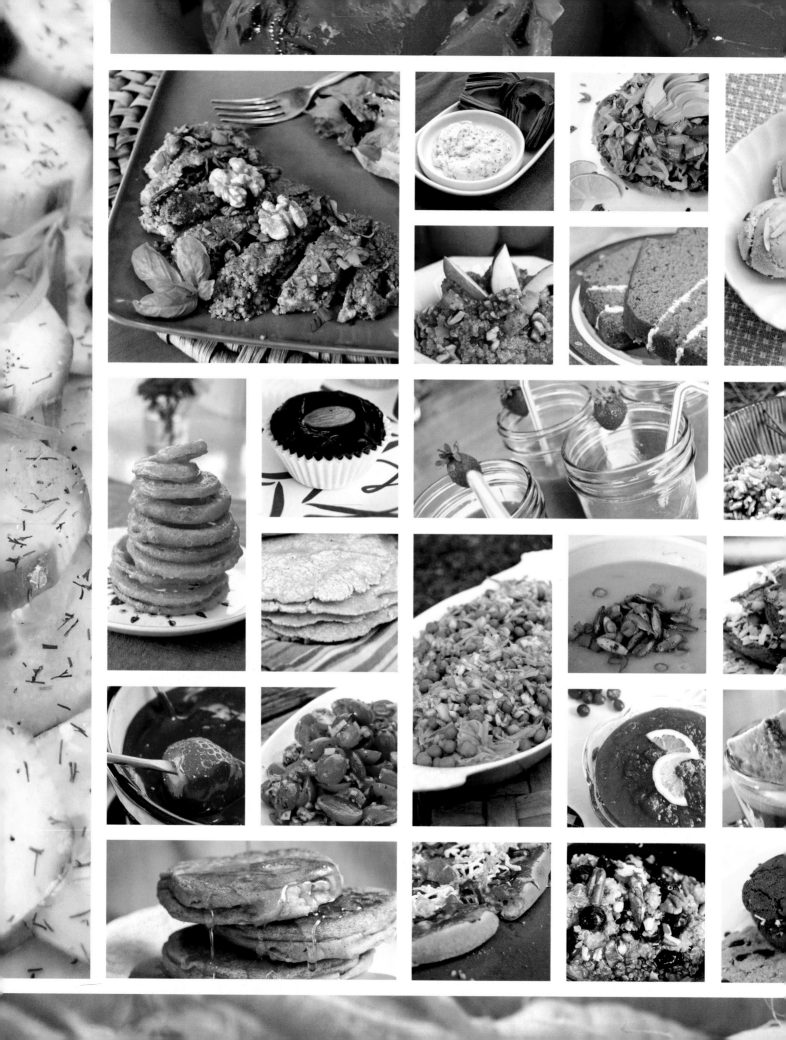

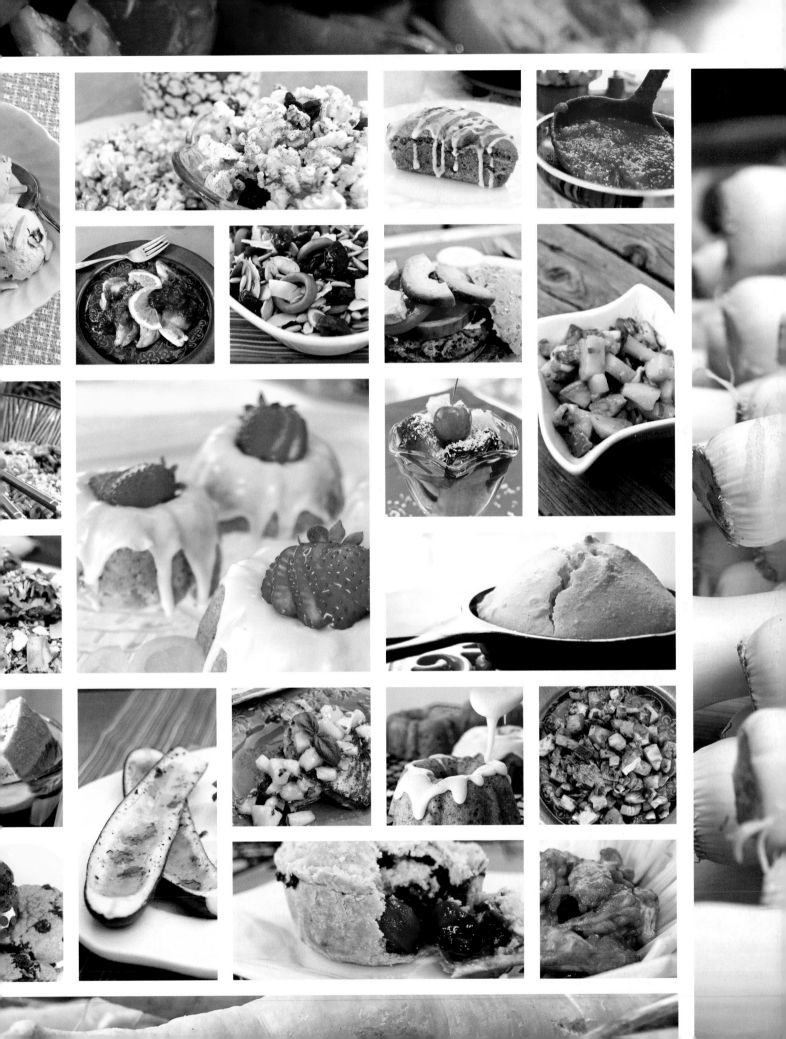

First Published in 2012 by Victory Belt Publishing Inc.

ISBN 13: 978-1-936608-71-3

Victory Belt ® is a registered trademark of Victory Belt Publishing Inc.
Printed in the USA
RRD 06-14

Table of Contents

7   Foreword

9   Acknowledgments

12   Preface

16   Introduction

20   A Word About "Healthy"

22   About the Book

25   Our Pantry and Resources for Products

27   Gluten-Free Flours and Starches

28   The Big Secret

29   Flour Substitutions

31   Natural Sweeteners

33   Oils and Fats

35   Dairy and Egg Substitutions

36   Eating Out and Cross Contamination

38   Tips For a Happier Kitchen

40   Make Ahead and Freeze

41   My Favorite Kitchen Tips

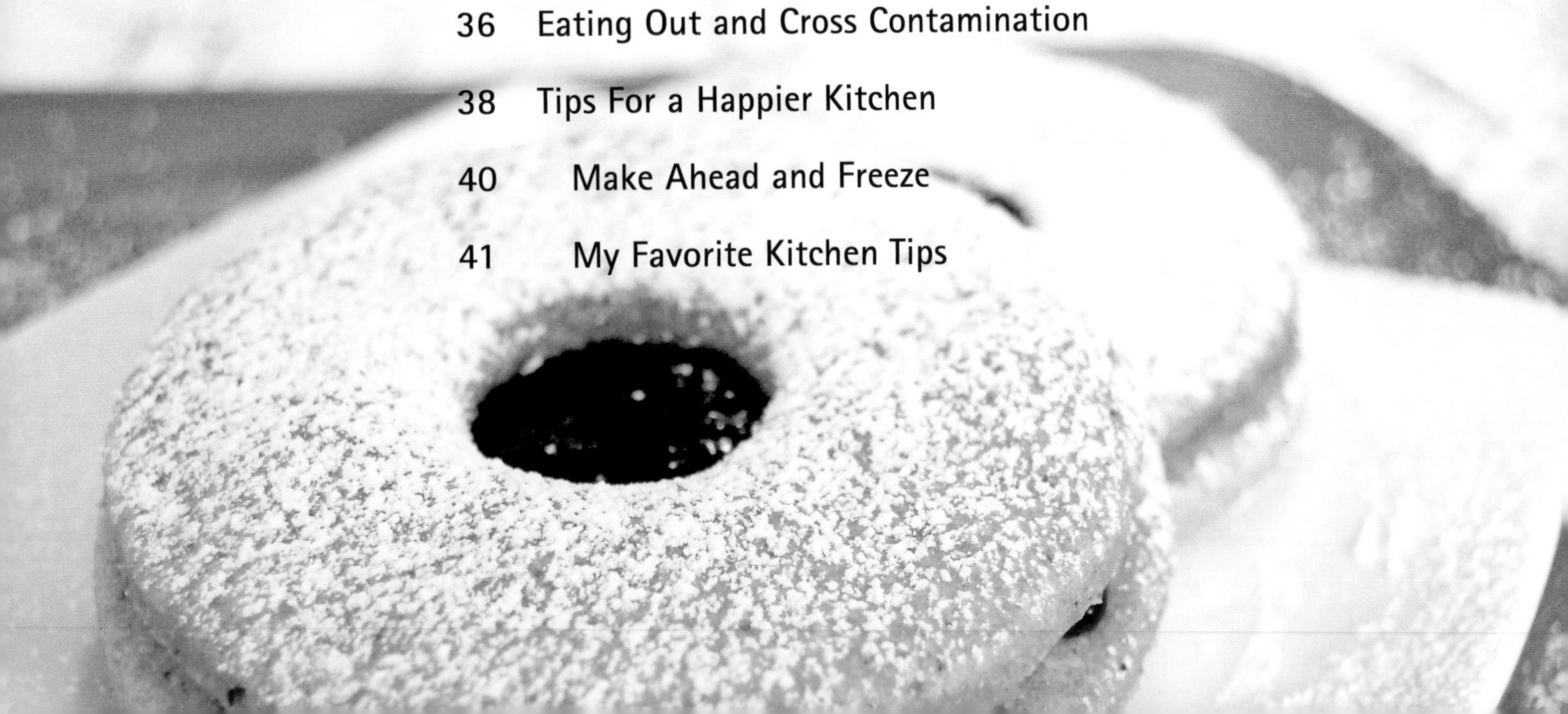

44   Recipes

46   Breakfasts

98   Entrées

200   Sides

246   Sauces / Rubs / Dressings / Misc.

272   Baking / Desserts / Snacks

394   Beverages

412 School Lunches

415 Ingredient Index

418 Recipe Index

426 Resource Index

428 Research Index

429 About the Author

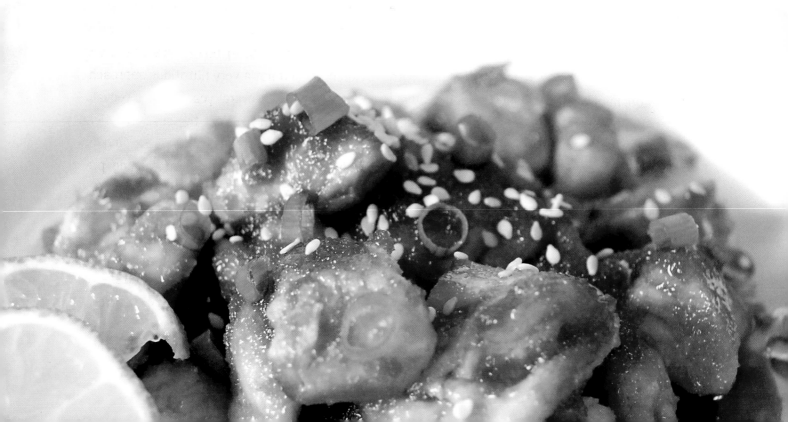

Foreword

By Nadine Grzeskowiak, the Gluten-Free RN

Food is powerful. It can be powerfully good in taste, texture, healthfulness, nutrition, and healing. Food is also powerful in an emotional sense. Close your eyes and think of food—what pops into your head? For many of us food is related to special people—like our grandmothers or an aunt that would spoil us with decadent confections we believed were somehow magical they tasted so good. Was your Uncle the go-to guy for the best barbeque chicken? Mine was. Food is associated with events like weddings, birthdays, Fourth of July BBQ picnics, and Sunday brunches. Gatherings, celebrations, family, and friends. The essence of our lives is in the food we eat.

I think back to all of my powerful associations with food and I get overwhelmed with emotion; happiness, fullness, love, and contentment. As a kid my life was *all* about food; hamburgers, ice cream, popcorn, hot dogs, roasts for Sunday dinners, lobster feasts on the back patio, popsicles, birthday cakes, penny candy from the neighborhood candy store, hot, fresh, homemade cookies and milk.

Even as I write this I am flooded with strong association and memories long put away in the deep sulci of my brain. Prior to finding out I am Celiac I would happily eat anything! I really believed I had an iron stomach. I am still sad I was brain fogged and delusional about food all those years. I just didn't know better; thankfully, now I do.

When I found out several years ago that I could no longer eat gluten my first response was—"What the heck is gluten?" When I found out gluten is wheat, barley, rye, and oats, I realized, *that's what I eat for breakfast, lunch, snacks, and dinner—followed by dessert.* What do I eat now? What else *was* there to eat? Panic set in.

What I started doing was simply replacing all my gluten-containing products with gluten-free products. This made sense to me at the time. What other options did I have? It didn't take long, however, to realize this was a very expensive and not a very nutritious approach.

For the past several years, I have reevaluated everything I eat. Is it the best food I can afford? Is it nutrient dense? Is it helping my body heal or is it hindering the healing process? Can I do better? Who can help me find answers to my questions?

Several years ago I met Tammy and have been blown away by her passion, determination, and creativeness in providing gluten-free food for her family. My initial exposure to Tammy's baking was in the form of an English muffin. Really? Gluten-free English muffins?

I'm from the East Coast so I thought, "Sure, I'll try your hockey puck." To my amazement that English muffin was amazing! Light, fluffy, with incredible texture and taste—not at all what I had learned to expect. "Bring me more!" I said enthusiastically with my mouth still full.

As I have talked with Tammy over the last few years, both of us have continued to evolve in our gluten-free eating and our lifestyles. She is the person I turn to regarding food questions, and concerns. It is fun to converse with Tammy regarding great tasting, gluten-free, dairy-free, and egg-free options for people of all ages.

You see, food *is* powerful, and hopefully powerfully good. For those of you new to the gluten-free lifestyle, learn from us. Tammy will help you avoid the pitfalls and obstacles as you start your own journey down a different food avenue. Read this book knowing the flours Tammy uses are *not* empty-calorie carbohydrates, but rather nutritionally dense. She has perfected each recipe to not only her high standards, but also to the high standards of her children. Every recipe has to pass the "kid test" in her own home.

Your life as you knew it is over as far as the food you used to consume. The thing you will miss the most is the convenience of picking up *anything* to eat. While that convenience is lost, you will gain your health, your brain, and—hopefully—a better life. It's worth it. Trust me, I am a nurse. I want you to feel better. Read Tammy's book and utilize her recipes. You will come to reconnect with food in a whole new way. Learn from her experiences and save yourself time, energy, and money in the long run. Cut to the chase and enjoy the new path you and your family are on. It is a great one!

Happy Cooking.
Happy Eating.
Happy Health.
Happy Life.
Bon Appétit!

Acknowledgments

First and foremost, a giant thank you to my husband, The Maniac. Had your immune system not turned on you, our kids would be sick and miserable, and I'd still be sitting in an office somewhere feeling unfulfilled and unmotivated. Without your unwavering support and motivation I would be an unhappy employee and not a struggling, stressed out, but very challenged, happy, and fulfilled entrepreneur. Thank you for always pushing and believing I could do more than I thought I was capable of. But mostly, thank you for being my husband and the most amazing father to our girls. I could have only dreamed you up, but somehow you came true.

Thank you to my two amazing, beautiful, funny, and perfect little people, Makenna and Rilee. You are the reason I smile, the reason I love, and the reason I exist. The joy you give my heart each time you smile and laugh can never be put into words. You are my favorite kitchen helpers and the best taste-testers any cook could ask for. Thank you for giving me the best job in the world—being your mom! I love you big baby and little baby (pronounced Elvis Style: "Bay-Beh")!

To my mom and dad for a lifetime of support in whatever I pursued. Thank you, Mom, for teaching me how to be a good mom, how to be patient, understanding, a good listener to my kids, and a supportive partner for my husband. You are an inspiration and I'm lucky to call you my mama. Thank you, Dad, for teaching me to camp, fish, and clean a trout. For teaching me I could do anything I wanted and achieve anything I set my mind to. Thank you for being a shining example of what to look for in a husband and partner and telling me to never settle. And for all of the sacrifices, night shifts, and long hours you worked to provide for your family, including selling your boat to pay for that last year of college. I still vow to buy you a boat someday!

To my sister for keeping me grounded and making me laugh at myself, even when I thought I was too cool to care. For inspiring me to be creative in the kitchen and for just being a great friend! And of course, a thank you to my "bother"-in-law, Tim, for making sure you expressed your opinion about some of my cooking experiments. And to my wonderful niece and nephew, who in my eyes will always be three and eight. So stop growing!

A big thank you to my mother- and father-in-law, Bill and Anne, for supporting all of our endeavors and for raising one amazing man whom I get to be married to! For that I will always be grateful. Even if your genes did pass along ADD and Celiac—but without which I never would have been able to write this book!

So again, thank you.

So many people have touched our lives and helped us in some way on our journey. I certainly travel in good company: My sis-in-law Misty, nephew Jake, my Aunt Harriette. And a special thank you to Erich Krauss and the Victory Belt Family, for listening to an idea and giving me the freedom and encouragement to run with it.

And a great big thank you to every customer of The Celiac Maniac who supported us from the first bite of that first English muffin; who tracked us down at farmers markets and showed up on our doorstep to buy a loaf of bread. You are the best, most loyal customers in the GF community!

I hope that this book provides you joy, comfort, a fully belly, a moment with your family, and perhaps a new keepsake recipe or two that you can pass on to your kids. My cherished recipes follow on these pages, and I'm so honored and excited to share them with all of you!

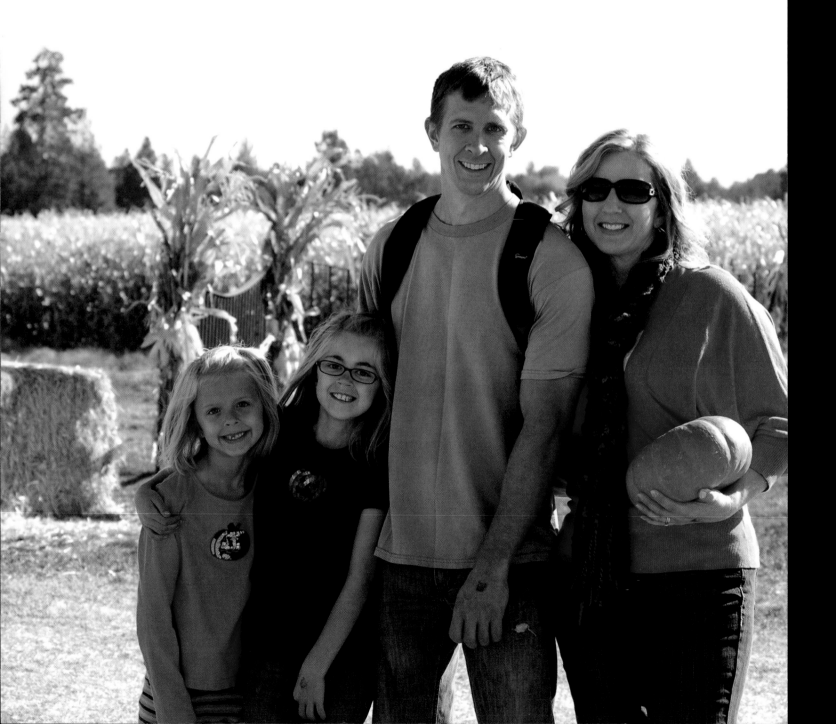

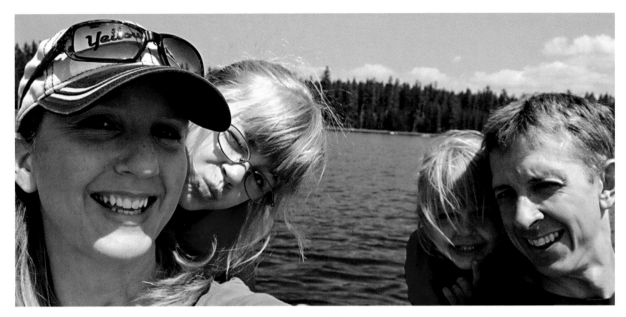

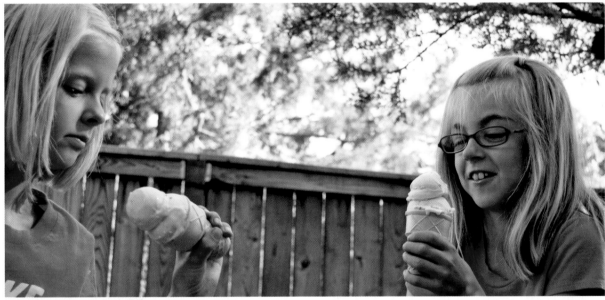

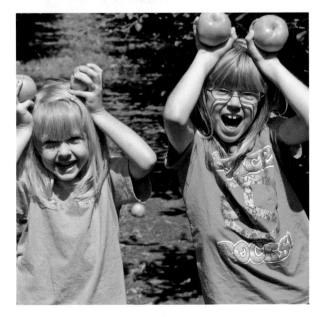

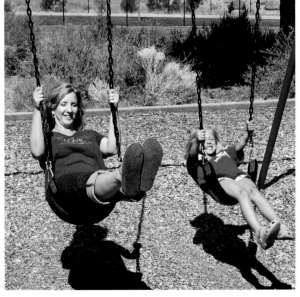

Preface

by Cain Credicott, "The Celiac Maniac"

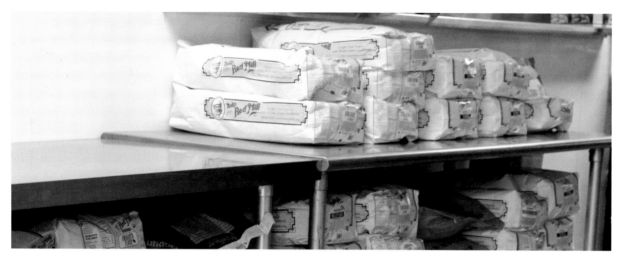

A few years ago, I was diagnosed with Celiac disease, as well as some pretty bad allergies to eggs and dairy. While initially it felt great getting that diagnosis and finally knowing what was wrong with me, that wonderful feeling quickly faded once I started to explore the gluten-free food options that were available at that time. Needless to say, I quickly started to worry about what I would actually be able to eat, and the depression began to settle in.

Like a lot of newly diagnosed individuals, I was disappointed time and time again at the gluten-free foods that I tried. Just about every single one was bland, dry, tasteless, and a pathetic attempt at recreating the "regular" version. There were several times that I figured I'd just have to suck it up and accept that these boring, flavorless foods were now my reality and what I would be eating from this point on. So much for actually enjoying my food.

It also didn't take me long to realize that the ingredient lists of just about every pack-

aged product started the same—white rice, tapioca or potato starch, and sugar. No wonder everything tasted the same, it was all made from the same ingredients! And what a pathetic line up of ingredients it was. How on earth was I supposed to heal my damaged gut when all of the gluten-free food I found was devoid of nutritional value? Short answer—I wasn't.

Fortunately for me, and now for you, my wife also recognized this, rolled up her sleeves, and started going crazy in the kitchen. In no time, Tammy was creating healthy, nutritious food that tasted absolutely amazing. It was a complete one-eighty from the other gluten-free foods I had been eating. These foods were moist, airy, flaky, and tasted just as good—if not better—than the "regular" foods I was used to. Not surprisingly, I wasn't the only one to think so.

In the spring after I was diagnosed, Tammy made some gluten-free, egg-free, dairy-free, soy-free, nut-free cookies for an event at our youngest daughter's preschool. The school

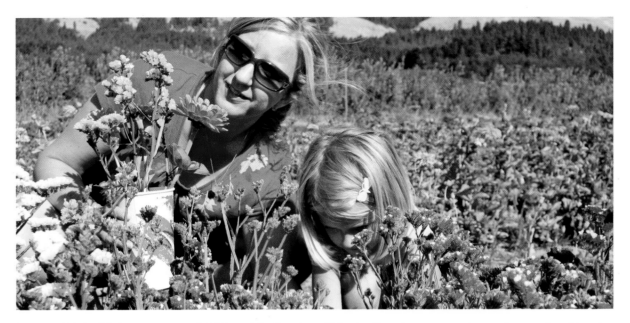

had a fairly high amount of kids with food issues, and she desperately wanted those kids to be able to enjoy a cookie. Apparently the kids did enjoy them, because the plate was empty when we left.

About a month later, my wife received a phone call from another mother at the school. The mom had spent some time tracking Tammy down to thank her for bringing something her own daughter could also enjoy. Normally her child was not able to participate in the same treats as the other kids, and it just about brought tears to her eyes that day when, because of the cookies Tammy made, she found that she could. She also told Tammy that her daughter liked the cookies so much, she wanted to buy some. With that, The Celiac Maniac bakery was born.

What started as a little gluten-free cookie production, selling frozen cookie doh-balls, quickly exploded into a full-blown wholesale bakery. Within months we were selling three different flavors of frozen cookie doh-balls, three different flavors of English muffins, pumpkin bread, banana bread, and pizza crust. Our products were quickly found in Whole Foods stores throughout the Northwest, local health food stores in Oregon and Washington, and local farmers markets, and we were shipping English muffins (our most popular product) all over the United States. We finally received so many requests from individuals for us to ship more stuff, we created some dry mixes—teff scones, pancakes, brownies, and batter mix. Those mixes were also incredibly well received and quickly found their way to store shelves and packages being shipped all over the country.

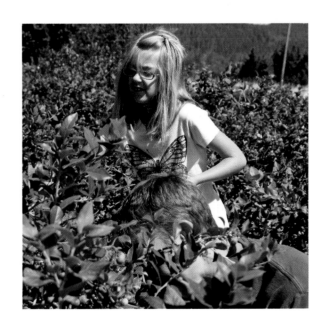

At events and product samplings, I would constantly hear the same three comments—"Wow, this doesn't taste gluten-free at all!" "I love that you're using different flours." "This tastes amazing!" It was an incredibly enjoyable time.

I spent most of my days selling and delivering the products to stores, speaking at local Gluten Intolerance Group meetings, hosting our booth at food fairs, and basically being the face of The Celiac Maniac. Because I was constantly out working to promote the bakery, people began to associate me as The Celiac Maniac. Tammy, however, was the real magic behind it all. She created every recipe, baked every product, and was the wizard behind the curtain. The secret to all her success was her two-pronged approach; every recipe had to be not only tasty, but also nutritious. She understood the fact that for someone with a damaged gut, it's critical to make every bite count and pack as much nutrition into each one as possible. She focused on flours and sweeteners that I had never heard of, determined to find a way to create healthy, gluten-

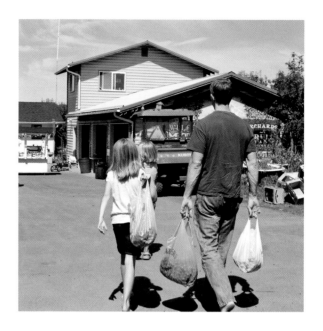

free, dairy-free, and egg-free options. People all over the country agreed—she was hitting the nail on the head.

But with stores constantly selling out of our products, there was no more opportunity for Tammy to be creative and come up with new recipes. She spent all of her time mass-producing our products. People were gobbling up everything we produced, and we were enjoying it, but we quickly realized we were not able to help as many people as we wanted to. It was a painful decision, but we finally decided to put the bakery on "pause" in order to focus on putting all of the knowledge and the recipes Tammy had made—and that people fell in love with—in a cookbook. This would enable her to reach far more people.

I hope you understand exactly what you're holding in your hand right now. This is not just another gluten-free cookbook. Not even close. It is the culmination of years of research, trial and error, and long hours standing over a hot oven. It's a labor of love. These recipes aren't starchy, white rice–filled sugar bombs with a pasty taste and color that

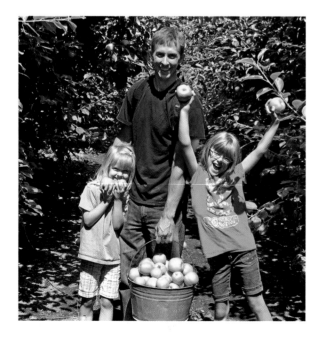

will shoot your blood sugar through the roof. They aren't reincarnations and reworks of the same old recipes you find in countless other books. Simply put, these recipes are some of the best I've ever seen, gluten-free or not, and I guarantee that thanks to this book, you'll be amazed at the gluten-free goodness you're pumping out of your very own kitchen. There's a reason why so many people fell in love with The Celiac Maniac—the recipes. And now you have those exact recipes here.

Thank you Tammy for realizing that you are, in fact, a magician in the kitchen. Thank you for recognizing the fact that you possess the amazing ability to take ingredients and create amazing-tasting food. Thank you for putting so much time, effort, and thought into creating recipes that I know will be loved by millions of people around the world. I know that you are amazing at what you do, and I can't tell you how happy it makes me knowing that now everyone else will know it too.

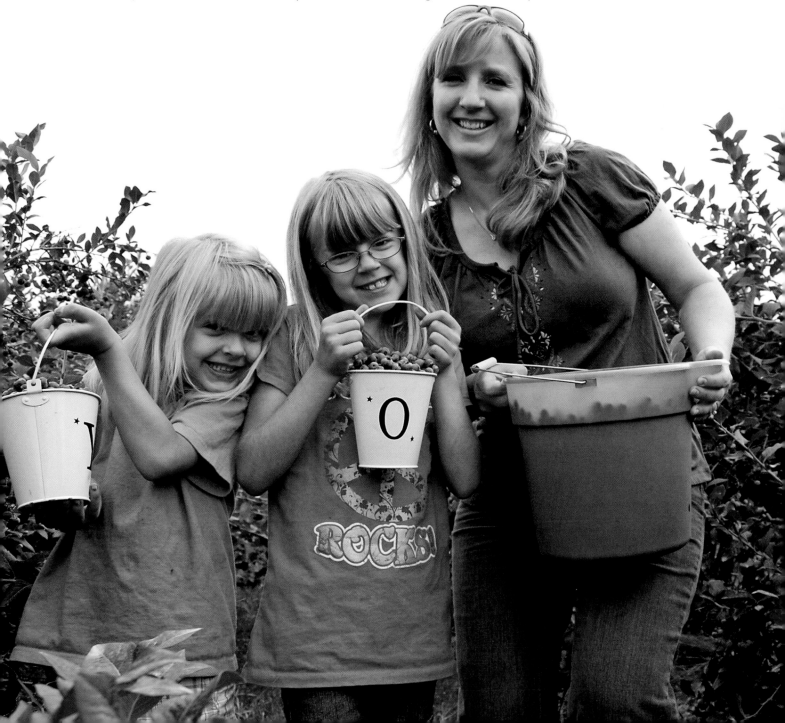

Introduction

My recent beginning:

My life got very complicated very quickly. A handful of years ago, the dynamic of my family life changed over the span of only a few months. Of course, now we recognize the signs that had been flashing by us for years, going unnoticed in our busy lives of full-time jobs and young kids.

In a five-month period my husband lost his job and was diagnosed with Celiac Disease (along with egg, dairy, and some random food intolerances), while my oldest daughter was having focusing problems in school, was diagnosed with ADD, and started a vision therapy program for some serious ocular issues. Meanwhile, my youngest suffered from dermatitis, severe dark circles under the eyes (anemia we are now convinced), and night terrors. Yep. Life was sunshine and rainbows.

I'm still not sure how we all survived that very stressful period. But we did survive and—I can honestly say now—thrived after the initial shock wore off. The rest of that year was spent trying to figure it all out. Why are the kids tired all the time? Are we sure it's ADD? Do we try Ritalin or natural methods? Why isn't the dermatitis going away? Why does she whine and cry all the time? And the big question—what the heck are we going to eat now?

The first few weeks after the celiac diagnosis, my husband went into overdrive, devouring as much information as he could to learn about the disease, how to heal, and what to eat. I cried. I cried because I felt helpless, and I cried mostly because I couldn't bake anymore.

After a time though, my genetics kicked in and my determination took over. I may wallow for a while, but it's never long lived, and I always come out the other side motivated and ready to move forward.

My husband's Tasmanian devil approach to learning about celiac earned him the name "The Maniac." He was definitely maniacal in his methods for acquiring and processing information! I soon realized the only way for us to live our best life was to face this head on, and I felt it was my job to make sure my family ate well and received as much nourishment as possible, both from food and from our family dynamic. I refused to have mealtime be something we avoided. Consuming meals together brings families closer. It can be a midweek meal or a celebration—either way, food is a big part of our lives.

But I knew after a week of trying to prepare separate meals for The Maniac, the kids, and myself that there were going to be issues with cross contamination. Pasta sticks to the strainer, it's impossible to clean every crumb off of the counter, and have you ever looked in a tub of butter or a jar of jelly? Crumbs everywhere! No. I knew that to keep The Maniac safe we'd all have to go gluten-free. This decision was made easier by the fact that we were now convinced that our kids had food allergies as well. Everywhere we researched was another connection between gluten, casein, artificial colors, nuts, etcetera, and the ailments of my husband and kids. It didn't take long to start

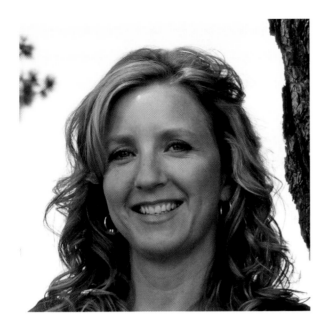

connecting the dots. Dermatitis? Food allergy. Night terrors? Food allergy. ADD? Food related. Aha! Throw in a light bulb moment of family genetics and we had ourselves an epiphany!

But what about me? I didn't have a food issue, I was sure of it! But a week after going gluten-free I had a headache nonstop, my stomach hurt, I was shaky, and not in the best mood. So I had a giant soft pretzel and I felt better within minutes. Great even! That's when I knew I had been having withdrawals. Gluten was my drug and I was detoxing. The funny thing about food issues, when you start to eliminate possible offending foods, the changes can be subtle to the point of unnoticeable. It's when you reintroduce a problem food that I think the true reaction becomes visible. I especially notice it with my kids.

Yes, the decision was made; we were in this thing together.

Now to just put it all into practice. But how? I was pretty sure at this point that my cooking would consist of air and water since everything else was off limits. Now it was my turn to be fanatical about researching gluten-free food, especially baking, every chance I had.

I was determined to bake again. And in time, I did! Not only was I baking, I was really enjoying gluten-free baking. It was like a puzzle, trying to figure out which ingredients worked well together and which ones didn't. I discovered that gluten-free baking was much more exciting and adventurous than traditional baking. There was a world of nutrient-dense flours out there to experiment with. Now I had choices! And every combination of flours turned out something just a little different, so I had the utmost control in what the finished product was like. I was crazy with power, and baked goods! So I started having other people try my results, and the response was overwhelming.

The bakery and our passion for wanting to help others deal with food-related issues started with taking cookies and snacks to my kids schools, so that any child with a food allergy could enjoy the same foods as their classmates and be safe. Pretty soon I had moms asking for recipes and wanting to buy cookies from me! It was then that I saw a need for quality, tasty foods that kids actually enjoyed and parents didn't mind providing.

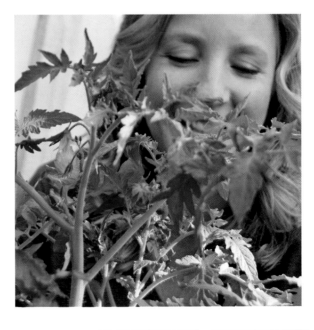

I knew I wanted to help more people, to provide something that made their lives a little better, a little easier. So The Celiac Maniac wholesale bakery was born, with a concept of producing frozen baked goods and doughs that people could thaw and eat or bake and eat. In about eighteen months we sold more than 30,000 English muffins and 10,000 cookie doh-balls. And in keeping with my mission of helping and reaching as many people as possible, I now share these recipes with all of you. Make them with your kids, your spouse, your mom, whoever! Just make them and enjoy the feeling of being in control of your life and your family's health. It's a big responsibility and I'd like to help.

The Very Beginning

I started baking at a young age. I remember many Sunday afternoons standing in our kitchen helping my mom scoop, mix, and stir our way to delicious peanut butter cookies, chocolate chip cookies, or maybe a peach cobbler.

In junior high school, I finally got to take a home-ec class! I had waited and looked forward to that class for years. Finally I was able to make and bake yummy goodies—at school. I was in heaven learning how to make biscuits, bread, and pies. Baking was my new obsession.

By high school, my mom surrendered her cookie baking duties to me as she said my big soft chewy cookies were better than her "hockey puck, burnt-bottom cookies." (Her words, not mine.) Aww, thanks, Mom! Coming from such a great cook, that was a huge compliment.

For a decade plus after that, I planned and schemed on different ideas for a bakery busi-

ness. My biggest hurdle seemed to be that I was not a morning person and bakeries had to start really, really early. I decided to keep thinking on that. So I continued to bake, mainly because I wanted to eat what I made. In college, some of my favorite evenings were spent making cookie dough with my roommate out of the few ingredients in our pantry—flour, sugar, eggs, and chocolate chips—and then talking for hours as we ate the dough by the spoonful. Apparently, someone forgot to tell me about the freshman fifteen.

After getting married to The Maniac, we tackled cooking and menu ideas together, always trying to keep things budget friendly and as healthy as we could. We did the same when we collectively decided to go gluten-free.

My cooking and baking in the gluten-free realm has been a result of trial and error, family memories, and lots of cravings! I'm a self-taught home cook who loves good food, and even more, loves food that is good for us. I'm not a chef, I've never been to culinary school, and I'm not a nutritionist. And while I've never received formal training, what I have done is conquer my fear of cooking and baking without

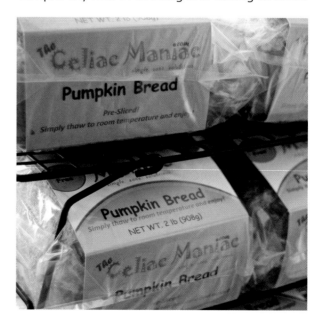

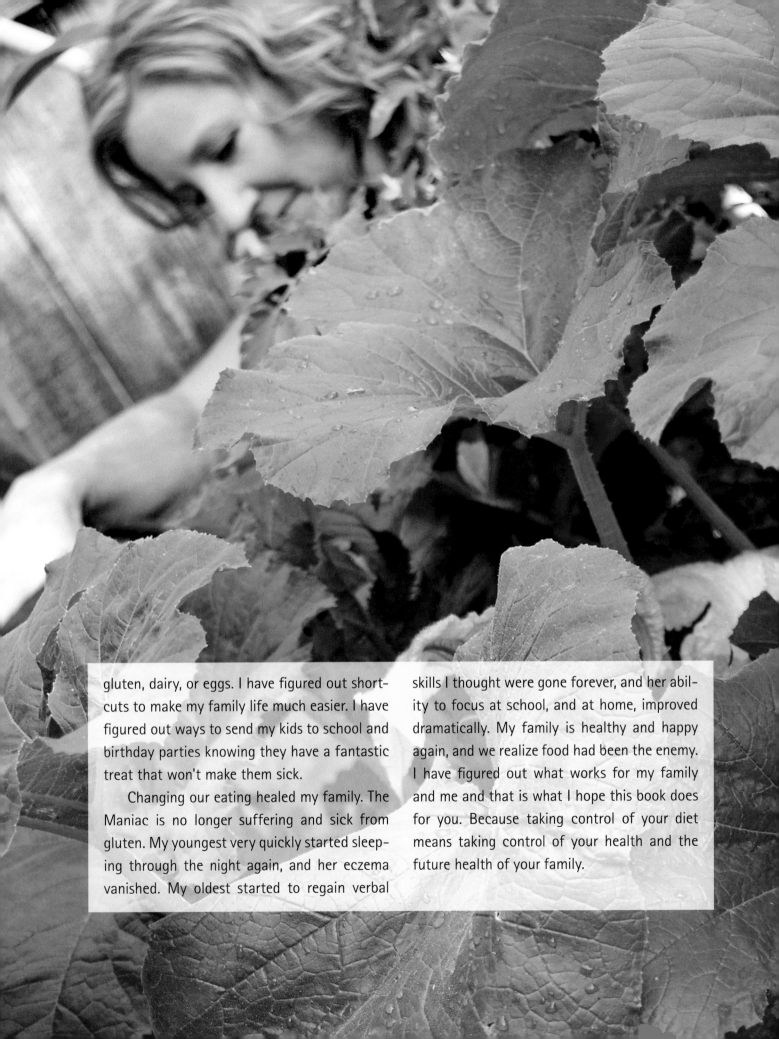

gluten, dairy, or eggs. I have figured out short-cuts to make my family life much easier. I have figured out ways to send my kids to school and birthday parties knowing they have a fantastic treat that won't make them sick.

Changing our eating healed my family. The Maniac is no longer suffering and sick from gluten. My youngest very quickly started sleeping through the night again, and her eczema vanished. My oldest started to regain verbal skills I thought were gone forever, and her ability to focus at school, and at home, improved dramatically. My family is healthy and happy again, and we realize food had been the enemy. I have figured out what works for my family and me and that is what I hope this book does for you. Because taking control of your diet means taking control of your health and the future health of your family.

A Word About "Healthy"

There are definitely recipes in this book that some may question as healthy. Is a chocolate chip cookie made with real brown sugar healthy? No, not if you eat an entire batch every week. But if you make it on a rainy Sunday with your kids and you enjoy a couple of cookies with them, yes. Very much yes! That is a healthy moment.

To me, "healthy" is all encompassing, not just low calorie. It means balance and moderation. It means having hot chocolate that I make from scratch so there are no trans fats or chemicals. It means making my own graham crackers and marshmallows once every summer so my kids can marvel in the joy of s'mores while we camp, without costing me $30 at the health food store and causing major stress on us and our finances. It also means having a fish fry or beer-battered onion rings with a homemade hamburger once in a while so my husband doesn't get sick from a careless chef at a restaurant.

Health is all of these things and how they play into your day-to-day life. So do we eat fried onion rings? Yes, sometimes. Do we eat them twice a week? Goodness no! Be mindful of indulgences, and don't make them an everyday occurrence. But do make your life enjoyable and less stressful by overseeing the food that your family consumes. Having the confidence and authority over your family's groceries, and therefore health, results in

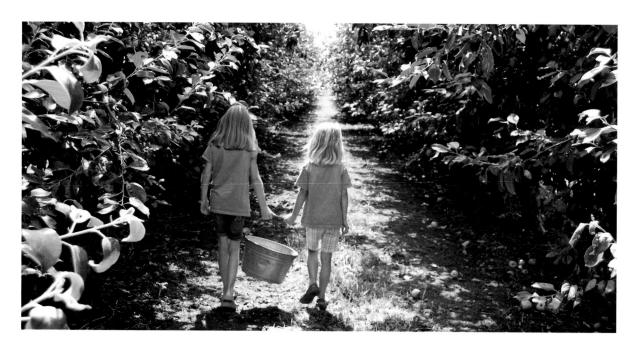

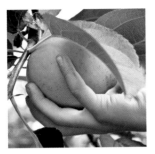
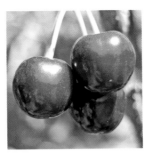

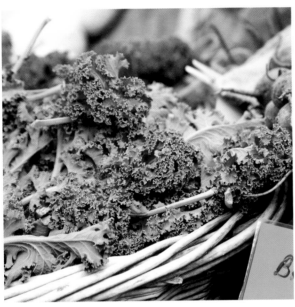

but nothing is added back. Nothing. You are eating straight carbs, which elevate blood sugar and wreak havoc on your body. Getting a gluten intolerance or celiac diagnosis should be a wakeup call. Your body is trying to tell you that it can't handle the bad stuff anymore and to clean things

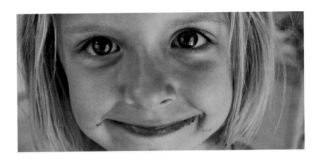

up. Your goal after going gluten-free should be to make every bite count, not to spend your time trying to replace all of the unhealthy foods you ate before going gluten-free.

Is it really necessary to have the same donut? I'm going to say no. Now, is it necessary to make a delicious but as-healthy-as-you-can birthday cake? You betcha. Family traditions are very important and only happen occasionally. A donut with your coffee every morning? Not so much.

As much as the media would like to convince you, the world of gluten-free isn't inherently healthy, but natural gluten-free foods generally are (meat, veggies, fruit, nuts, seeds). Gluten-free isn't the miracle cure, but it is on the "path" to a healthier you. And while this book is not entirely free of sugar and starch, it is limited, so I call it a rest-stop along the path to better health. I call my cookbook a transitional tool for those taking a step away from a "Gluten-Free—Standard American Diet" into "the healthy gluten-free life." This journey to health and good eating is transitional and incremental; *The Healthy Gluten-Free Life* is another stair step in the right direction!

happier tummies and less worry on you. And that will benefit your health just as much as a carrot stick!

This book and my recipes were created as part of a journey to good health. I see a lot of people who find out they have gluten issues go from eating a nutritionally empty Standard American Diet to eating a nutritionally empty gluten-free diet. If your doctor tells you not to eat white processed foods before celiac, why on earth would you eat white processed foods after being diagnosed? You can eat just as badly on a gluten-free diet as you did before, and in many cases, worse.

Although the white pasta and bread you had before going gluten-free had the nutrients stripped out, at least they were added back in (enriched). When you eat all of the wonderful GF products on the store shelves made primarily with white rice flour, sugar, and potato starch, guess what? It's stripped of all nutritional value,

About the Book

My Kitchen Philosophy

My kitchen philosophy is simple, real, budget friendly, efficient, and family friendly. When it comes to the meals in this book, real food is at the heart of the recipes. I don't make a lot of fuss with most meals because I want to spend time with my family after school and on the weekends. I like to premake everything I can to help with efficiency. I premake sauces and stocks, and I even freeze meats along with the marinade so I can just thaw and cook! For this reason I've included many make-ahead meals and tips on saving time.

My view of recipes is that they give me great ideas to play with. So please, use my recipes as a base—a jumping-off point to create your own meals and your own flavors. Get creative! Find inspiration in other cookbooks and on the Internet. I always tell people to not re-create the wheel here. People have been gluten-free for years, so search the Internet and look for ideas. Take regular recipes and ask yourself what you can change to make them allergy friendly. Yes, maybe you can't make the gluten-filled crust, but the seasonings and sauce may work wonderfully!

My approach to baking is to make tasty, texturally pleasing treats as healthy as I can. Sometimes that means I reduce the sugar drastically; sometimes I replace it altogether, depending what the final result will taste like. If no one will eat it, then it wasn't worth the time or ingredients. On the other hand, most traditional baking recipes call for way more sugar than is really needed. And the trend with gluten-free baking isn't much better. Lots of sugar and lots of starches are what everyone thinks they need to make food taste good. Not so.

When it comes to gluten-free flours, there is a reason most cookbooks and recipe sites use an all-purpose flour blend. It's easy, and a bit of a crutch. Knowing that a cookie has a different texture than a cupcake, and then altering your recipes to reflect that difference is challenging. Mixing a large amount of starches with white rice flour, and then using it to replace wheat flour in every recipe, seems easier—except in most instances it isn't the same, and now you've wasted a lot of flour and money on a concoction you won't use again.

The fact is you can't replicate wheat flour exactly, no matter how hard you try. All-purpose flour mixes are not consistent with all recipes, so you're left with the unpredictable, inedible results and the price tag. The only time you can fudge this outcome is if you're using lots of butter and eggs in your baking. Once you take those tried-and-true methods out of the picture, your façade of great taste and texture fades away.

But don't worry, I have done all of the trial and error work for you! In each recipe, I've created a balance between flour and starch that is tasty and nutritious. No all-purpose flour mix here. For cookies, the ratio has more flour and less starch because you don't need the rise or the super-chewy factor. For cakes, the ratio is about half flour and half starch due to the need for rise and a lighter texture. For yeast breads, the ratio has less flour and more starch and xanthan gum, which provides the stretch and chew we desire when eating a nice piece of French bread. This is one reason why yeast breads should be a rare treat, not an every-meal accompaniment.

Recipe Format

I have a method to my madness, really. I don't like recipes that give ingredients out of order. Especially in baking, you almost always combine dry ingredients, combine wet ingredients, and then add the two together. As a result, this is how I listed the ingredients in the recipes. Logically.

So for example, in a cookie recipe you may see organic evaporated cane juice under wet ingredients, even though it's dry, but this is because it is creamed with coconut oil or nondairy butter, which is part of the wet ingredient process. You still with me? Basically, I've grouped ingredients where they belong so recipes make sense while you're making them and you don't get lost. Trust me, you'll thank me later.

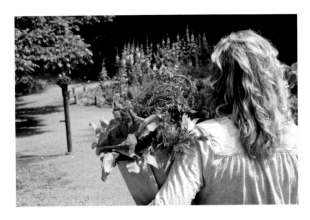

Nutrition Info

I didn't include nutritional information because I'm not a dietician or nutritionist. This is not my area of expertise, and it would be irresponsible for me to try and provide that information without the background to do it properly. That said, I do believe that foods should be enjoyed in moderation. If you're really concerned about the fat grams of a food or meal, then you probably shouldn't be eating it in the first place, or you should be eating a very small amount. Do you worry about the calories in a carrot stick? A treat is a treat and should be handled as such. We are not baking broccoli, we are creating the occasional indulgence.

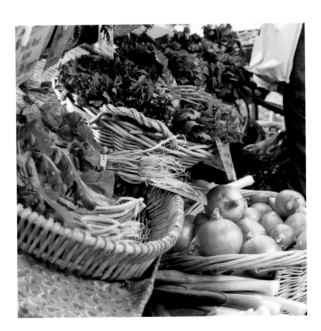

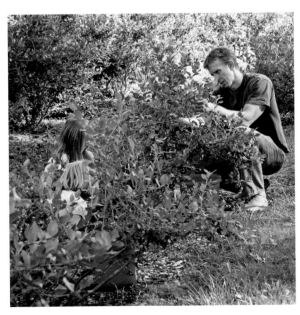

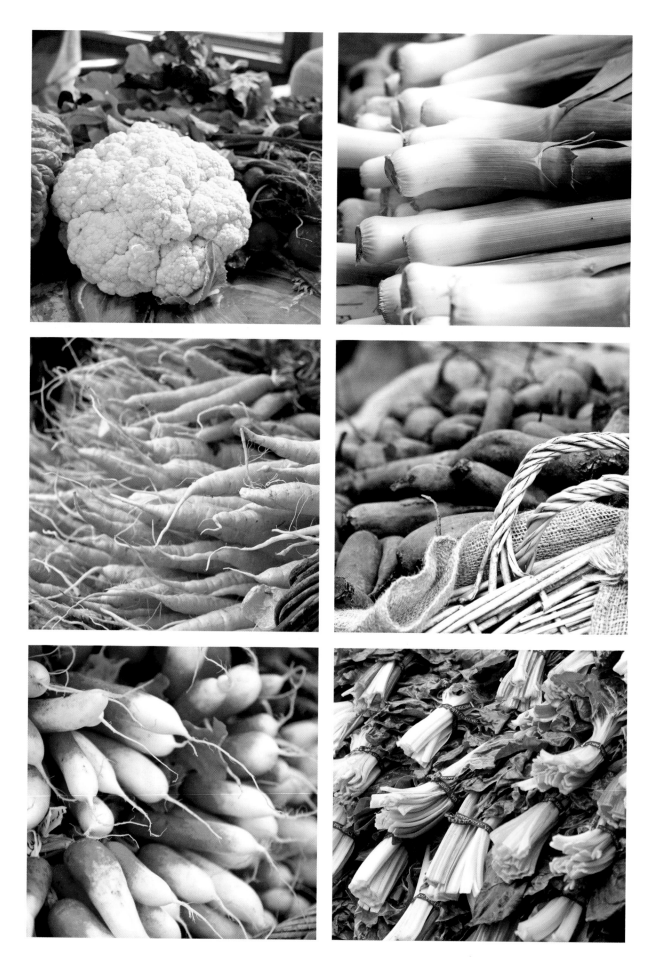

24   About the Book

Our Pantry and Resources for Products

With all the recipes and my ingredient recommendations, always assume they are organic and as close to unprocessed as possible. Always try to get ingredients that are close to their original state. And please do not use imitation vanilla flavoring, as it is simply chemicals made to taste like vanilla. Buy pure vanilla extract every time. I know organic can be spendy, so if needed, cut a corner or two on produce that contains less harmful pesticides, otherwise known as the Clean 15 list by the Environmental Working Group. But always buy organic for the produce that contains the highest levels, The Dirty Dozen.

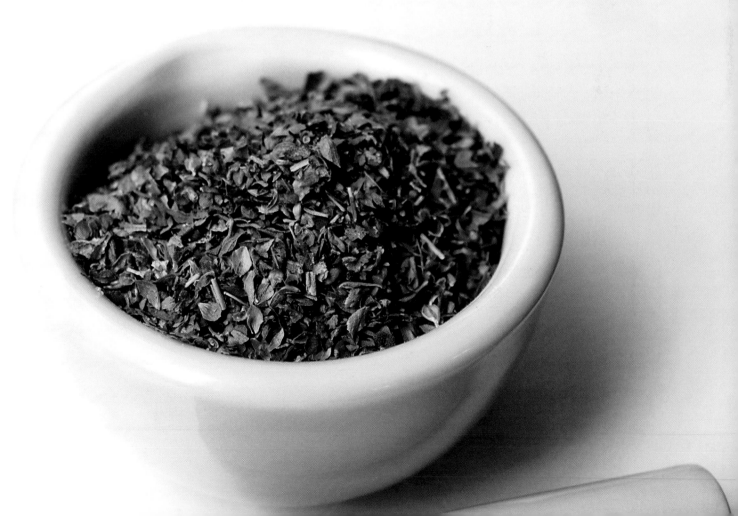

EWG's Shopper's Guide to Pesticides in Produce

Dirty Dozen Buy these organic	Clean 15 Lowest in Pesticide
1 Apples	1 Onions
2 Celery	2 Sweet corn
3 Strawberries	3 Pineapples
4 Peaches	4 Avocado
5 Spinach	5 Asparagus
6 Nectarines – imported	6 Sweet peas
7 Grapes – imported	7 Mangoes
8 Sweet bell peppers	8 Eggplant
9 Potatoes	9 Cantaloupe – domestic
10 Blueberries – domestic	10 Kiwi
11 Lettuce	11 Cabbage
12 Kale/collard greens	12 Watermelon
	13 Sweet potatoes
	14 Grapefruit
	15 Mushrooms

Our Pantry and Resources for Products

Gluten-Free Flours and Starches

In GF baking, if there is only one flour, it almost always overpowers the taste of the whole dish. A blend of flours balances flavor and texture, giving a more pleasing, neutral taste, while still maintaining nutrition.

Therefore, a lot of my recipes call for two (sometimes three) flours, plus starches. While at first glance this may seem like too much trouble, it's not when you consider how many recipes you've tossed because of graininess and bad taste. The recipes included are wholesome, filling, and taste great because of flour blending. But I always recommend playing with recipes, so please feel free to substitute your own flours of choice and see if you like it! Maybe you love the taste, texture, and ease of only using brown rice flour in certain baked goods, so give it try and do what works for you. Below, I've provided some information on a few of my favorite flours, and a couple of my not so favorite.

Teff

A staple in the Ethiopian diet, teff is the smallest grain in the world. Nutritional info: 14% protein, 78% carbs, and 8% fat. Teff is an excellent source of essential amino acids, especially lysine, which is usually deficient in most grains. It contains more lysine than barley, millet, and wheat, but not quite as much as rice or oats, and it is an excellent source of fiber, iron, calcium, and potassium. Teff contains a good amount of phosphorus, magnesium, aluminum, copper, zinc, boron, and thiamin, making it a great choice for gluten-free baking.

Sorghum

Labeled as the third most important cereal crop in the United States (between wheat and corn) and the fifth most important in the world, sorghum may have unique health benefits due to high antioxidant levels. The sorghum wax surrounding the grain may be beneficial to heart health, and according to the Whole Grains Council (www.wholegrainscouncil.org), sorghum may inhibit tumor growth and certain varieties may protect against diabetes and insulin resistance. And since it is also a rich source of phytochemicals, sorghum may help manage cholesterol. Sorghum provides a great texture in gluten-free baking without being heavy or grainy, plus its flavor is fairly neutral.

Amaranth

Amaranth contains about 30% more protein than cereals like rice and sorghum. It is a good source of lysine, fiber, iron, magnesium, phosphorus, copper, and manganese, but it is not a complete source of essential amino acids. It can be strong in flavor if used alone, but gives a great nutritional boost and nice flavor to baked goods in small amounts.

Brown Rice Vs. White Rice

The milling and polishing that converts brown rice into white rice destroys:

- 67% of the Vitamin B3
- 80% of the Vitamin B1
- 90% of the Vitamin B6
- Half the Manganese
- Half the Phosphorus
- 60% of the Iron
- All of the fiber and EFAs

Again, white rice flour is stripped of almost all nutrients, but none are added back in by being "enriched" the way white flour (wheat flour) products are. If we've always known that enriched wheat products were heavily processed and not good for us, and we were supposed to be consuming whole grains instead, why would anyone on a gluten-free diet consume 99% of their grains from white rice flour? This simply illustrates how bad most processed gluten-free products are on the supermarket shelves, since they are basically worse than the worst gluten-filled processed junk. We have a very long way to go to make manufacturers aware that they need to improve their products. Simply being gluten-free is not good enough, and we all should be demanding higher-quality products.

Soy

Soy is another hotly debated topic, but with risk factors including elevated hormone levels, it's just not worth it for me. Animal studies suggest that eating large amounts of soy can have potential harmful effects on female fertility and reproductive development.[1, 2] Studies also suggest a high soy intake is associated with a low sperm count.[3] Another study suggests that soy-based supplements might affect the efficacy of breast cancer treatment with aromatase inhibitors.[4] When all of this is coupled with the fact that soy is highly allergenic, I don't use it in any form, except for the occasional fermented GF soy sauce or Bragg liquid aminos.

Oats

Whether oats are safe for those sensitive to gluten remains undecided. But since it is the only grain that is limited in consumption quantity by gluten intolerance groups and several doctors, I don't feel comfortable using oats, even certified gluten-free oats. A study has shown that oats are not safe for all patients with celiac disease, and that some of the patients with celiac disease had the same molecular reaction to oats that other patients had to wheat, barley, or rye.[5] Be careful when deciding to consume oats, and if you do, make sure they come from a quality source and are certified gluten-free.

The Big Secret

Now, I'm going to let you in on a *big* secret that no one tells you in any of the GF forums or books . . . *flours and starches are not the same thing!* Everyone talks about the ratio of flours in a recipe, and they include starches in that equation. This causes unnecessary confusion for people and prevents them from learning. Whole-grain, gluten-free flours are heavier, denser, and more nutrient rich because they are the grain ground into powder. But starches, like potato and tapioca, are the actual starches of those roots, extracted, dehydrated, and then ground. It's not the whole plant. Flours give a recipe its core structure and create the consistency of the dish. Starches are accessories that add lift, body, and chew. Flour is flour, starch is starch. Once you understand that any gluten-free baking recipe needs to be a combination of some flour and some starch, you are on your way to great gluten-free baked goods!

Ready for another secret no one tells you in the gluten-free community? Potato starch and tapioca starch are not the same and cannot be used interchangeably. Shocking, I know. I mean, how many gluten-free cookbooks have you read that state you can substitute one for the other? I'm here to tell you, don't do that, because you will have a gummy mess if using tapioca alone and a fairly dry, crumbly result if using potato starch alone.

Potato starch tends to add lift and lightness, but will dry baked goods faster than tapioca. Tapioca adds a little lift, good chew, and a nice crumb, but tends to be more "wet" than potato. That's why if you use all tapioca in a recipe, you get a denser, almost wet and gummy product. A good rule of thumb is to start with half potato and half tapioca. I make adjustments depending on the final result I want. For example, if I wanted to make a more delicate sugar cookie, for the starches I would use a little more potato than tapioca. This is because while I want lighter and tender (potato), I don't want heavy and chewy (tapioca). If that recipe was for a chocolate chip cookie, I'd use half potato and half tapioca because I want it chewier.

You will also notice that I don't do percentages or ratios for flours because I generally don't care to break out my scientific calculator while baking a cookie. Too complicated! Now, I'm going to fill you in on a little trick that works almost flawlessly. If you're trying to convert a non-gluten-free baking recipe to gluten-free (as long as it's not primarily made of eggs, like a quiche or soufflé), *take the amount of wheat flour called for in the recipe and divide it in half. The first half will be made up of one or two gluten-free flours you choose, and the other half will be starches.*

So, for example, a recipe calls for 2 C regular wheat flour. I would use 1 C of flours (maybe ½ C sorghum and ½ C teff) and then 1 C starches (maybe ½ C potato and ½ C tapioca). Starting a recipe with half flour and half starch is a great jumping-off point and works well for a lot of baked goods.

As you get more comfortable, you can play with that formula. I tend to use a little more of the flours and less of the starches to increase the nutrient factor. But don't get hung up on percentages! Start changing your formula by ¼ C here and ¼ C there to see what you like. From that point, you can adjust recipes further, depending on your tastes. This little trick is great for getting you started on a recipe without stressing out. Try it. If you like it, keep it. If the texture isn't quite right, now you can adjust your flours, starches, or any combination of the two. As an example, I created my teff scones to be heartier and denser, so that's why it calls for more flour than starch. One taste and you'll see why they've been a customer favorite ever since!

Flour Substitutions

When I list a combination of flours in a certain recipe, it is the optimum combination that results in the best taste and texture. It usually has a nice nutrition boost as well. You can interchange *sorghum, brown rice, and teff flours* at any time, but this will usually alter the recipe slightly. Again, the combinations given were tested and created to provide the best taste and texture for each recipe. For example, if a recipe calls for 1 C sorghum and 1 C brown rice, you can use 2 C brown rice, but the texture will be slightly heavier and the flavor may be heartier.

With that said, it is important to be creative! Interchanging those flours won't be a deal breaker in any of these recipes by any means. However, I always think it's a good idea to make a recipe as instructed the first time, so you understand how to make it and how it's supposed to turn out. Then subsequent attempts can be altered so you can see and taste the differences. This is also a great way to learn how different gluten-free flours taste and feel in recipes. But for ease of what you may have on hand or cost restrictions, you can certainly interchange any of those three flours.

I do also use *millet* and *amaranth* flours. Millet gives a great, light, cakelike texture to baked goods, but I have found it to be very strong in flavor, so I have to limit its use in recipes. When you see it called for in a recipe in the book, it is because of the boost in texture it provides (it is quite nutritious too!), but it will be called for in smaller quantities. It provides a specific function in the recipe, so I do not recommend replacing it with any other flour. If absolutely necessary (you're in the middle of a recipe and realize just then you don't have millet, but you have brown rice), then you can substitute and the recipe will not fail. However, it may not be the exact texture the recipe was designed for.

Amaranth is another stronger-flavored flour that I use to boost flavor and nutrition in recipes. The trick with amaranth is that you can remove it from a recipe and replace it with sorghum, teff, or brown rice with no changes, but you cannot substitute any of those three with amaranth because the flavor is so strong.

To really understand the role individual flours make in a recipe, I highly recommend trying each flour firsthand with your finger. Line up your flours, stick your finger in one at a time, and taste each one. You may want to rinse your mouth in between to taste each with a clean palate. Feel the texture of each. Is it grainy or powdery? How about the flavor? Is it mild or earthy or bitter? Now, write them down and rank them in taste and texture so you can refer back at any time when creating recipes. After doing this taste test, I knew I would never use only brown rice for a delicate vanilla cupcake recipe because of its heavier, grainer texture. To me it was a flour that needed to be disguised with other textures, such as in a cookie. Here are my personal flour rankings:

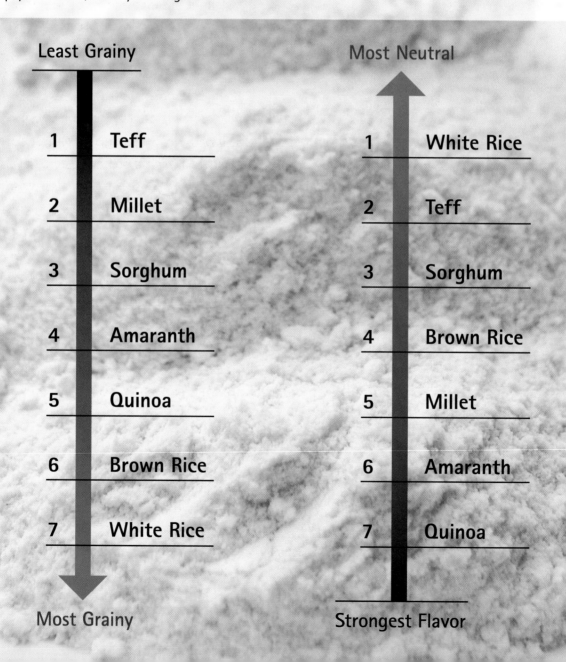

Least Grainy		Most Neutral	
1	Teff	1	White Rice
2	Millet	2	Teff
3	Sorghum	3	Sorghum
4	Amaranth	4	Brown Rice
5	Quinoa	5	Millet
6	Brown Rice	6	Amaranth
7	White Rice	7	Quinoa
Most Grainy		Strongest Flavor	

So in summary, my arsenal of flours consists of:

1) Teff
2) Brown Rice
3) Sorghum
4) Amaranth
5) Millet
6) Quinoa

And for starches:

1) Potato Starch
2) Tapioca Starch
3) Arrowroot Starch (as a thickener)

And for alternative "flours" that aren't really flours:

1) Coconut Flour
2) Almond Meal

Note that I use coconut flour and almond meal, and that I've placed them in a separate category. I don't count these as a flour because they don't generally taste or act like a typical flour or starch. Coconut is high in fiber and strong in flavor, so I usually use it in small amounts to add fluffiness and to help retain moisture in recipes. Almond meal is simply ground almonds and is higher in protein but doesn't bind the same as a flour or starch. I use it in recipes that go well with a little almond flavor or need a rougher texture.

For resources on where to buy flours, see page 426.

Natural Sweeteners

This topic can be very touchy for some folks, and it can certainly be a confusing one. Part of the debate regarding sweeteners involves the glycemic index (GI). The GI is a numerical scale used to indicate how fast and how high a particular food can raise our blood glucose (blood sugar) level. However, it's important to keep in mind that it's not the GI alone that leads to the increase in blood sugar. Equally important is the amount of food that you consume. The concept of the GI combined with total intake is referred to as "glycemic load." For example, although an entire candy bar has a relatively high GI, eating a small piece of that candy bar will result in a relatively small glycemic response. This is because your body's glycemic response is dependent on both the type and the amount of carbohydrate consumed.[6]

Another factor to consider is fructose, which has a low GI of about 19. It used to be recommended for use by diabetics due to its small effect on blood glucose levels. However, due to the possibility that excessive consumption of fructose may be a factor in some diseases, including metabolic syndrome and insulin resistance, products containing high levels of fructose have been discouraged.[7] Fructose promotes dyslipidemia (high blood cholesterol levels), decreases insulin sensitivity (blood glucose levels rise and may cause health issues), and increases visceral adiposity (organ fat, it's what gives that beautiful looking beer belly look) in overweight adults.[8] Fructose can cause nonalcoholic fatty liver disease and induce insulin resistance in humans, may accelerate the development of type 2 diabetes, doesn't acutely stimulate leptin, may not trigger normal satiety (you don't know you're full), and may elevate blood pressure.[9, 10]

Agave

Agave is one of the most popular "natural" sweeteners on the market today. But most forms of agave currently sold are heated—and heated agave is extremely high in fructose (4,919 mg fructose vs. 442 mg glucose in 1 oz). If you can find truly natural, raw agave, it is better and actually has more glucose than fructose (274 mg fructose vs. 333 mg glucose). The problem is that even some of the agave syrups being sold as "raw" really aren't, as they are heated above 118 degrees F during processing. And if you're using "raw" agave in baked goods that are heated to 350+ degrees, then the syrup is no longer raw and it will be much higher in fructose. This is why we don't use agave in our home and why you won't see it in any of the recipes here. Of course, as with anything concerning your body, if you love agave and want to use it, you can certainly use it to replace the sugar or other sweeteners called for in the book.

Pure Maple Syrup

Maple syrup is a fairly benign sweetener with potential health benefits, and it is very low in fructose (only about 2%). When compared to honey, maple syrup contains less sugar, 17 times more calcium, 11 times more magnesium, 6½ times more zinc, and 4 times the potassium. However, it should be noted that the sugar and mineral content in maple syrup can vary depending on the tree it is taken from and the time of year/day/location the syrup is produced.

I often use pure maple syrup as a sweetener in my baking because of its great flavor and high level of sweetness. Being that it's a liquid and very sweet tasting, I don't have to use as much to get the level of sweetness I desire in baked goods, which helps in not compromising the texture. I also like it because it has been heated in order to actually create the syrup, so it does not deteriorate during the baking process.

Organic Honey

Honey has been shown to possess antibacterial and antimicrobial properties, and it may help protect against cardiovascular disease as well. Honey has the potential to help decrease plasma glucose in diabetics (though it's also been shown to increase hemoglobin A1c levels in diabetics), and it has been shown to increase vitamin C concentrations, B-carotene, and serum iron levels in humans. Honey has also been shown to lower triglycerides and fasting blood sugar levels. And while it has a high fructose level, studies have shown that substituting honey for fructose may protect against the pro-oxidative effects of the fructose. Theoretically, the fructose in honey may be less problematic for those with fructose issues.

Not all honey is created equal, so it is important to shop around. Translucent honey, found in traditional bear containers at your supermarket, doesn't have the same health benefits as raw honey, again because of the over-processing. Whenever possible, try to find raw, organic honey, as it will have the maximum health benefits. I have also found that certain types of honey, such as clover honey, tend to have a stronger flavor than I prefer, and therefore I avoid using it in cooking and baking. I absolutely love Really Raw Honey because the neutral flavor is beyond any other honey I've tried.

Coconut Nectar

Coconut nectar is a very low glycemic liquid sweetener derived from the sap of the coconut blossoms, and it naturally contains vitamins, minerals, amino acids, and other nutrients (including vitamin C). It has a low fructose content (anywhere from 7% to 10% depending on who you ask) and is minimally processed at a low temperature, just enough to remove excess moisture and let the sap thicken. You can use coconut nectar as a cup-for-cup replacement for other liquid sweeteners. Compared to traditional brown sugar, coconut nectar has 20 times the amount of nitrogen, 26 times the phosphorus, 15 times the potassium, 10 times the zinc, and 1½ times the amount of iron.[11]

And when they take the coconut nectar and air dry it down to its crystalline form, you get coconut crystals, which can be used like traditional sugar. It is also low glycemic and nutrient rich. And since both sweeteners are completely unrefined, unbleached, non-GMO, gluten-free, and still contain key vitamins and minerals, they are both well used in my kitchen.

Organic Evaporated Cane Juice

(organic powdered sugar/organic brown sugar)
Evaporated cane juice does not undergo the same degree of processing that refined white sugar does and therefore, unlike refined sugar, it retains more of the nutrients found in the sugar cane. But unlike honey and maple syrup, there is no research that shows definitive health benefits of sugar cane. There is research showing that overconsumption of over-processed cane sugars is associated with such debilitating conditions as adult-onset diabetes and colon cancer.

The bottom line for me is this; I don't care for the amount of processing that most cane sugars endure, nor am I happy with study after study that shows its dangers to health. But I do know that most of this is based on overconsumption. So while I do use organic evaporated cane juice in some recipes, I always reduce the amounts significantly while still maintaining the integrity of the dish, because sometimes, nothing else works quite the same. An example

is making a great buttercream frosting. While I can remove the dairy, artificial colors, and trans fats, it is difficult to achieve a delicious frosting that can stand up and not melt off without organic powdered sugar.

For other recipes, I have replaced sugar with maple syrup, raw honey, or coconut nectar. In any case, feel free to replace any sweetener with one of your choice. Do not worry about replacing a dry sweetener with a liquid. My rule of thumb is that for each ½ C of dry sugar, I use ¼ C to ⅓ C of liquid sweetener.

In short, "sugar" is "sugar" when it comes to our bodies and the amount we choose to consume in our everyday diets. Sweets, no matter what form they come in, should be limited. I don't recommend consuming twenty cookies in a day made from evaporated cane juice, just as you also shouldn't eat as many containing honey. Please be mindful of indulgences; have them infrequently, but enjoy and savor the moments that you do. Then move on.

Oils & Fats

Oils and fats are another source of debate among health conscious cooks. When we first started our bakery, canola oil was our fat of choice because of its neutral flavor, low cost, and decent Omega 6:3 ratio. But after learning that it's difficult to find non-GMO canola oil, coupled with the insane processing it takes to make it suitable for consumption, canola oil is not something we use anymore. Coconut oil is by far our fat of choice for cooking and baking. I'm not going to get into great detail as to why saturated fat isn't the enemy like so many sources would like us to believe. But if you'd like more information on this topic, please take a look at www.marksdailyapple.com, or www.mercola.com. While I recommend using coconut oil in most of the recipes here, you can certainly substitute with your favorite high-heat oil for cooking or neutral oil for baking.

Canola Oil

Canola oil is made from the rapeseed and is low in saturated fat and high in monounsaturated fat. It has a decent Omega 6:3 ratio of 2:1 and a high smoke point of 470 degrees. However, about 80% of rapeseed crops grown in Western Canada are Genetically Modified Organisms (GMOs). The production method of canola oil is slightly shorter than the time it takes to read *War and Peace*, and it involves things like hexane "bleaching" and deodorizing.[12] All of this is necessary partly because wild rapeseed contains large amounts of erucic acid, a known toxin. But thanks to GMOs, the plant that is now used to produce canola oil is bred to contain less than 2% erucic acid, a level not believed to cause harm to humans. At least, that's what we're being told for now.

Coconut oil

Coconut oils are all made from the meat (white flesh) of a mature coconut. Water, fiber, and proteins are removed from the flesh of the coconut to obtain the oil. All coconut oil, once these constituents are removed, is stable at room temperature. This oil is more stable than any other oil because it is predominantly composed of medium-chain fatty acids, which are "saturated" by hydrogen atoms and resist oxidation and, therefore, rancidity. Coconut oil is an excellent source of medium-chain fatty acids (MCFAs), easily digestible, and is sent directly to the liver where it's converted into energy rather than being stored as fat. It can help stimulate the body's metabolism and is very high in lauric acid (the predominant type of MCFA in coconut oil), which can help strengthen the immune system.

Because of these health benefits, along with the decadent and satisfying nature of coconut oil, I use this oil for most of my cooking and baking. I like to keep more refined coconut oil for savory cooking because the flavor is neutral and it has a higher cooking temperature. I also keep raw coconut oil on hand for the higher lauric acid profile and a slightly coconutty flavor, which enhances many desserts and veggies. Plus, it makes a great moisturizer and smells yummy!

I have found that, depending on the brands of flours and types of liquids used in some recipes, coconut oil can be very light and not as viscous as a heavier oil like olive. So in some instances, I like to add a tablespoon or two of olive oil to a recipe to help with moisture levels. Coconut oil, like real butter, can give you a light, flaky texture, which you may not want in a chocolate chip cookie, for example. In this instance, just add a tablespoon of olive oil and it helps keep it on the chewy side.

Organic Palm Shortening

Palm shortening is a great addition to many baked goods because it's colorless, odorless, and neutral in flavor. It's produced from palm oil by removing some of the unsaturated fats, which firms it up. Spectrum Organics, my preferred shortening, processes their organic palm shortening by extracting it with manual pressing, then refining it without chemicals. The palm oil is then whipped using nitrogen to give it that light but solid consistency. It is non-hydrogenated, however, which makes it light years better than traditional shortenings. In any instance where you would use traditional shortening for optimal flakiness or texture in a baked good, organic palm shortening can be used instead, with better results than nondairy butters.

Dairy and Egg Substitutions

Everyone's first reaction to not being able to bake with dairy and eggs is "How?" Well, it's quite simple really. You don't need them. Really. I have found that eggs are completely unnecessary in most baking, except of course those dishes that rely entirely on eggs for consistency like a quiche.

Try looking at it from a scientific standpoint. What is butter? Fat. Therefore, we replace butter with another fat like coconut oil or a nondairy butter substitute such as Earth Balance Soy Free Butter or Vegan Buttery Sticks. What is an egg? That one can be trickier, but generally it is a binder and adds liquid and rise to a recipe. Flax meal (ground flax seeds) mixed with hot water; room temperature applesauce with baking powder; and even simpler, warm water, all provide excellent moisture and even activate baking powder for rise in most baking recipes.

When creating recipes, if I know I have sufficient baking powder for lift and I'm using flax meal mixed with hot water (or applesauce with baking powder) for binding and lift, but the dough is a bit dry, I simply add warm water until it is right. That's it. Having your liquids very warm helps kick that baking powder into action, which gives your baked item lift and air bubbles while it bakes, which is what we want!

Ready for another GF secret? You don't need commercial egg replacer in gluten-free baking! Ask yourself this, *what is egg replacer, anyway?* Generally the ingredients are: potato starch, tapioca starch, calcium lactate, calcium carbonate, citric acid, sodium carboxymethyl-cellulose, and methylcellulose. Well, if you're already using potato starch and tapioca starch, you certainly don't need a duplicate of those in a recipe. Calcium lactate is basically a form of baking powder; calcium carbonate is used as baking soda. I don't really want to ingest carboxymethylcellulose or methylcellulose (thickeners/emulsifiers), and since we are using a gum to help bind our ingredients, they aren't needed anyway.

Egg replacer is useful in vegan baking where eggs are removed but wheat flour is still being used. In this instance, you're not adding any starches because the wheat flour has everything it needs on its own. So when you remove the eggs, the recipe loses leavening. Adding starch and extra baking soda/baking powder via commercial egg replacer helps replicate that lift. But egg replacer isn't necessary in gluten-free baking when you are using starches and baking powder and baking soda. And since this is almost always the case, please do not waste anymore time or money on commercial egg replacers.

Eating Out and Cross Contamination

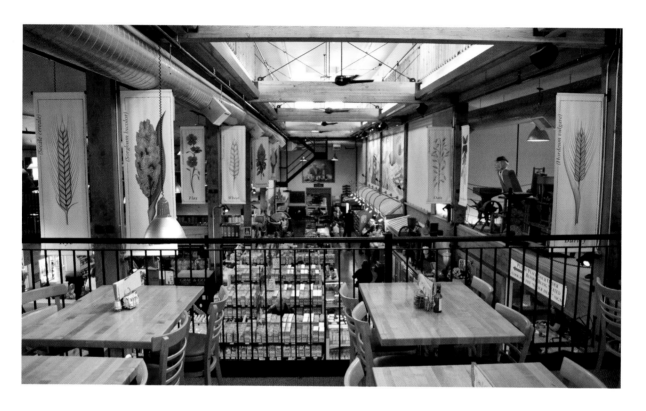

Cross contamination is a real problem for those with intestinal damage because if you are exposed to gluten, even in tiny amounts, it repeatedly damages the villi in the small intestine. Your family must support you by being gluten-free at home, or at the very least, with those products that present the biggest problems—flour and pasta. Flour can stay in the air for as long as twenty-four hours and cover every inch of a kitchen, seeping its way into drawers and coating place settings and napkins. It is impossible to remove all traces of flour once it is used, no matter what anyone tries to tell you. This holds especially true for food production. If you eat a cupcake from a bakery that bakes traditionally as well as gluten-free, you will get gluten in your cupcake. It doesn't matter how often they clean or what order they bake, the flour gets everywhere and there is no way to control it.

So tell your family I said that they need to help you and be supportive! Going gluten-free is healthier for them in the long run, and safer for you now and down the road. Your life depends on it. Statistics show that those with celiac disease who are exposed to gluten have a significantly higher chance of dying from various causes such as heart disease and cancers. It's just not worth it.

Eating out is another danger zone. So here are some tips:

1. Pick places you trust, that are accommodating, helpful, and courteous. Preferably where the owner has food allergies as well so they are aware of the dangers.

2. If you ask questions about gluten-free foods at a restaurant, how they are prepared and so on, and your server asks, "What's gluten?" walk out. If the server doesn't know the basics, it means no training has occurred at that establishment and no safety procedures are in place. Run.

3. Ask questions about their procedures for handling gluten-free orders. Then the next time you go in—ask again. Restaurants change food-handling procedures, menu items, and suppliers constantly, so what was safe a month ago may not be safe now. Don't assume anything, ever.

4. Research restaurants on the web before you travel. Many restaurants offer menus online and advertise if they are gluten aware. Also, make sure to check the restaurant search on the Gluten Intolerance Group's website for those establishments that have participated in their Restaurant Awareness Program. Visit: http://www.gluten.net/find-a-restaurant-search.aspx

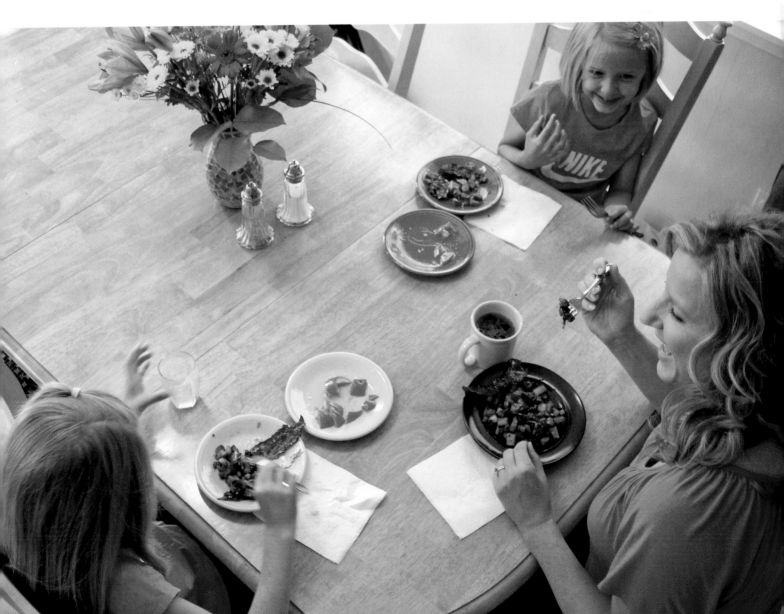

Tips for a Happier Kitchen

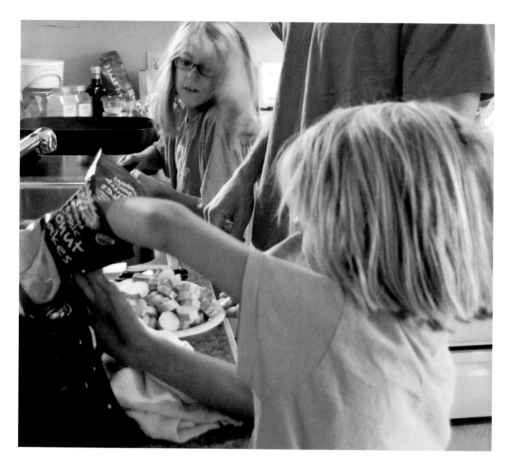

One of the reasons our retail products were so popular was because they were convenient and cost-effective. Our loaves of quick breads were sliced and had wax paper inserts to keep slices from sticking together once frozen. That way, you could remove a slice or two at a time without thawing the entire loaf, therefore preventing waste. Our cookie dough was mixed and scooped into individual dough balls, then frozen. Again, this was to prevent the waste of baking an entire batch of cookies that dry out quickly. Frozen cookie dough balls could be removed from the freezer one or ten at a time and then baked immediately—no need to thaw! Plus, of course, our dry mixes, which enabled customers to save time during baking by grabbing a premixed selection of ingredients. And while this sounds wonderful, the convenience has a price. We all know the cost of gluten-free retail products! But you can now use all of the tricks we used in our retail products in your own kitchen—saving time and money!

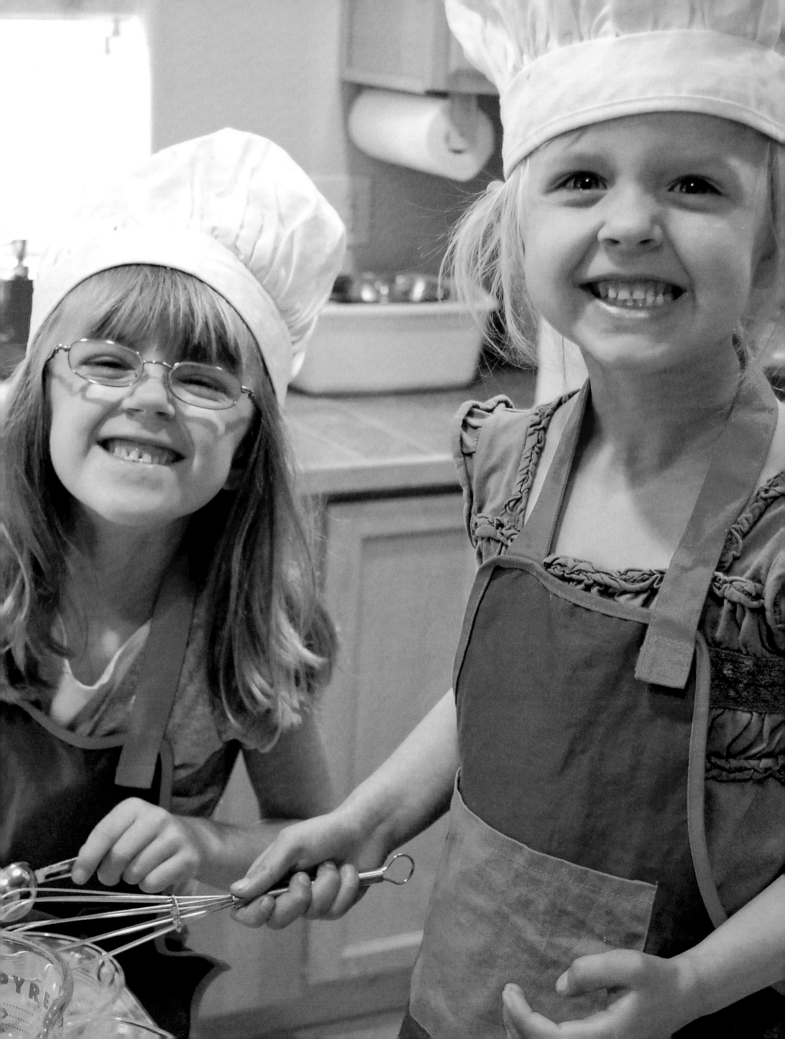

Make Ahead and Freeze:

- Meals—Many meals in this book can be prepped ahead of time and then frozen until ready to use. For example, for the Raspberry Chicken (p. 108) you can make the sauce, then place chicken breasts and sauce in a freezer bag. Just thaw and cook when you're ready! Modeled after many of those dinner-prep businesses, but without the price tag and food allergies! Look for tips and options at the bottom of the recipe pages to see ways you can create make-ahead meals.

- Dry Mixes—One of the biggest hurdles in the GF kitchen is having the time and energy to mix all of those flours and dry ingredients needed to bake. This is why prepackaged mixes, both traditional and gluten-free, have become so heavily used. I encourage you to save your money and control the ingredients you use by making dry mixes yourself. With any recipe for baked items, simply place all dry ingredients in a zip-top bag, shake to combine, and then store until needed. I usually store a dry mix in my pantry for quick use, and then make extras that are stored in the freezer to keep ingredients fresh. If frozen, just let the dry mix come to room temperature before using. My favorite recipes for utilizing this make-ahead method are:

  - Cookies
  - Cakes
  - English Muffins
  - Pancakes
  - Brownies
  - Scones
  - Batter Mix
  - Quick Dinner Rolls

- Doughs and Crusts—You can par-bake pizza crusts so they are ready to top and bake anytime you'd like! For pizza crusts, see recipe instructions for par-baking and freezing the crusts (p. 192). I like to make as many as I can in an afternoon to keep the freezer stocked.

- I also like to premake doughs so I can bake on demand. For cookie dough, simply mix dough as usual, and then scoop any leftover dough into cookie-size balls, place on a baking sheet, and freeze. Store frozen cookie dough balls in a freezer zip-top bag until you're ready to bake. No need to thaw the dough! Just bake from frozen. But you will probably want to press down the dough balls halfway through baking with a spatula to make them a little less "round" at the end. Still tasty, but resembles a golf ball. If you're feeling less energetic, just pack cookie dough into an airtight container and freeze. To use, simply thaw until soft enough to scoop the dough. Then scoop and bake as usual. I've even used this method for scones. Make the dough, add your fruit, then pack the dough into an airtight container and freeze. Simply thaw until soft, scoop, and bake according to recipe directions.

- Freezing Baked Goods—If you have leftover baked goods, freeze them for another time. Don't feel you have to eat an entire pan of brownies in two days before they dry out! For loaves of bread, slice and then place wax paper between slices. Wrap in plastic wrap, place in a freezer-safe zip-top bag, and freeze. This way, you can remove however many slices you need later, without thawing the entire loaf and wasting ingredients! For brownies, cookies, muffins, and such, I like to freeze them in airtight containers and then place them in freezer zip-top bags once frozen to preserve space in the freezer. Now you can grab a single brownie for a snack or a couple of blueberry muffins for breakfast. Just heat and eat!

My Favorite Kitchen Tips:

1. Microwave or bake a few potatoes at the beginning of the week. They should be soft, but still firm. Refrigerate until needed on a busy morning. Just dice and brown in a skillet—they cook in minutes. Add some ham and avocado for a quick, healthy breakfast!

2. Precook breakfast meats like sausage, bacon, and homemade sausage patties ahead of time. Cooking them at the beginning of the week and refrigerating for midweek breakfasts saves time. Just heat and eat.

3. On the go in the morning? Try a smoothie made with fruit and coconut milk. Or how about a breakfast burrito, made with teff or brown rice wraps and filled with sausage veggie hash (p. 56)?

4. Meal plan, meal plan, meal plan! Use a calendar to plan meals ahead of time. Keep a notepad next to it for grocery lists and hit the store just once a week. Stop spending quality weeknight time in the checkout line!

5. Utilize that freezer! Stock up on sale meats, purchase half of a cow, whatever is in your budget, but pack that freezer when you can so you are able to grab it when you need it. Make sure to look at your menu for the week and take out what meats you will need in advance. My rule of thumb is three days of meats at a time. For larger roasts and whole chickens, it takes about three days to fully thaw in my fridge.

6. One of the biggest complaints about eating right is the time it takes to cook meals. One of the easiest tricks to speed up cooking for a midweek lunch or weeknight dinner is to cut that steak or chicken breast into bite-size pieces before sautéing for quick cooking. You can have a wonderfully tender, flavorful steak (bite size!) in about five minutes. You can't even make it to the drive-thru in that amount of time. Look for many bite-size recipes in this book.

7. Use fresh herbs when called for to get optimum flavor. But in a pinch, a little dried herb can replace the fresh. Remember, you need much less of a dried herb because the flavors are more concentrated.

8. While I always encourage experimenting with my recipes to find what works for you, I do recommend trying these recipes as written first, so you have a starting point for what it should be like. Adjust as needed after that.

9. Chop onions and peppers once a week and freeze small portions in zip-top bags. Use in stir-fries, crock pot meals, and so on for quick veggie add-ins. For that

matter, you can chop fruit for smoothies and veggies and put them in the freezer for later use. Spend one afternoon a month doing this and your weekdays will be wonderful and glorious! At least when it comes to meal prep.

10. Save asparagus ends, leek ends, and so on in a zip-top bag in the freezer and use when you need to make vegetable stock.

11. Keep mason jars filled with carrot sticks, pepper slices, celery sticks, and such on a low shelf in the fridge (we like a lower shelf in the door) for your kids to have access to. You will be amazed at how many veggies they eat when you grant them free access to these snacks whenever they want, without asking! They think they're so cool.

12. Freeze leftover smoothies in Popsicle molds for nutritious, effortless after-school treats that you can feel good about. Or how about breakfast smoothie popsicles? The kids will think you're the coolest parent ever for giving them ice cream for breakfast, but you'll know it's nutritious!

13. Freeze lemon rinds to use when you need lemon zest. If you have to use a fresh lemon and don't need the juice, squeeze the juice anyway and freeze it in ice cube trays. When you need lemon juice in a sauce, just add the cube or melt first in the microwave.

14. Keep peeled ginger pieces in the freezer. Frozen ginger lasts longer and is easier to grate.

15. Barter with venders at your local farmers market for fresh veggies and meat. You never know when they will trade produce for a service you can provide. For example, we have traded our baked goods for mountains of organic produce.

16. Stock up when the sales happen! May and October are Celiac Disease Awareness Months, so find those health food stores that put everything GF on sale and load 'em up!

17. Freeze leftover coconut milk to use in baking later on.

18. Slice apples and sprinkle with a little cinnamon for snacking at school or at home. If they turn a little brown, no one will know because of the cinnamon... and it tastes like apple pie!

19. Don't throw those brown bananas in the trash! Freeze in zip-top bags to add to smoothies or use in banana bread recipes. Frozen and then thawed overripe bananas are the best-kept secret to moist, flavorful banana bread.

20. Utilize your local Gluten Intolerance Group and other allergy support groups. You can get free samples (before you blow the money on something you don't like), share recipes, access lots of books, and get support from those going through the same issues. But be careful when listening to advice from fellow meeting goers. Opinions are like mouths—everyone has one, and they may not always be speaking the facts. Make sure to verify information before you utilize the advice with your family.

21. Buy gluten-free flours in bulk (i.e., 25 lb bags) and store in the freezer in airtight containers. If cost is an issue, try contacting someone in your local GIG group to go in with you and split large purchases. But don't buy any items in the bulk bins at grocery stores. People share the scoops with other items that may contain gluten, and stores don't always clean bins before changing their contents. Your gluten-free rice may be in the same bin that had pasta last month.

22. Don't refrigerate leftover baked goods. Either freeze or store at room temperature, covered. Refrigerating sucks the moisture out quickly and makes them too dry to enjoy.

23. Flax Meal—use only organic golden flax seeds that have been refrigerated. Freshly grind for each recipe, or if you bake a lot, grind a cup or so at a time and store in an airtight container in the fridge for up to three weeks.

24. Get those kiddos in the kitchen!

    a. Get a hand-operated food chopper (like Pampered Chef Food Chopper). Small hands can help with chopping lots of veggies without the risk of cutting off fingers.

    b. Keep a pair of extra-long tongs on hand. Kids can help stir, flip, or toss without getting too close to hot stoves and pans.

    c. Keep a pair of kid-safe scissors in the kitchen drawer for little ones. They can use them to safely chop herbs like basil leaves, parsley, cilantro, chives, and green onions.

    d. Probably my kids' favorite kitchen chore is pounding chicken breasts or other cuts of meat. Place meat in a zip-top bag, seal (making sure air is taken out), and let the kids go at it with a wooden kitchen mallet. Just make sure to keep other little hands out of the way and let them know when it's flat enough . . . you don't want that chicken breast to disintegrate.

    e. Get a few pieces of kid-size equipment. Purchasing one extra-small frying pan and a small spatula just for the kids gives them the confidence to handle the tools safely. Now let them make some breakfast!

25. My favorite kitchen tools

    a. Tongs

    b. Electric skillet

    c. Slow cooker

    d. Griddler or George Foreman indoor grill with removable plates

    e. Digital meat thermometer

    f. Scissors

    g. Mason jars

    h. Glass lock food containers

    i. Freezer

    j. Size 12 (2¾) oz ice cream scoop

    k. Parchment paper

    l. Celtic sea salt (fine and coarse)

    m. Restaurant quality aluminum sheet pans (half and quarter sheet)

    n. Cooling racks, oven safe preferably

    o. Magic Bullet food blender

    p. Lodge enameled Dutch oven

    q. Lodge cast-iron skillets

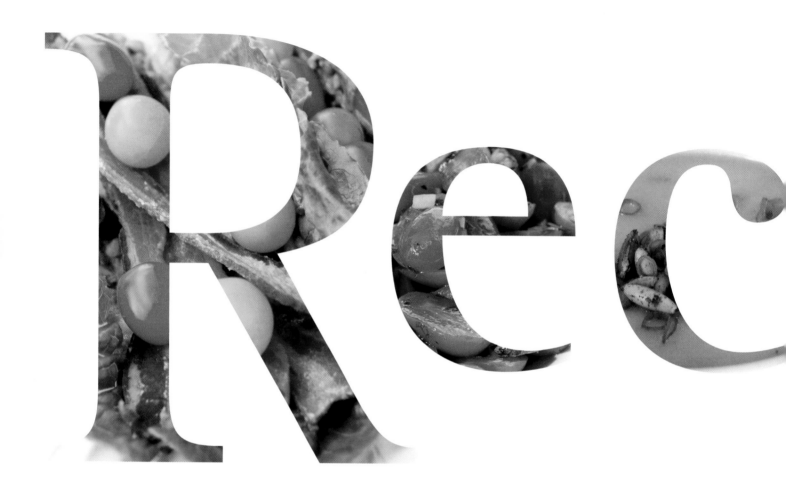

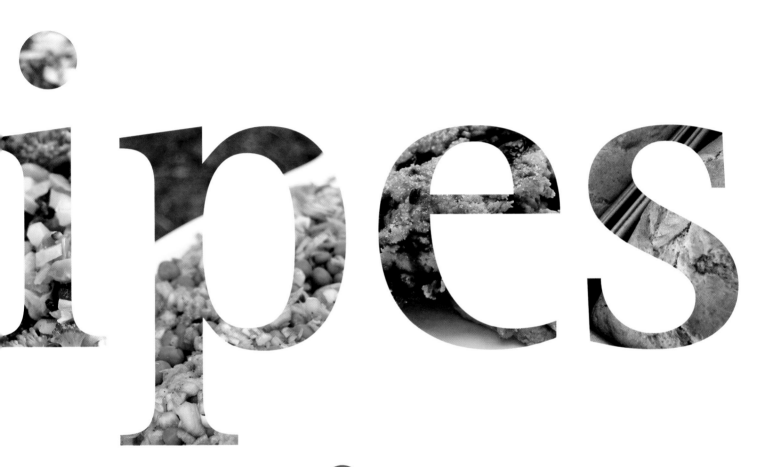

Breakfasts

Entrées

Sides

Sauces/Rubs/Salad Dressings

Baking/Desserts/Snacks

Beverages/Smoothies

School Lunch Ideas

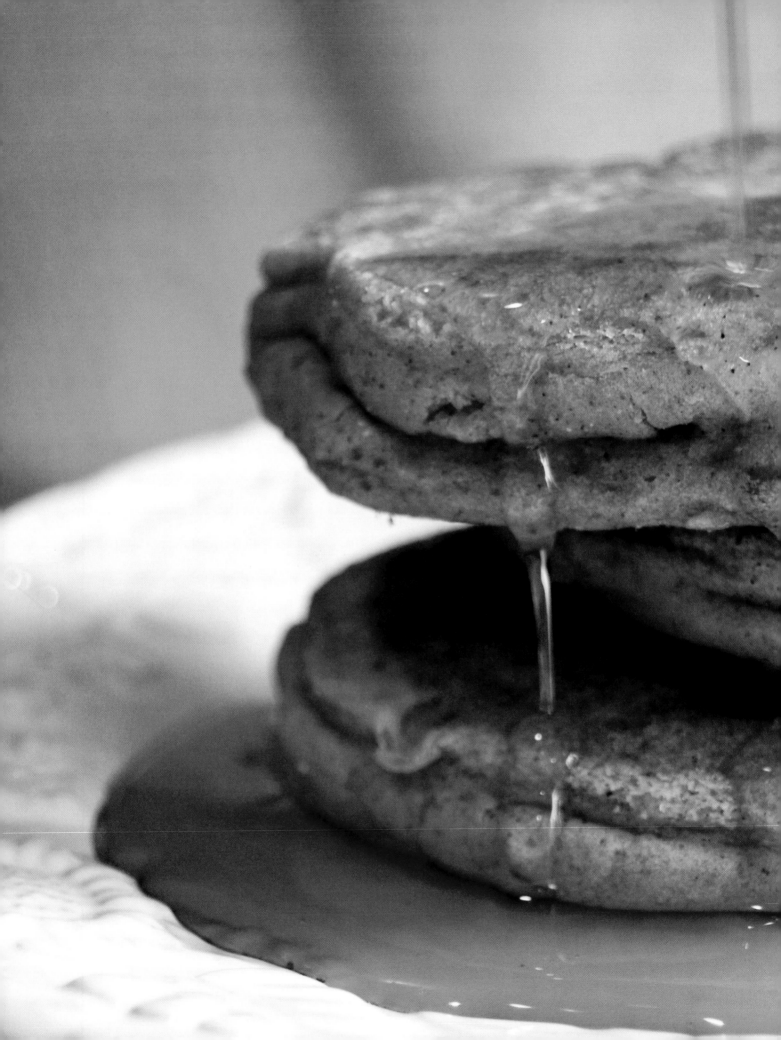

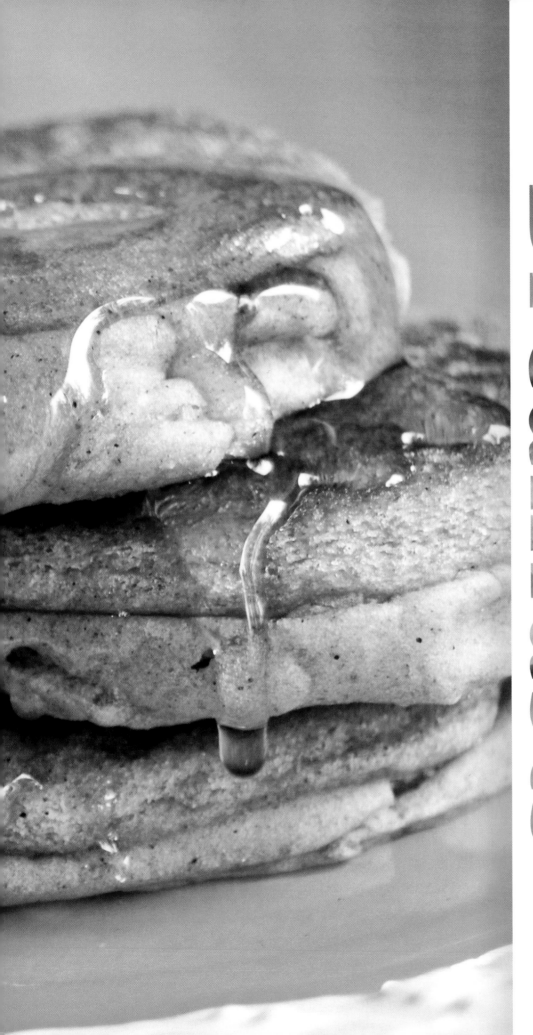

Breakfasts

Vanilla Honey Quinoa
with Strawberries and Almonds

I tried for a while to get my family to eat quinoa as a side dish to many dinners. But no matter how I seasoned it, everyone said "eh," and it was left on the plate. Then one glorious morning The Maniac, being in his usual morning rush, threw together some leftover quinoa and frozen strawberries, warmed it in the microwave and, wow! It makes frequent appearances at our breakfast table, especially on those cold winter days. Make sure to add the strawberries and all of the juice. It seeps into the quinoa, making it beautiful and delicious!

1	C (250 mL) water
½	C (90 g) organic quinoa, rinsed
~	Pinch of sea salt
1	tsp pure vanilla extract
2	tsp raw organic honey
½	C (75 g) frozen organic strawberries, thawed (keep the juice)
2	Tbsp toasted almonds, coarsely chopped

1. Bring water, quinoa, and salt to a boil. Turn to low and simmer, uncovered, until quinoa is tender and water is absorbed, about 15 minutes. Remove from heat, stir in vanilla extract, and cover with a lid and let rest for 5 minutes.
2. Fluff quinoa with a fork, spoon into bowls.
3. Drizzle honey over quinoa and add strawberries with their juice to each bowl. Sprinkle tops with almonds and serve!

Option:

For a creamier quinoa, add a little bit of nondairy milk to the bowl before serving.

Makes 2 servings

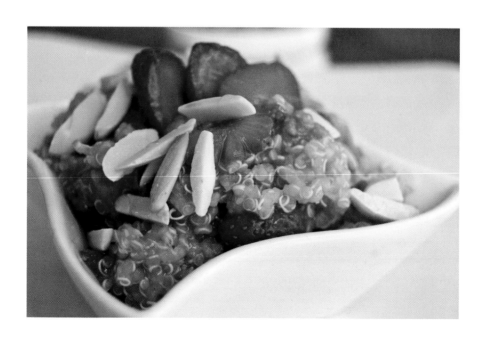

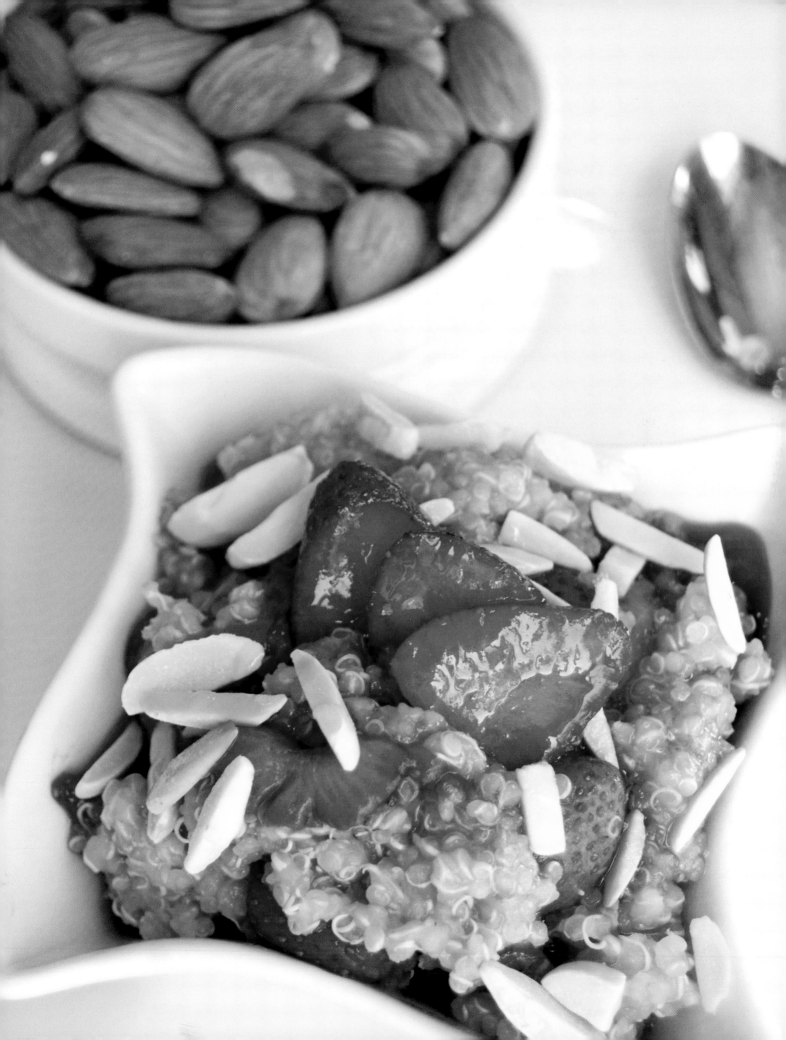

Apple Cinnamon Quinoa

I love the combination of apples and cinnamon with crunchy walnuts for breakfast. Satisfying yet still light, this bowl of goodness will keep everyone running full steam ahead well into lunchtime!

1¼	C (300 mL) water
½	C (90 g) organic quinoa, rinsed
~	Pinch of sea salt
½	medium organic apple (Granny Smith or Pink Lady work well), diced
½	tsp cinnamon
2	Tbsp chopped raw walnuts

1. Bring water, quinoa, salt, and diced apples to a boil in a medium saucepan. Turn heat to low and simmer, uncovered, until done and water is fully absorbed, about 15 minutes. Remove from heat.
2. Cover and let rest for 5 minutes.
3. Fluff quinoa with a fork. Spoon into bowls and top with a sprinkle of cinnamon and a few walnuts. Enjoy!

Option:

Try adding a little nondairy milk of choice to your quinoa for a creamier breakfast treat!

Makes 2 servings

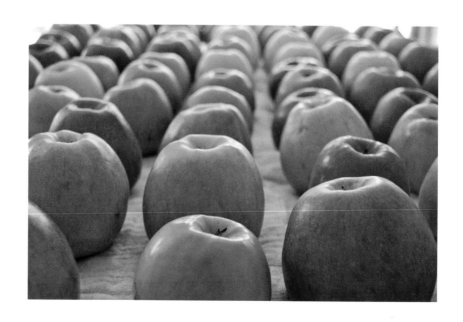

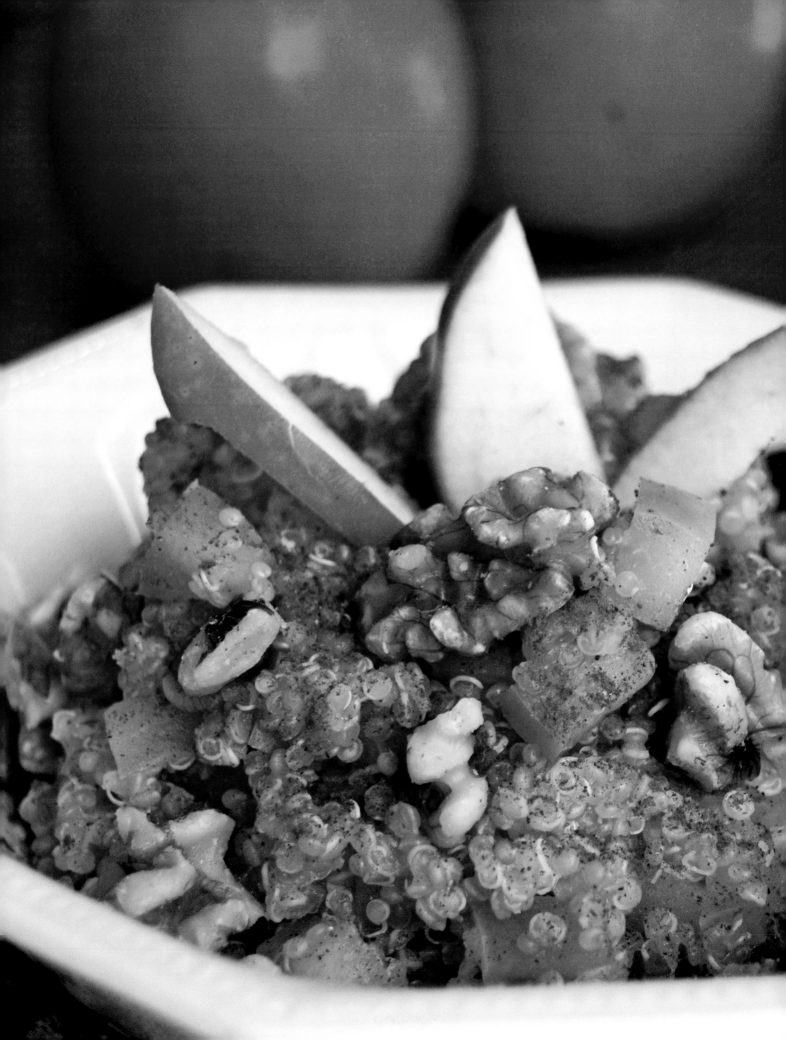

Brown Sugar and Cinnamon Quinoa

You will notice as you cook your way through this book that there are no recipes containing oats. This is because oats can be troublesome for many people who cannot tolerate gluten. So I knew on our first snowy morning after going gluten-free, that I had to figure out a way to recreate my favorite oatmeal, and fast! This did the trick, and surprisingly, it's also my kids' favorite way to eat quinoa, with the proof shown in their empty bowls time and time again. I hope you enjoy it too!

1	C (250 mL) water
½	C (90 g) organic quinoa, rinsed
~	Pinch of sea salt
1	Tbsp organic brown sugar
½	tsp cinnamon
2	Tbsp organic raisins
1	Tbsp roasted salted sunflower seed kernels
¼	C (60 mL) nondairy milk

1. Bring water, quinoa, and salt to a boil. Turn to low and simmer, uncovered, until quinoa is tender and water is absorbed, about 15 minutes. Remove from heat and cover with a lid and let rest for 5 minutes.
2. Fluff quinoa with a fork; spoon into bowls.
3. Sprinkle even amounts of brown sugar, cinnamon, raisins, and sunflower seeds onto each bowl of quinoa.
4. Pour in milk and serve!

Makes 2 servings

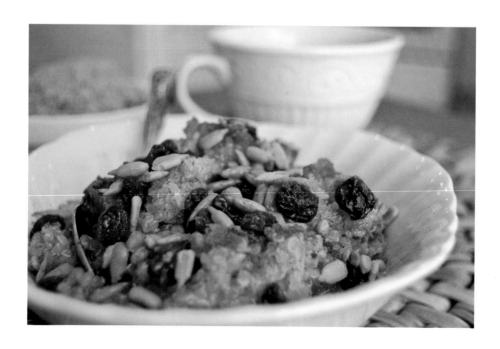

Breakfasts

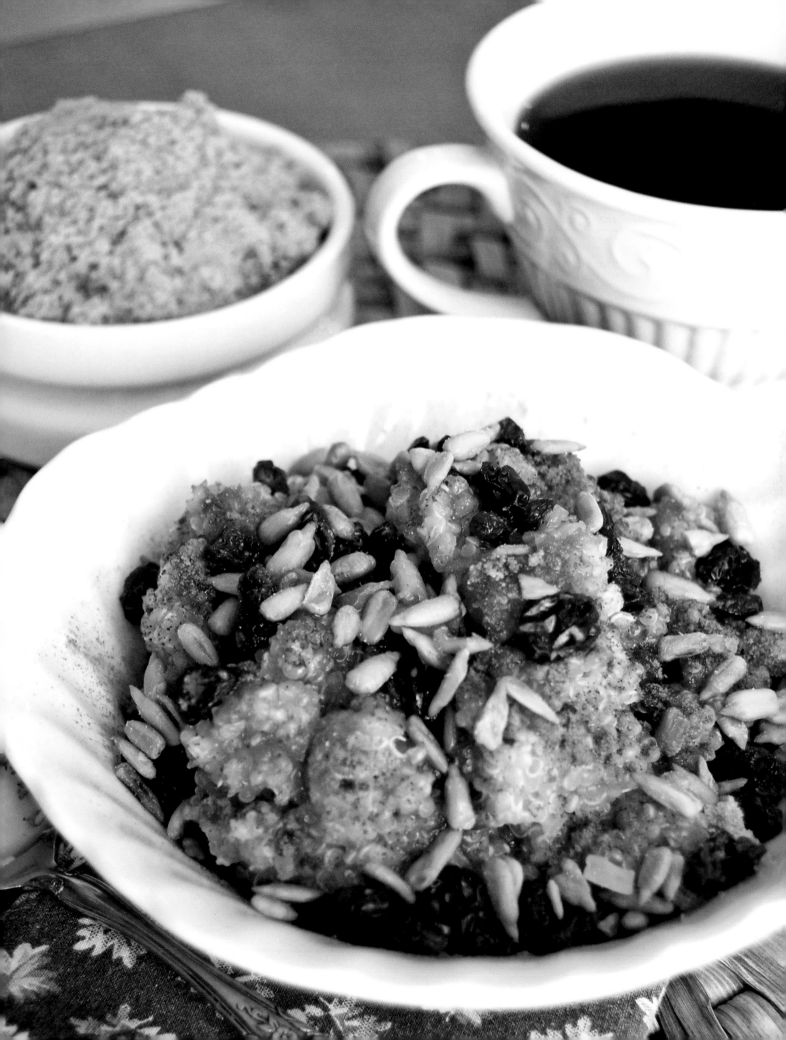

Maple Pecan Quinoa with Blueberries

Juicy blueberries really turn this bowl of warm cereal into something special. Not only is it incredibly tasty, but the juices turn the quinoa into an explosion of purple and blue that you don't usually see in a typical breakfast cereal, unless it's chock-full of those pesky artificial colors. Let's just stick with the high-protein quinoa and antioxidant-rich blueberries because nature did just fine on its own, don't you think?

1	C (250 mL) water
½	C (90 g) organic quinoa, rinsed
~	Pinch of sea salt
2	Tbsp pure maple syrup
½	C (75 g) frozen organic blueberries, thawed (keep the juice)
2	Tbsp chopped raw pecans

1. Bring water, quinoa, and salt to a boil. Turn to low and simmer, uncovered, until quinoa is tender and water is absorbed, about 15 minutes. Remove from heat and cover with a lid and let rest for 5 minutes.
2. Fluff quinoa with a fork; spoon into bowls.
3. Drizzle maple syrup over quinoa and add blueberries with their juice to each bowl. Sprinkle tops with pecans and serve!

Option:

For a creamier quinoa, add a little bit of nondairy milk to the bowl before serving.

Makes 2 servings

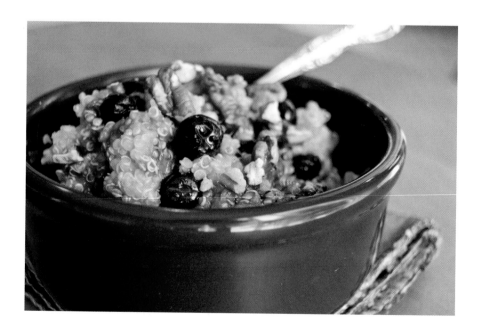

Breakfasts

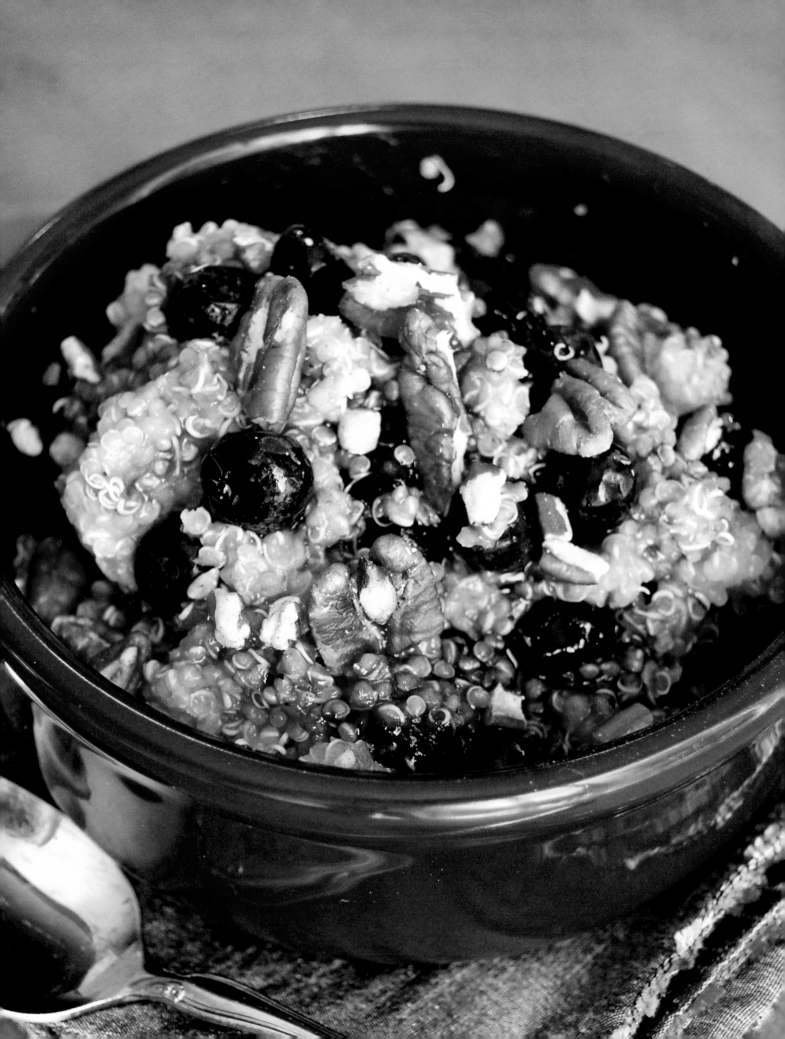

Sausage Veggie Hash

This is a powerhouse breakfast to kick off your day like no other. Lots of protein, energizing carbs, and healthy fat from avocados will keep you feeling satisfied all the way to lunchtime. And if you're always rushing during your weekday mornings like my family is, check out my tips on cutting cooking time for this breakfast to get you out the door in a flash. No more "skipping breakfast" excuses! I like to use an electric skillet for this one. One pan to clean, the potatoes brown without sticking, and it all fits nicely without overcrowding, causing steam cooking to occur. No soggy veggies please!

1	Tbsp coconut oil
¾–1 lb (450 g)	of your favorite GF breakfast sausage. Links or bulk work fine.
1	small organic yellow onion, diced
2	medium organic russet potatoes, scrubbed clean and diced
3	medium organic zucchini, scrubbed, sliced in half lengthwise, then cut into ¼-inch slices
½	of a medium avocado, sliced

1. In a large electric skillet or nonstick frying pan, heat 1 Tbsp oil.
2. Add sausage and cook until done and no longer pink.
3. Remove from skillet. If using links, go ahead and cut them into bite-size pieces (kitchen scissors work great for this). Set aside and keep warm.
4. Add onions to the skillet. Cook for 1 minute.
5. Add potatoes. Cover and cook until browned and soft, about 12 minutes.
6. Add zucchini and cook for about 5 minutes, or just until softened.
7. Add sausage back to pan, stir to combine.
8. Serve bowls full of hash, topped with sliced avocado.

Tips for Fast and Easy Weekday Mornings:

~Precook sausage the night before, or at the beginning of the week for a couple of midweek breakfasts. Store in the fridge until ready to use. Then when needed, just heat sausage in skillet and proceed with remaining instructions. Cut 10 minutes out of your morning routine!

~Microwave potatoes ahead of time, or the night before using, just until softened. Store in the fridge until ready to use. To use, just dice and brown them. Saves about 10 minutes of cooking time!

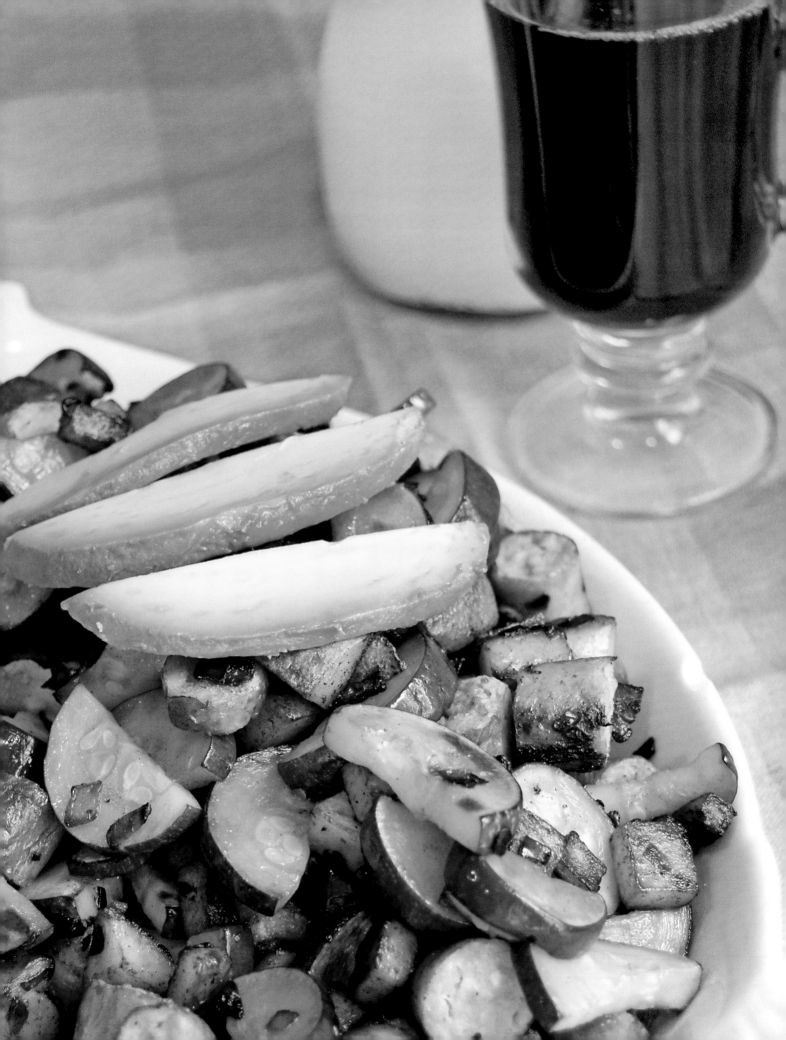

Blueberry Crumb Muffins

Oh how I love blueberry muffins and how I love this recipe! Wonderfully soft muffins with fragrant blueberries and a sweet, crispy topping. What could be better? And I love that they freeze well so I always have some on hand for a quick breakfast.

Dry Ingredients:

- ¾ C (90 g) teff flour
- ¼ C (30 g) millet flour (your secret muffin ingredient!)
- ½ C (60 g) sorghum flour
- ½ C (60 g) potato starch
- ½ C (60 g) tapioca starch
- ½ tsp xanthan gum
- ½ tsp sea salt
- 2 tsp baking powder
- ½ tsp baking soda

Wet Ingredients:

- ¾ C (180 mL) coconut oil
- ⅔ C (130 g) organic evaporated cane juice (or you can use ⅓ C sugar and ⅓ C raw organic honey)
- 2 tsp pure vanilla extract
- ½ C (120 mL) organic applesauce mixed with ½ tsp baking powder
- ⅔ C (160 mL) warm water

Add In:

- 1 C (150 g) frozen or fresh organic blueberries

Crumble Topping:

- ⅓ C (60 g) packed organic brown sugar
- 2 Tbsp brown rice flour
- 2 Tbsp potato starch
- ¼ C (20 g) crunched GF cornflakes or GF crisp rice cereal
- ½ tsp cinnamon
- 3 Tbsp melted coconut oil

1. In a medium bowl, whisk together dry ingredients. Set aside.
2. In a stand mixer blend wet ingredients, except water, until combined.
3. Slowly add dry ingredients to the wet, and mix on low until mostly incorporated. Add warm water, a little at a time, until the dough is moist and thick, but still capable of being "poured" into the muffin cups like a traditional muffin batter. It's OK if you don't use all the water, or if you need to add a touch more.
4. Fold in blueberries.
5. Mix crumble topping in a small bowl with a fork until crumbly.
6. Scoop muffin batter into greased or paper-lined muffin pans.
7. Add about 1 tsp of topping to each muffin, spreading evenly.
8. Bake in a 350° oven for about 25 minutes or until a toothpick inserted in the center springs back to the touch and comes out clean.

Tip:

These muffins freeze wonderfully. Cool completely and freeze in an air-tight container. To use, thaw at room temp and heat in the microwave to warm.

Makes about 18

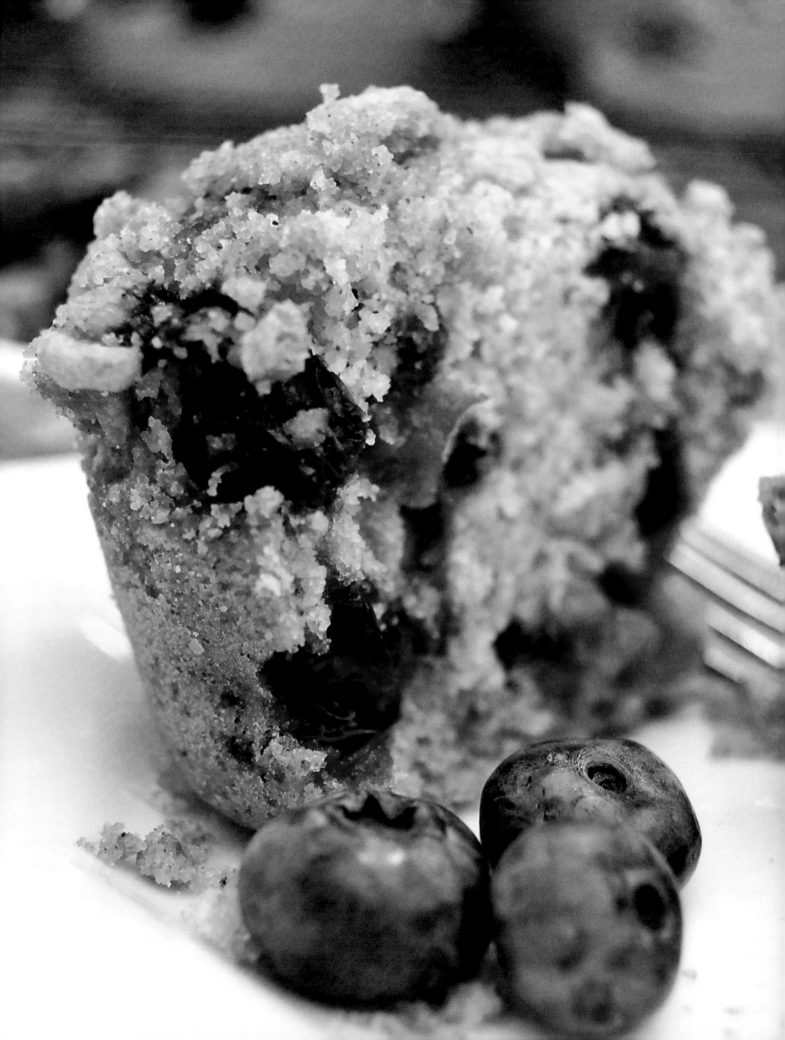

Apple Crisp Muffins

These muffins were a big seller at events for our bakery, partly because they look delectable with the crispy topping, and partly because they taste so amazing! You won't believe how soft and spongy they are. Plus, the great taste of tart apples with the sweet brown sugar topping will make you feel like you're eating dessert for breakfast!

Dry Ingredients:

¾	C (90 g) teff flour
¾	C (90 g) sorghum flour
½	C (60 g) potato starch
½	C (60 g) tapioca starch
½	tsp xanthan gum
½	tsp sea salt
3	tsp baking powder
½	tsp baking soda
1	tsp cinnamon

Wet Ingredients:

¾	C (180 mL) coconut oil
⅔	C (130 g) organic evaporated cane juice (or you can use ⅓ C sugar and ⅓ C raw organic honey)
2	tsp pure vanilla extract
⅔	C (160 mL) warm water

Add In:

1	C (150 g) Pie Apples, recipe (p. 358)

Crumble Topping:

⅓	C (60 g) packed organic brown sugar
2	Tbsp brown rice flour
2	Tbsp potato starch
¼	C (40 g) chopped pecans
½	tsp cinnamon
3	Tbsp melted coconut oil

1. Whisk dry ingredients together. Set aside.
2. In a stand mixer, mix wet ingredients, except water, until mixed.
3. Slowly add dry ingredients to the wet, mix on low. Add warm water, a little at a time, until the dough is moist and thick, but still capable of being "poured" into the muffin cups like a traditional muffin batter. It's OK if you don't use all the water, or if you need to add a touch more.
4. Fold in pie apples.
5. Mix topping in a small bowl with a fork until crumbly.
6. Scoop muffin batter into greased or paper-lined muffin pans.
7. Add about 1 tsp of topping to each muffin, spreading evenly.
8. Bake in a 350° oven for about 25 minutes or until a toothpick inserted in the center springs back to the touch and comes out clean.

Tip:

These muffins freeze wonderfully. Cool completely and freeze in an airtight container. To use, thaw at room temp and heat in the microwave to warm.

Makes about 18

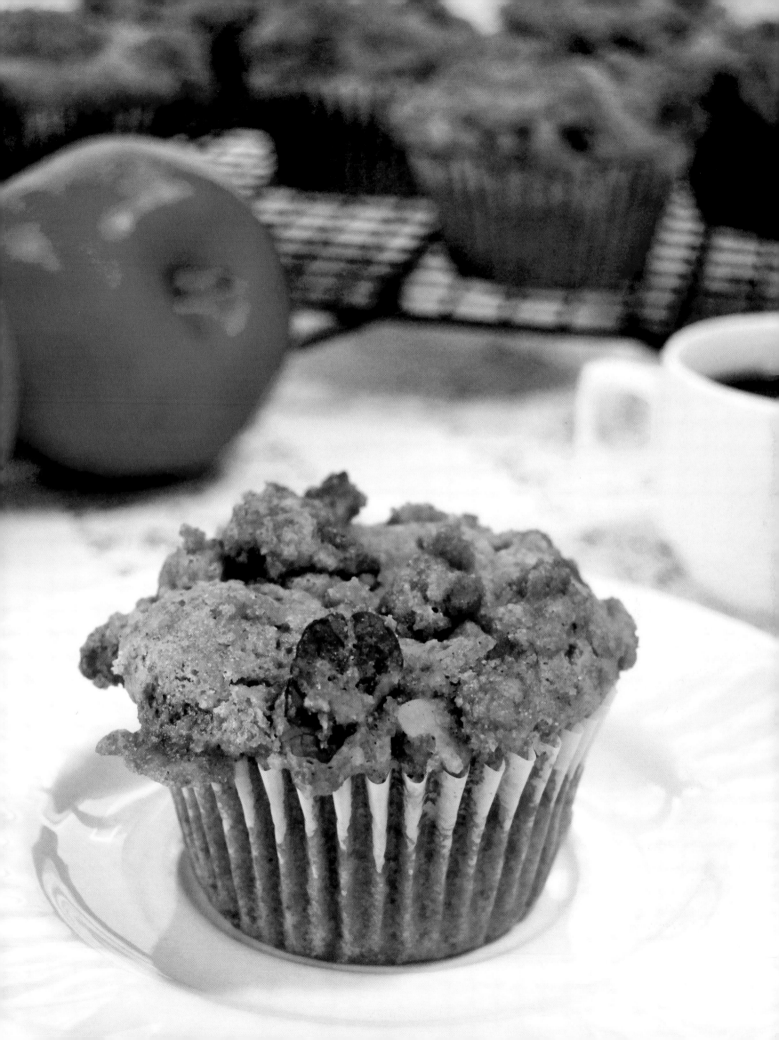

Morning Glory Muffins

Hearty and filling, these flavorful muffins really hit the spot for breakfast or anytime. If you're so inclined, you can frost these muffins with my buttercream frosting (p. 326) and tell everyone they're carrot cake cupcakes. I promise I won't tell, and no one will know the difference!

Dry Ingredients:

¾	C (90 g) brown rice flour
¼	C (30 g) teff flour
½	C (60 g) potato starch
½	C (60 g) tapioca starch
½	tsp xanthan gum
1	Tbsp cinnamon
2	tsp baking soda
1	tsp baking powder
½	tsp sea salt

Wet Ingredients:

¼	C (60 mL) raw organic honey
½	C (120 mL) coconut oil
½	C (90 g) packed organic brown sugar
1	Tbsp pure vanilla extract
¼	C (60 mL) organic applesauce (room temperature)
⅔	C (160 mL) warm water

Add Ins:

½	C (50 g) shredded organic unsweetened coconut
¾	C (110 g) chopped walnuts
2	large organic carrots, grated
2	small organic apples, peeled, cored and grated
¾	C (110 g) organic raisins

1. Whisk dry ingredients together. Set aside.
2. In a stand mixer, blend honey, oil, and brown sugar together until combined.
3. Add vanilla and applesauce, mix until incorporated.
4. Slowly add dry ingredients to the wet, mix on low. Add warm water, a little at a time, until the dough is moist and thick, but still capable of being "poured" into the muffin cups like a traditional muffin batter. It's OK if you don't use all the water, or if you need to add a touch more.
5. Fold in coconut, walnuts, carrots, apples, and raisins until incorporated.
6. Bake in a 350° oven for about 25 minutes or until a toothpick inserted in the center springs back to the touch and comes out clean.

Options:

~Try adding grated zucchini for some added moisture and nutrition.

~Add a little orange zest and replace the water with orange juice for added flavor!

Makes about 18

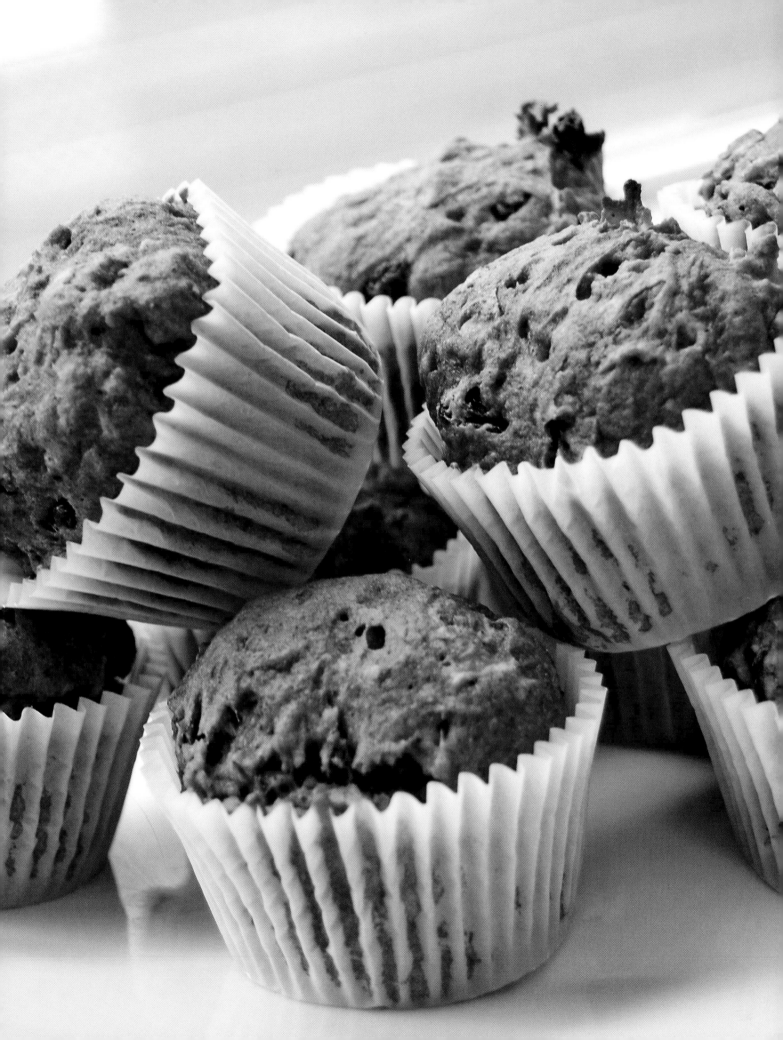

Hammin' It Up Morning Scramble

Who needs eggs to have a scramble? Pick your favorite breakfast meat, veggie, and potato and scramble away! This is our favorite weekday breakfast because it's fast, filling, and super-nutritious. OK, the kids don't really care about that part, but they do LOVE how it tastes, and I love that their tummies are full for school with lots of protein and vitamins. To help keep this meal super-quick, make sure to precook potatoes the night before or on the weekends.

1	Tbsp coconut oil
1	C (150 g) organic cooked sweet potato cubes
1	C (150 g) cubed GF ham
1	C (150 g) organic spinach leaves, chopped

1. Heat oil in a large skillet over medium heat. Add potatoes and cook until slightly browned.
2. Add ham and heat through, about 4 minutes.
3. Add in chopped spinach, stir and remove pan from heat.
4. Serve immediately.

Serves 2

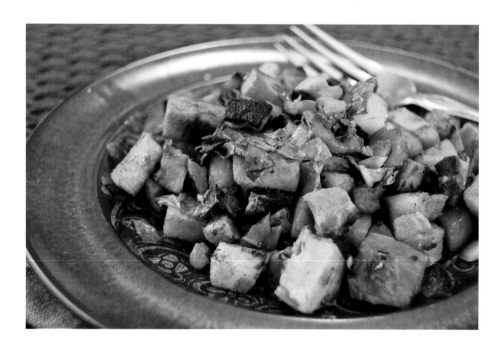

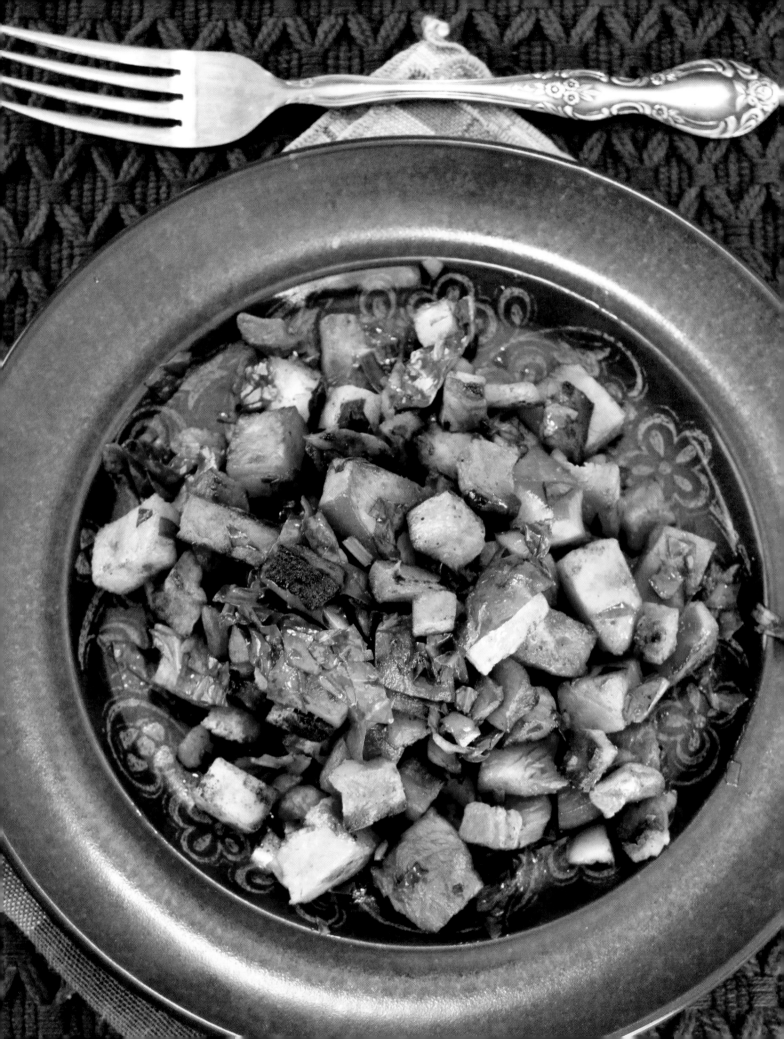

Pancakes

These pancakes are not for the faint of heart. Created as a hearty, fill your tummy, feel good about sending your kids out to tackle the day, walking barefoot in 5 feet of snow uphill both ways to get to school, kinda pancake. These are not your standard, starts with a "B" and ends with an "ick!" kinda pancake. Your tummy and your family will thank you. Plus, there are plenty for leftovers, which freeze extremely well. Just reheat in the microwave or toaster oven. Serve with your favorite real maple syrup, dust with cinnamon and sugar, or try the delicious Blueberry Syrup on the following page. Simple breakfast with no "ick" just "Mmmm!"

Dry Ingredients:

1½	C (180 g) sorghum flour
¼	C (30 g) teff flour
½	C (60 g) potato starch
¼	C (30 g) tapioca starch
2	tsp baking powder
1	tsp baking soda
1	tsp sea salt
1	tsp xanthan gum

Wet Ingredients:

⅓	C (80 mL) coconut oil
1½	C (350 mL) nondairy milk mixed with 1 Tbsp apple cider vinegar
1½	C (350 mL) warm water

1. Whisk dry ingredients in a mixing bowl.
2. Add oil, milk mixed with vinegar, and warm water. If you'd like, you can also add 2 Tbsp of your favorite sweetener such as raw honey or maple syrup.
3. Whisk together until well blended and all lumps are incorporated. If batter seems too thick, add a few Tbsp of warm water until desired consistency. Batter should be the same consistency of regular pancakes.
4. Heat griddle or large nonstick electric skillet to 350°. Brush lightly with oil.
5. Pour pancake batter, using a ¼ C measuring cup, onto hot skillet. Cook until golden brown and it starts to bubble. Flip and continue to cook until golden brown and cooked all the way through. About 3 minutes per side.

Options:

~After you spoon the batter onto the hot skillet, sprinkle fresh blueberries on each pancake. Cook as directed.

~For a special Valentine's treat or any special occasion, how about Chocolate Pancakes? Simply add ½ C cocoa powder and 3 Tbsp of your favorite sweetener and increase the warm water to 2 ¼ C. Top with warm syrup and raspberries or strawberries.

~For a heartwarming Christmas breakfast (or anytime), try Gingerbread Pancakes. Add 1 Tbsp cinnamon, 1½ tsp ground ginger, ½ tsp nutmeg, and 2 Tbsp of your favorite sweetener and proceed as directed. Delicious with real maple syrup and a sprinkle of powdered sugar!

Tip:

Want pancakes but out of milk? For this recipe you can use warm water in place of the milk (in addition to the water already called for). Still add the vinegar, just add it with the water.

Makes plenty for 4 plus leftovers

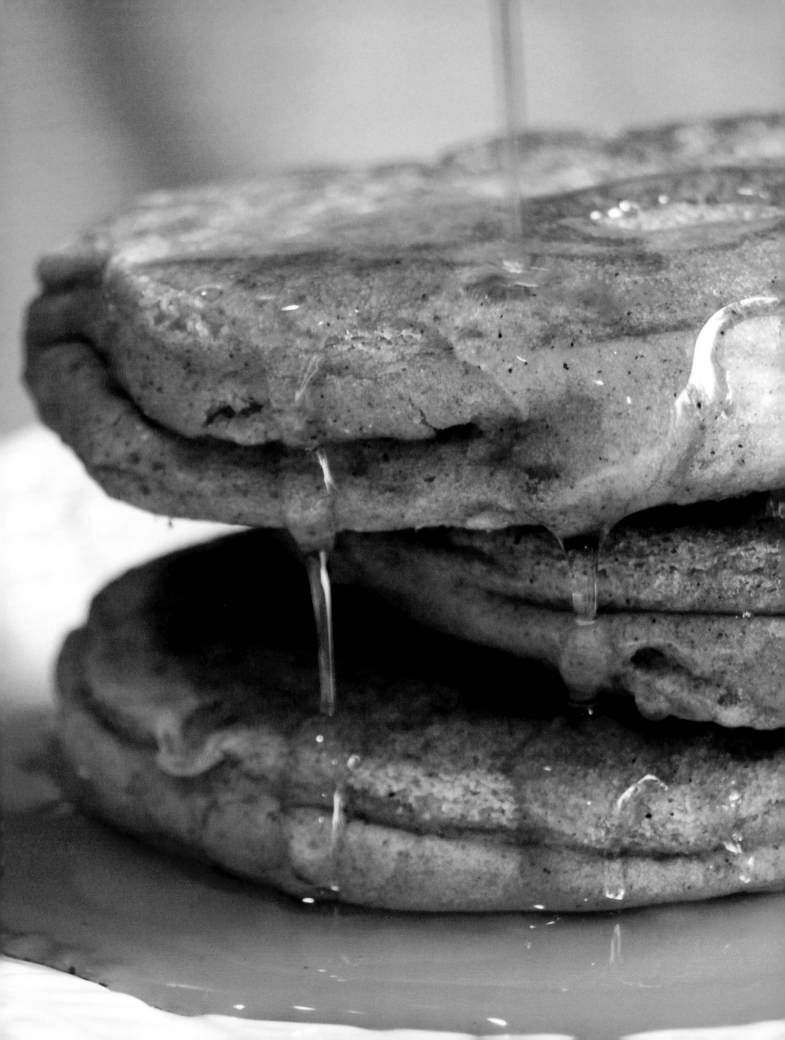

A Better Blueberry Syrup

This syrup is so easy you'll even make it on a busy Monday morning! Most syrups are filled with excess sugar, but this one really lets the blueberries do all the talking. Store leftovers in the fridge for more pancakes or waffles on the weekend.

2	C (300 g) frozen organic blueberries
¼	C (60 mL) organic 100% apple juice
1	Tbsp raw organic honey
~	Small squeeze of organic lemon juice

1. Heat all ingredients over medium heat until berries are thawed and sauce comes to a slight boil.
2. Simmer, on low, uncovered about 15 minutes until sauce thickens and reduces a bit.
3. Let cool 5 minutes before serving.

Makes about 2 Cups

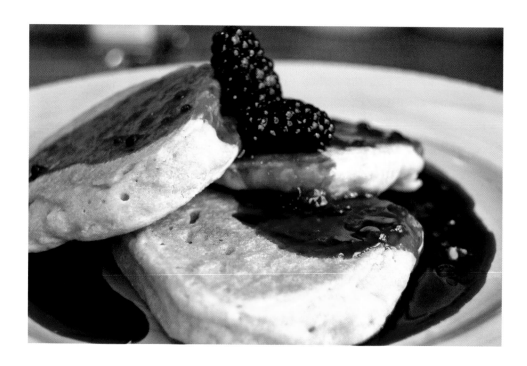

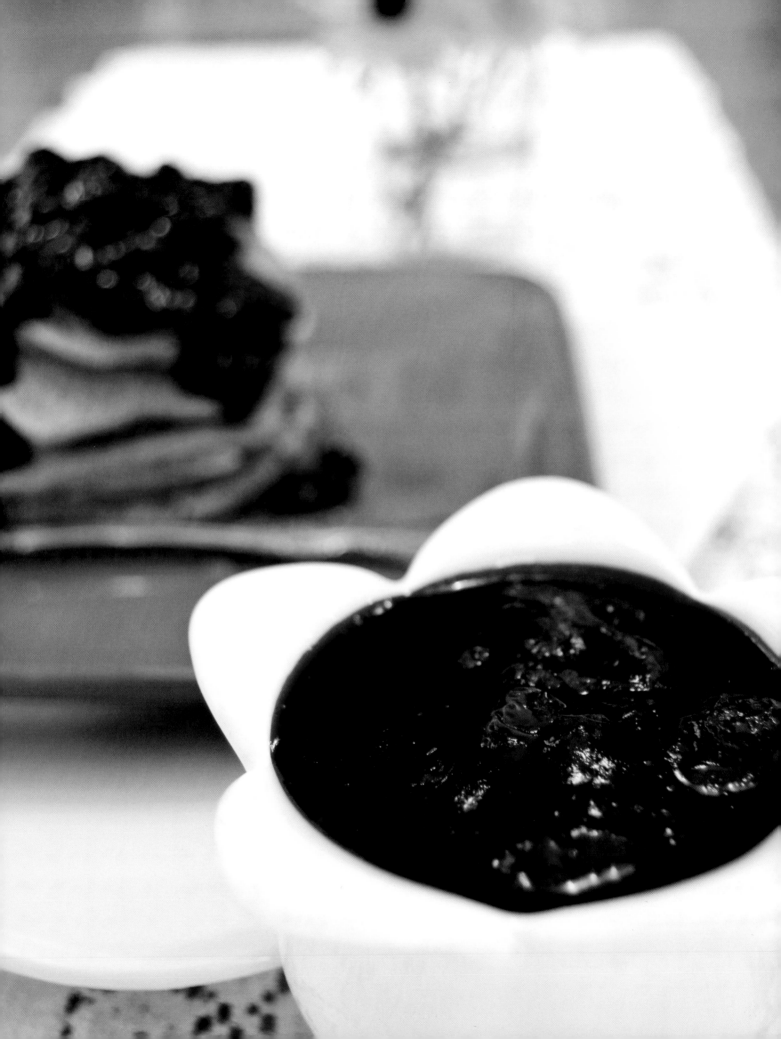

Quick Breakfast Sausage

A great breakfast, including high-quality protein, is essential for having sufficient energy to tackle your day and stave off hunger. But too many processed meats aren't good for us, even if they are uncured, since they generally still have higher sodium. This quick sausage is a great alternative without all of the preservatives or sodium that most breakfast meats contain. Plus it's quick to throw together in the morning, which means we actually all make it out the door well fed and ready to tackle the day. Feel free to either substitute ground pork for the beef, or combine half and half for even better flavor! In addition to buying from local farms, I like to use meats from US Wellness Meats, an online supplier of top quality, grass fed meats. US Wellness Meats is a family owned business that sells humanely raised animals that offer exceptional taste, quality, and health benefits at very reasonable prices.

1	lb (450 g) grass-fed ground beef (US Wellness Meats)
1	Tbsp raw organic honey
2	tsp dried parsley
1	tsp marjoram
1	tsp granulated onion
1	tsp paprika
1	tsp fennel seeds
½	tsp sage
½	tsp sea salt
¼	tsp turmeric
~	Freshly ground pepper
1	Tbsp coconut oil

1. In a medium bowl, mix all ingredients except for coconut oil.
2. Form into approximately 3-inch-wide patties.
3. Heat coconut oil in large skillet over medium heat.
4. Place patties in skillet, evenly spaced.
5. Cook 2–3 minutes or until really brown and caramelized; flip and cook for another 3 minutes. Serve.

Option: Italian Sausage

Add the following to the above ingredients and proceed with step 1:

~1 Tbsp Italian Seasoning
~2 tsp granulated garlic
~additional 1 tsp granulated onion
~⅛ tsp cayenne

Makes 8 patties

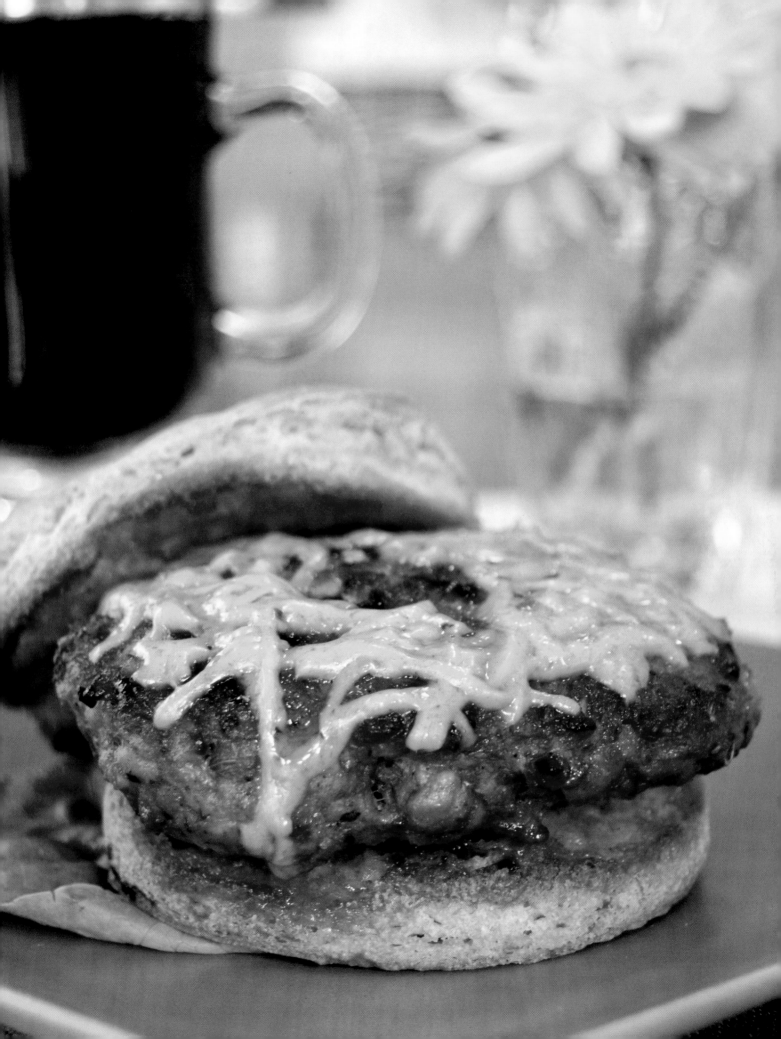

Teff Scones

I created this scone to have an alternative breakfast treat... and because I love scones. I do. All scones. Equally! Give me a lemon, a blueberry, a round one, a triangle one. Doesn't matter. A little bit crumbly, a little bit moist, the scone is the quintessential breakfast accompaniment. And by using teff flour, this scone delivers a great punch of protein, fiber, iron, and lysine. Who knew a scone could be filling and nutritious? Just add coffee, a Sunday morning, and a little James Taylor in the background, and you've got yourself the start to a great day!

Dry Ingredients:

1½	C (180 g) teff flour
1	C (120 g) sorghum flour
1½	C (180 g) brown rice flour
½	C (60 g) potato starch
½	C (60 g) tapioca starch
2	tsp xanthan gum
1	tsp cinnamon
1	tsp baking powder
½	tsp baking soda
¾	tsp sea salt

Wet Ingredients:

1	C (240 mL) coconut oil, melted
¾	C (150 g) organic evaporated cane juice (or ½ C [120 mL] honey or maple syrup)
1½	tsp pure vanilla extract
1¼	C (300 mL) coconut milk (or other nondairy milk of choice)

Add in:

2	C frozen or fresh fruit of choice

1. Whisk together dry ingredients.
2. In a stand mixer, mix oil and sugar together; add the vanilla.
3. Alternate adding the dry ingredients and the coconut milk to the sugar/oil mixture until all of the dry ingredients and milk have been used. Mix well. The dough will be very thick, but should be moist and hold together. If the dough is crumbly, add 1–2 Tbsp warm water and mix briefly, until incorporated.
4. Add 2 C frozen fruit of choice and mix briefly to incorporate. Don't mix too long or the fruit will break apart and your mixer will whine because the dough is so thick! You can also knead the fruit into the dough by hand.
5. Scoop dough into approximately 2½-inch balls, or about the size of a baseball (I use a 2¾ oz ice cream scoop), and place on parchment-lined cookie sheets.
6. Press down on dough balls firmly with the palm of your hand to flatten slightly, making approximately 3½- to 4-inch discs. Press more frozen fruit into tops of scones if you see some bare spots that need more yumminess. Lightly sprinkle organic evaporated cane juice over tops of dough discs.
7. Bake at 350° for about 25 minutes (a little less if using smaller dough balls), rotating baking sheets once after 15 minutes. When they are done, the edges should be ever so slightly browned and the center firm but giving to the touch.

Options:

~You can make the dough ahead of time! Simply follow steps 1–4, and then place dough in a freezer-safe container/tub and place in freezer for up to 6 months. To use, simply thaw on counter until soft enough to scoop, then proceed with steps 5–7.

~You can also freeze the individual scone dough discs (follow steps 1–6) so you can bake a fresh scone any time you'd like! Just thaw a scone (or two or three!) on a parchment-lined cookie sheet until the oven preheats to 350°. Then bake as directed above (step 7), lower cooking time to about 22 minutes. Less scones in the oven means a slightly reduced cooking time.

~Or, you can bake all of the scones as directed, then place cooled scones in a freezer-safe container and freeze for up to 2 months. To enjoy, simply thaw to room temperature, or defrost in the microwave a few seconds at a time until thawed and slightly warm...Don't you just love options!

Makes about 16 scones

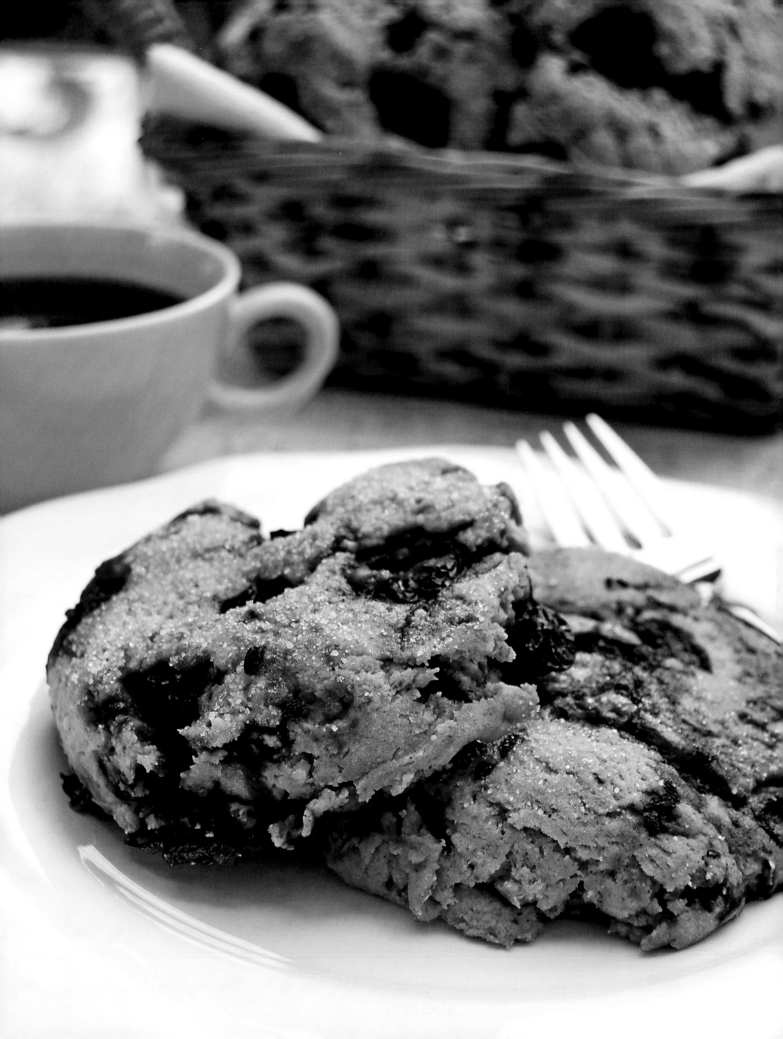

Strawberry Walnut Scones

The tender crumb, coupled with the light crunch of walnuts, in these scones makes them unbearably good. The even better news? The walnuts pack an Omega 3 punch, the strawberries vitamin C, and the whole-grain flours a nice dose of fiber, iron, and B vitamins. Now that's a way to start the day! And get creative with these scones. Try almonds with raspberry jam, or pecans with blackberry or cherry preserves. The flavor combinations are endless, so have some fun!

Dry Ingredients:

- 1½ C (180 g) ground walnuts (about 2½ C [225 g] whole walnuts ground in a food processor)
- ¾ C (90 g) brown rice flour
- ½ C (60 g) sorghum flour
- ¼ C (30 g) teff flour
- ½ C (60 g) potato starch
- ½ C (60 g) tapioca starch
- 2 tsp xanthan gum
- 1 tsp cinnamon
- 1 tsp baking powder
- ½ tsp baking soda
- ¾ tsp sea salt

Wet Ingredients:

- ¾ C (180 mL) coconut oil, melted
- ¾ C (150 g) organic evaporated cane juice (or ½ C [120 mL] honey or maple syrup—and reduce milk by ¼ C [60 mL])
- 1½ tsp pure vanilla extract
- 1 C (240 mL) coconut milk or other nondairy milk of your choice
- 1 jar of your favorite organic no-sugar-added strawberry fruit spread

1. In a mixing bowl, whisk together dry ingredients.
2. In a stand mixer with a paddle attachment, blend oil and sugar. Add vanilla.
3. Alternate adding dry ingredients and milk until both are used. Mix on high until well blended, about 1 minute. Dough will be very thick.
4. Line baking sheets with parchment paper. Scoop dough into balls and place on baking sheets. Dough balls should be about 2¼ inches in diameter.
5. With a teaspoon dipped in cold water (so it doesn't stick) press in the center of each dough ball, making a deep well.
6. Fill each well with 1 tsp strawberry jam. Sprinkle with additional sugar if desired.
7. Bake at 350° for 23–25 minutes, until tops are just becoming golden and the dough springs back to the touch.
8. Cool completely on wire racks and enjoy! Freeze any leftovers in airtight containers for about 2 months. To thaw, simply leave covered scones on the counter to thaw to room temp.

Options:

See Options for teff scones on previous page for freezing and making ahead.

Makes 14

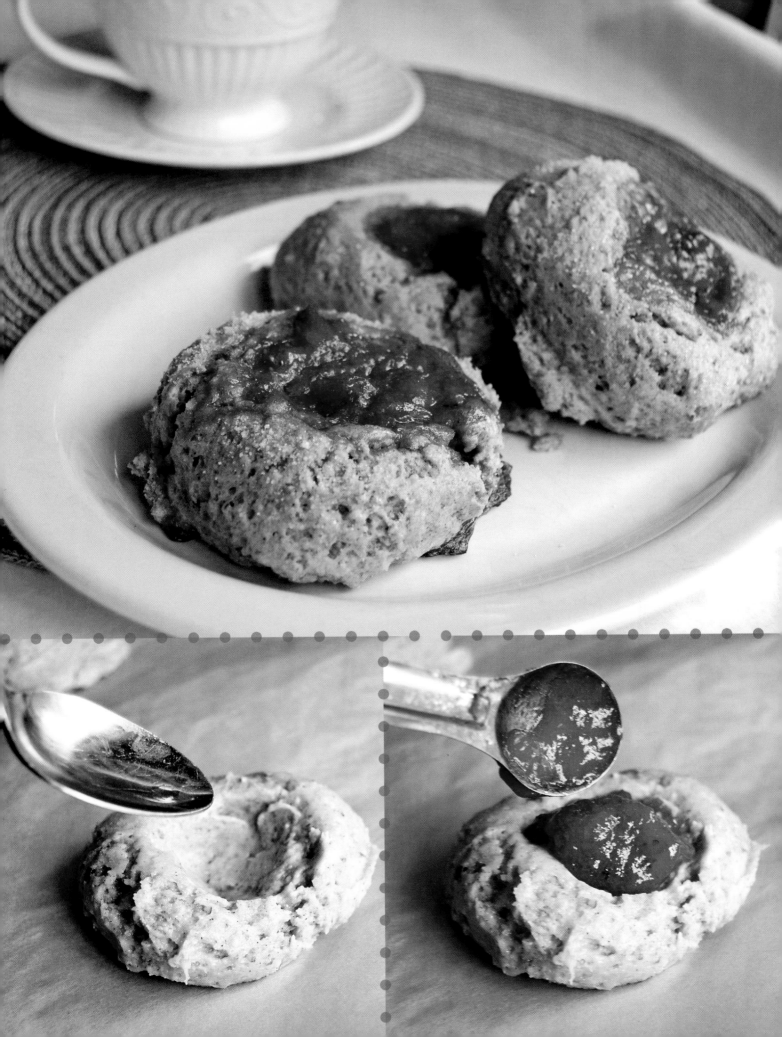

Apple Cinnamon Scones

Sweet, tart apples, crunchy pecans, and a delectable maple glaze. Ahhhh, that and a cup of coffee pretty much describes my happy place.

Dry Ingredients:

1½ C (180 g) teff flour

1   C (120 g) sorghum flour

1½ C (180 g) brown rice flour

½   C (60 g) potato starch

½   C (60 g) tapioca starch

2   tsp xanthan gum

1   tsp cinnamon

¼   tsp nutmeg

1   tsp baking powder

½   tsp baking soda

¾   tsp sea salt

Wet Ingredients:

1   C (240 mL) coconut oil, melted

¾   C (150 g) organic evaporated cane juice (or ½ C honey, or ½ C maple syrup)

1½ tsp pure vanilla extract

¾   C (180 mL) coconut milk (or other nondairy milk of choice)

Add In:

1   C (250 mL) Pie Apples (p. 358)

1   C (150 g) coarsely chopped pecans

1. Whisk together dry ingredients.
2. In a stand mixer with a paddle attachment, mix oil and sugar together. Add the vanilla and mix to combine.
3. Alternate adding the dry ingredients and the coconut milk to the sugar/oil mixture until all of the dry ingredients and milk have been used. Mix well. The dough will be very thick, but should be moist and hold together. If the dough is crumbly, add 1–2 Tbsp warm water and mix briefly, until incorporated.
4. Fold in the pie apples and pecans.
5. Scoop dough into approximately 2½-inch balls, or about the size of a baseball (I use a 2¾ oz ice cream scoop), and place on parchment-lined cookie sheets. Or spoon dough into a Lodge cast-iron wedge pan and smooth tops with a spoon.
6. Press down on dough balls firmly with the palm of your hand to flatten, making approximately 3½- to 4-inch discs.
7. Bake at 350° for about 25 minutes (a little less if using wedge pan—check for doneness at the 18-minute mark). The edges should be ever so slightly browned and the center firm but giving to the touch when they are done.
8. Cool scones on a wire rack. Once cooled, frost with Maple Glaze (p. 383).

Note:

See freezing options for the Teff Scones (p. 72) to make these tasty treats last even longer!

Makes about 16 scones

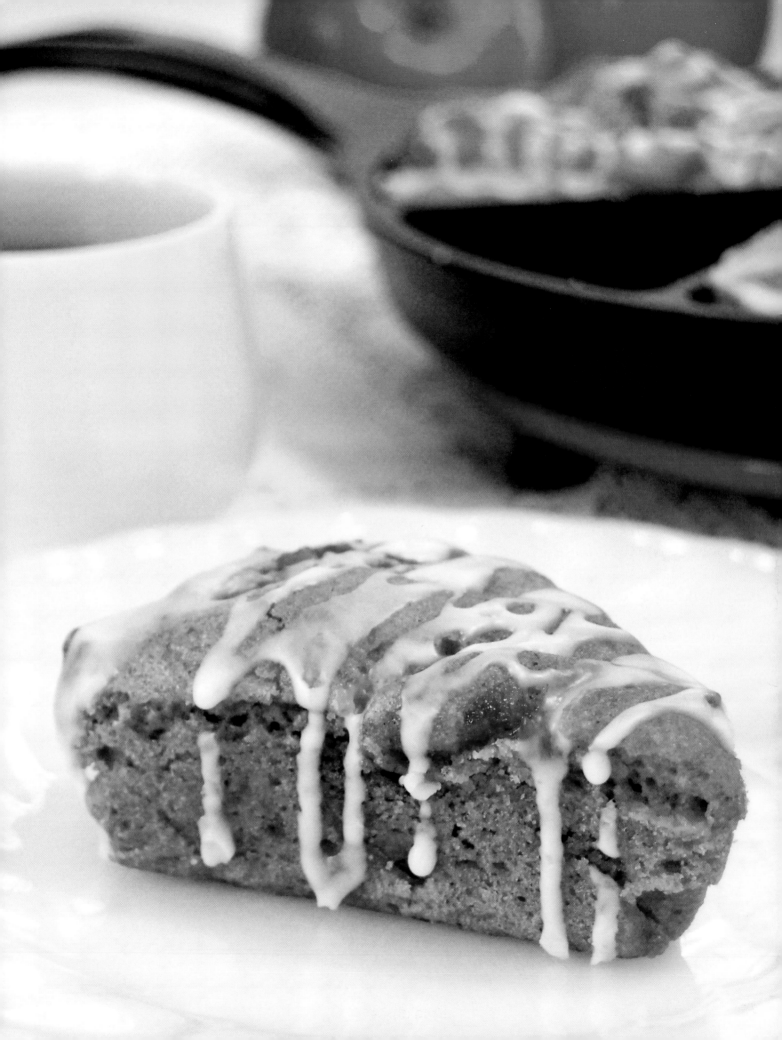

Breakfast Stack

If you've never tried beef bacon, I highly encourage you to give it a whirl. It's delicious and smoky like regular bacon, but a little heartier than pork. Delicious! Trader Joe's carries one that I like, and you can also order it through US Wellness Meats. Combined here with spinach and tomato, you've got yourself a filling, nutritious, egg-free breakfast!

8	**oz (230 g) package uncured beef bacon**
2	**C (85 g) organic baby spinach**
1	**large organic tomato, thick sliced**
~	**Nondairy cheese**
~	**Olive oil**
~	**Sea salt**
~	**Freshly ground pepper**

1. Cook bacon according to package directions.
2. On a parchment-lined baking sheet, lay spinach leaves into 4 even piles.
3. Layer bacon on top of spinach.
4. Add 1 slice tomato to each.
5. Sprinkle with cheese.
6. Drizzle tops with olive oil, salt, and pepper.
7. Broil for about 5 minutes, until tomato starts to brown and cheese is bubbly.

Serves 4

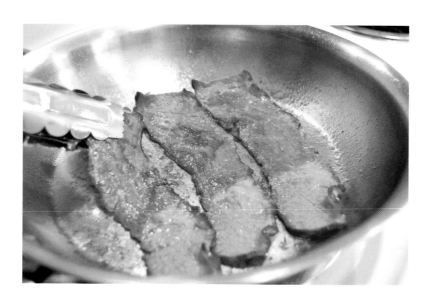

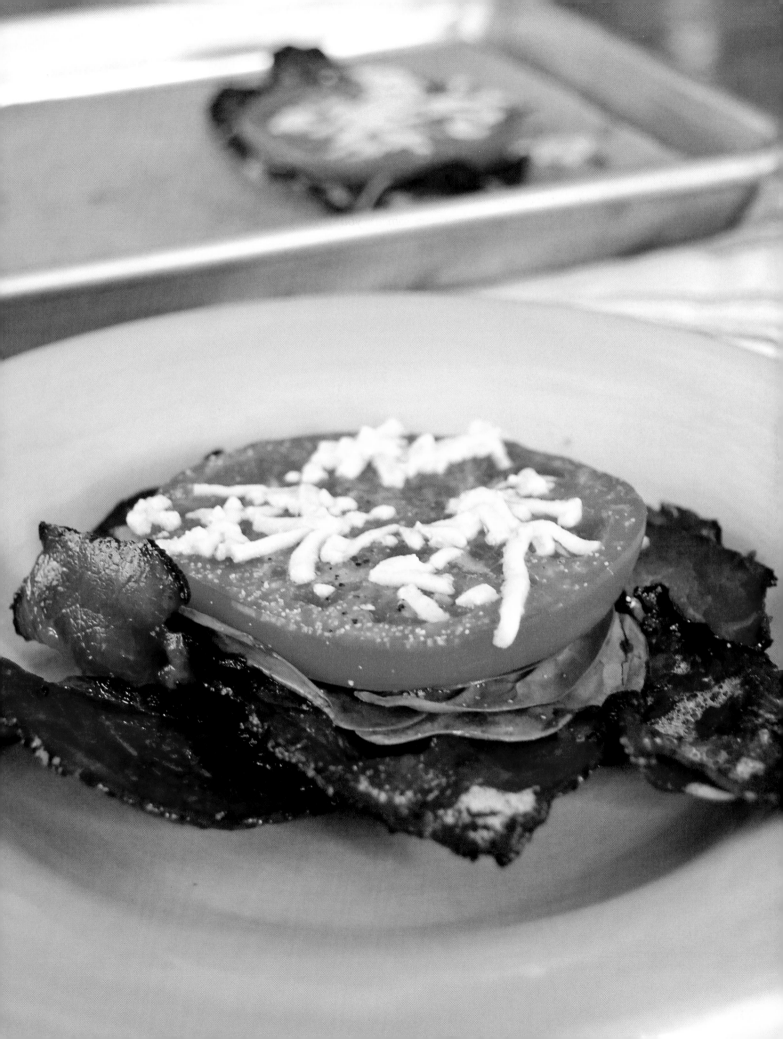

Jellied Biscuits

Years ago, long before food allergies were an everyday thought in my head, I happened upon a little bakery that made these gorgeous flaky drop biscuits with a tasty pool of jam and sugar sprinkled on top. It was the perfect blend of flaky, buttery, and sweet. I loved it so much, I spent the next year experimenting with recipes to try and duplicate it. I finally mashed all of the trial and error together to create a pretty darn close replica of that wonderful biscuit. Then I got married, had children, and everyone changed my life forever... including in terms of food. I happened across my old biscuit recipe one day, ready to throw it out since I couldn't use it anymore, when I decided it was time to recreate some of my old favorites. So here it is! I'm happy to say, while it isn't oozing with butter—not necessarily a bad thing—it is oozing with flaky, sweet goodness. Great with coffee on Sunday morning!

Dry Ingredients:

½   C (60 g) sorghum flour

½   C (60 g) brown rice flour

½   C (60 g) potato starch

½   C (60 g) tapioca starch

1   tsp xanthan gum

2   tsp baking powder

½   tsp sea salt

½   tsp cream of tartar

Wet Ingredients:

½   C (120 g) organic palm shortening, chilled (I like Spectrum brand)

1   Tbsp raw organic honey

¾   C (180 mL) canned lite coconut milk, chilled

Add Ons:

⅓   C (80 mL) of your favorite GF jelly or jam

2   Tbsp melted coconut oil

~   Organic evaporated cane juice

1.   In a medium bowl, whisk together dry ingredients.

2.   With a pastry cutter, cut shortening into dry ingredients until pea-size crumbs form.

3.   Add honey and milk to crumb mixture and stir with a fork just until mixed.

4.   Drop by rounded spoonfuls onto a parchment-lined baking sheet.

5.   Make an impression in each biscuit with your thumb or a spoon. Fill each with 1 tsp jelly.

6.   Brush tops with melted coconut oil. Sprinkle with sugar and bake in a 400° oven for 15–20 minutes or until biscuits are browned on top.

Makes 9–10

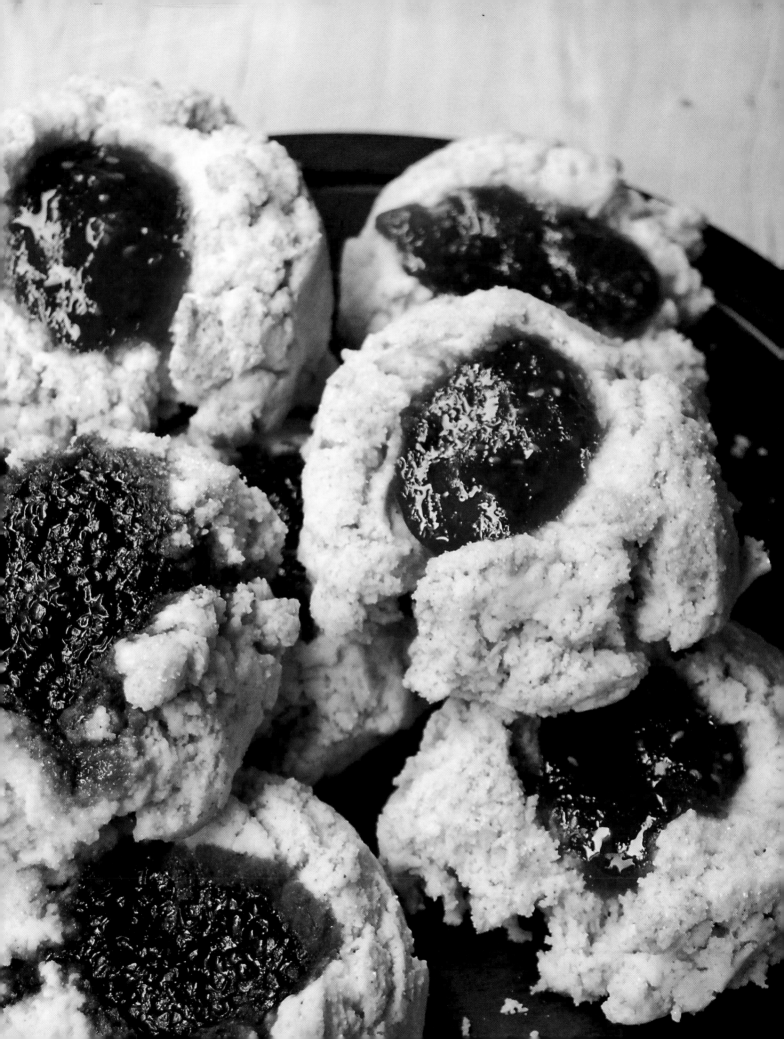

Banana Crumb Coffee Cake

This recipe was originally inspired by a photo and recipe in Good Housekeeping. And while the recipe looks nothing like the original, the fact that a completely forbidden recipe could inspire such goodness should provide hope for all gluten-free cooks! I'm a firm believer in looking at all sources for kitchen inspiration, so don't write off a favorite family recipe because you don't think you can convert it. Maybe down the road when you've learned more and feel more confident, you can tackle the challenge. Until then, make this cake!

Cake:

Dry Ingredients:

½	C (60 g) sorghum flour
¼	C (30 g) teff flour
½	C (60 g) potato starch
¼	C (30 g) tapioca starch
1	tsp xanthan gum
1	tsp baking powder
½	tsp baking soda
¼	tsp sea salt
¼	tsp cinnamon

Wet Ingredients:

¼	C (60 ml) coconut oil (or nondairy butter)
¼	C (45 g) packed organic brown sugar
2	Tbsp raw organic honey
¼	C (60 mL) organic unsweetened applesauce mixed with ½ tsp baking powder (mix right before adding to bowl)
1	C (250 mL) mashed, very ripe organic bananas (the darker the better!)
2	tsp pure vanilla extract

Topping:

½	C (75 g) toasted, chopped pecans
¼	C (40 g) organic unsweetened shredded coconut, toasted
2	Tbsp brown rice flour
2	Tbsp potato starch
¼	C (45 g) packed brown sugar
1	Tbsp raw honey
¼	tsp cinnamon
2	Tbsp coconut oil (or nondairy butter), melted

1. To prepare topping, combine all ingredients except for oil. Add oil and mix with a fork until crumbly. Set aside.
2. For the cake: Whisk together dry ingredients. Set aside.
3. In a stand mixer, blend together the wet ingredients until combined.
4. Slowly add in dry ingredients until incorporated. Mix on high for 30 seconds to mix well.
5. Pour batter into a greased 9-inch cake pan, smoothing top to make it level.
6. Sprinkle with crumble topping.
7. Bake in a 350° oven for 50–55 minutes or until toothpick inserted in center comes out clean.
8. Cool on a wire rack before serving.
9. Store leftovers in an airtight container for up to 2 days or wrap well before placing in airtight container and freeze for later use. To thaw, simply set on the counter for 1 hour.

Options:

~Try blueberry! Use ½ C applesauce in place of bananas and mix in 1 C fresh blueberries.

~How about a pumpkin coffee cake? Replace 1 C bananas with 1 C pureed pumpkin (canned pumpkin). Add in a pinch of nutmeg for a great fall treat!

Breakfasts

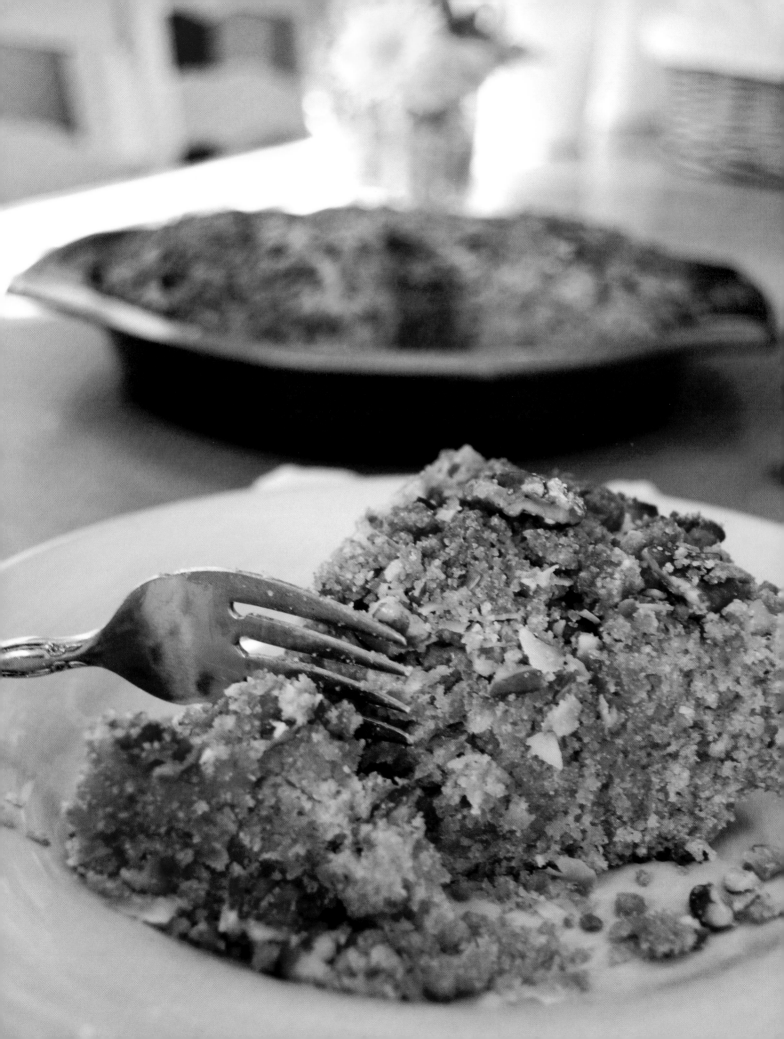

Homemade Chorizo

I love the flavor of chorizo, but we stopped eating it for a long time because I couldn't find any brands that were safe. Most of the time, I couldn't get any allergy information at all, which is a no-go for us. When in doubt, don't eat it. Then my mom found an old recipe card in her stash with this spicy, flavorful recipe. So thank you to whoever gave this to her many, many years ago; we enjoy it very much. And I think you will too!

1	lb (450 g) grass-fed ground pork (you can also use ground beef but it's not quite as authentic)
¾	tsp sea salt
2	Tbsp chili powder
1	clove garlic, crushed
1	Tbsp white wine vinegar
1	tsp cumin
~	Black pepper to taste
~	Red pepper flakes to taste

1. Mix all ingredients together in a medium bowl. Cover and let sit in the refrigerator overnight so flavors blend.
2. The next morning, shape meat into patties and cook until browned and done, or cook crumbled and serve with your favorite breakfast sides.

Serves 4

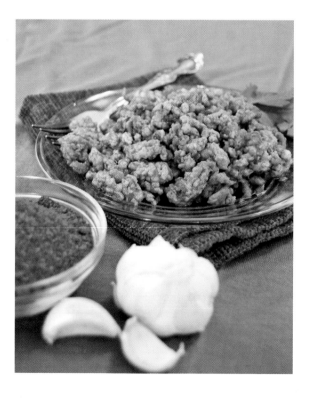

Breakfasts

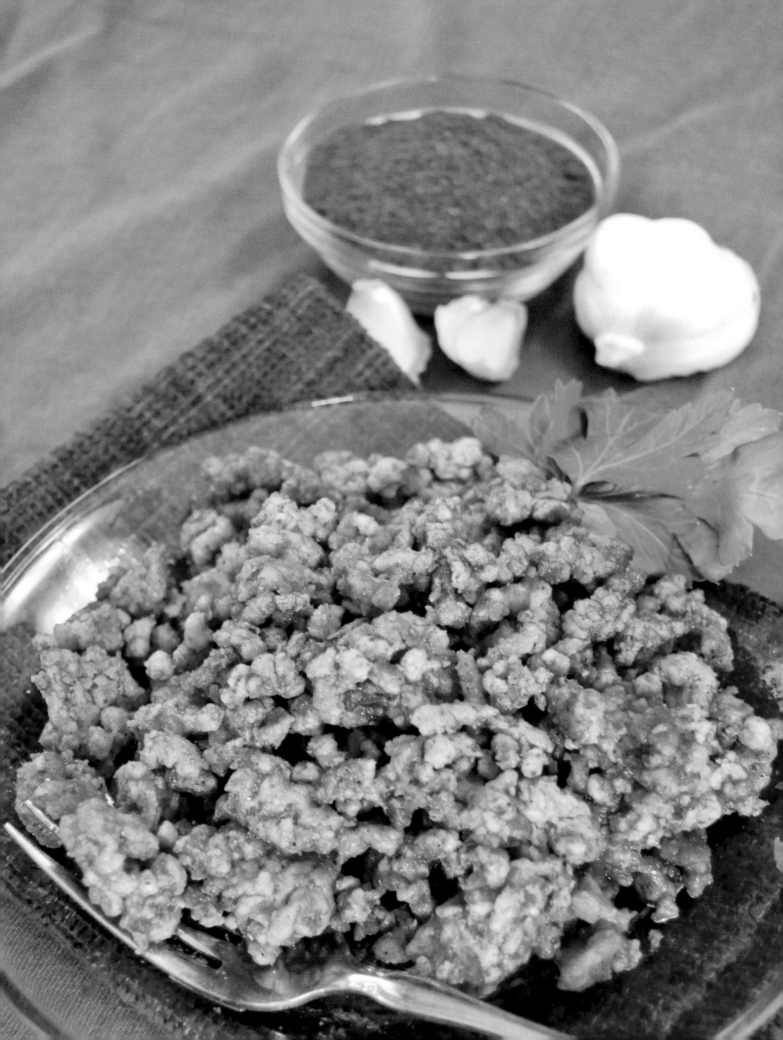

Waffles

Yummy, crispy waffles make for a wonderful weekend breakfast. Make a few extra, freeze them, and you've got wonderful weekday breakfasts available in minutes! Have I mentioned how much I love my freezer? For time and money savings, you can't beat making your own and freezing them for another day. Just pop them into the toaster!

Dry Ingredients:

½	C (60 g) sorghum flour
½	C (60 g) teff flour
½	C (60 g) potato starch
¼	C (30 g) tapioca starch
¼	tsp xanthan gum
1	tsp baking powder
½	tsp sea salt

Wet Ingredients:

1	C (240 mL) coconut milk or nondairy milk of choice
2	Tbsp organic unsweetened applesauce
¼	C (60 mL) coconut oil, melted
1	C (240 mL) warm water

1. In a large bowl, whisk together dry ingredients.
2. Add wet ingredients to the dry ingredients and whisk until batter is smooth. Batter will be like traditional waffle batter, not too runny, not too thick.
3. Scoop batter (I use ¼ C) into heated waffle iron and cook according to manufacturer's instructions and waffles are crisp and slightly browned on the edges.
4. Serve with yummy Blueberry Syrup (p. 68), or perhaps a smear of sunbutter and maple syrup.

Options:

How about chocolate waffles? Add ½ C cocoa powder and 3 Tbsp honey or maple syrup to the batter.

Makes 12 squares

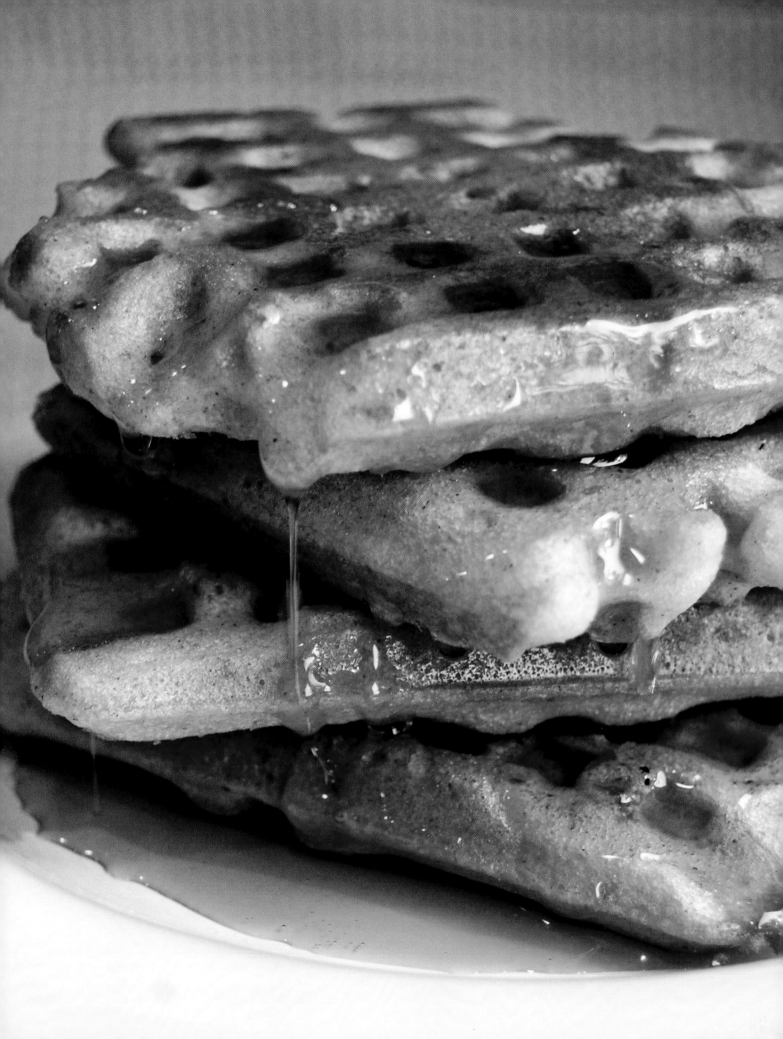

Famous Celiac Maniac English Muffins

There isn't much to say about this recipe, except make them. Enjoy them. Revel in the joy of having bread again. Lose yourself in those nooks and crannies you thought only existed in gluten-filled English muffins. Then make more. Give them to friends and family and share the goodness. An entire wholesale bakery business was built on this one recipe. Now I pass it on to you.

Yeast Mixture:

4	C (950 mL) water
⅓	C (80 mL) raw organic honey
1	rounded Tbsp active dry yeast

Dry Ingredients:

2	C (240 g) sorghum flour
1¼	C (150 g) brown rice flour
½	C (60 g) teff flour
1½	C (180 g) potato starch
⅔	C (80 g) tapioca starch
1½	Tbsp xanthan gum
1	Tbsp sea salt

Wet Ingredients:

⅔	C (160 mL) coconut oil, melted
1	Tbsp raw apple cider vinegar
⅓	C (80 mL) hot water

Makes 24 muffins

1. Whisk together dry ingredients, set aside.
2. Preheat oven to its lowest setting, or on "warm," about 150°-170°.
3. Heat water in the microwave for about 2 minutes, or until temperature is around 100°-110°. Add honey and yeast, mix gently to combine. Set aside in a warm place, like on top of the stove or in the microwave, to proof and become frothy, for 4-5 minutes.
4. Line 2 half sheet pans with parchment paper. Place 12 English muffin rings on each pan. Spray rings with nonstick cooking spray.
5. In a stand mixer fit with the paddle attachment, mix dry ingredients, yeast mixture, and wet ingredients. Blend on high for 2 minutes to fully incorporate. Dough should be the consistency of a very wet bread dough. Almost like a thick muffin batter.
6. With a 2¾ oz scoop (about ⅓ C), scoop dough into muffin rings. Dough should be just below the top of the rings.
7. Fill a bowl with cold water. Dip a metal spoon into water and, with quick strokes, press down dough in each ring to smooth tops.
8. Place baking sheets in oven (place oven racks on the 2nd and 4th position in oven). Let muffins rise for about 15 minutes, or until dough reaches just above the tops of the rings.
9. Raise oven temperature to 425°. Bake muffins for 40 minutes, rotating trays after 25 minutes of baking. Tops should be browned and muffins will sound hollow when you tap lightly on the tops.
10. Cool for 15 minutes on trays. Then remove muffins from rings to cool completely on wire racks.
11. Once cool, use a fork to pierce the sides of the muffins all the way around, until muffin pulls apart.
12. Enjoy freshly baked, or place in freezer-safe zip-top bags to use later. To enjoy from frozen, simply split apart and place in toaster until nicely toasted.

Options:

~Toast and top with vegan butter and cinnamon and sugar for the classic cinnamon toast you remember.

~Toast lightly, top with GF ham and dairy-free cheese, toast again to melt cheese, and enjoy grilled ham and cheese again!

~Toast lightly, let cool, and use as a sandwich bread or hamburger bun!

Note:

If 24 muffins are too many to bake at once for you, the recipe can be cut in half easily.

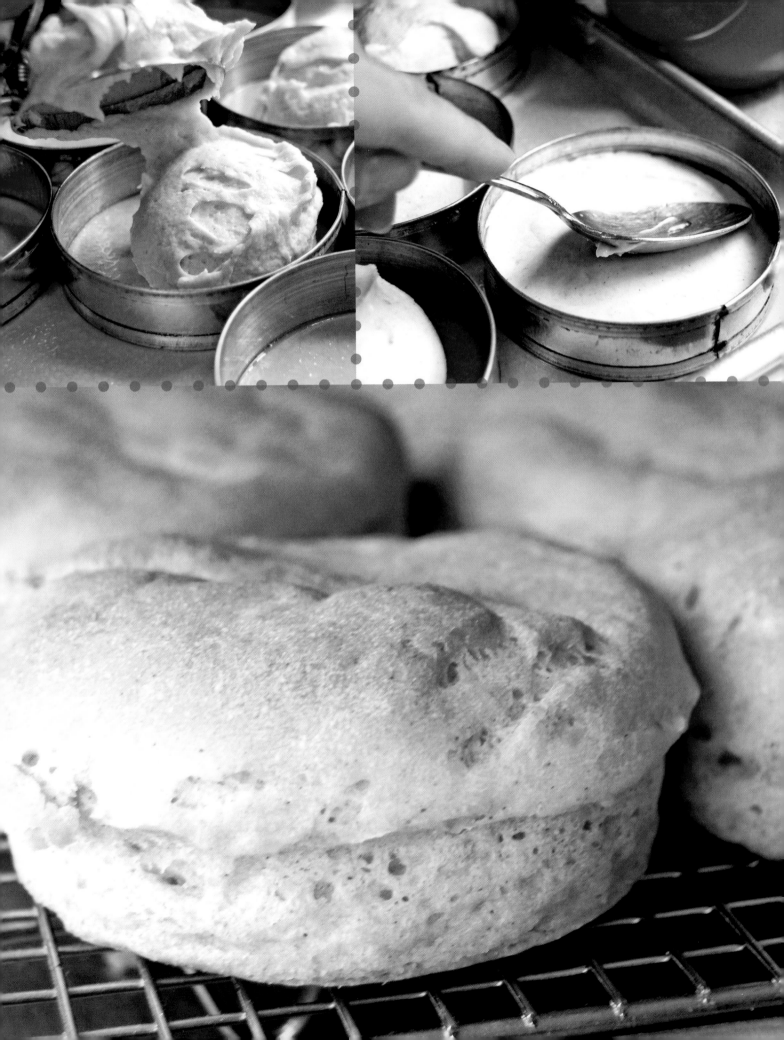

Cinnamon Raisin English Muffins

The same wonderful taste, texture, and nooks and crannies of our original English muffins, but with the slightly sweet, cinnamon-y and raisin-y taste of your favorite cinnamon bread of the past. There has been an ongoing debate with our bakery customers as to which muffin is best... original or cinnamon raisin? Which one do you like best?

Yeast Mixture:

4	C (950 mL) water
⅓	C (80 mL) raw organic honey
1	rounded Tbsp active dry yeast

Dry Ingredients:

2	C (240 g) sorghum flour
1¼	C (150 g) brown rice flour
½	C (60 g) teff flour
1½	C (180 g) potato starch
⅔	C (80 g) tapioca starch
1½	Tbsp xanthan gum
1	Tbsp sea salt
1	Tbsp cinnamon

Wet Ingredients:

⅔	C (160 mL) coconut oil, melted
1	Tbsp raw apple cider vinegar
⅓	C (80 mL) hot water

Add Ins:

¼	C cinnamon sugar blend (Mix ½ C organic evaporated cane juice with 2 Tbsp cinnamon. Use any leftovers for topping pancakes, plain English muffins, etc.)
1	C (150 g) organic raisins

1. Whisk together dry ingredients, set aside.
2. Preheat oven to its lowest setting, or on "warm," about 150°-170°.
3. Heat water in the microwave for about 2 minutes, or until temperature is around 100°-110°. Add honey and yeast, mix gently to combine. Set aside in a warm place, like on top of the stove or in the microwave, to proof and become frothy, for 4-5 minutes.
4. Line 2 half sheet pans with parchment paper. Place 12 English muffin rings on each pan. Spray rings with nonstick cooking spray.
5. In a stand mixer fit with the paddle attachment, mix dry ingredients, yeast mixture, and wet ingredients. Blend on high for 2 minutes to fully incorporate. Dough should be the consistency of a very wet bread dough. Almost like a thick muffin batter.
6. Add raisins and mix slightly.
7. Gently fold in cinnamon/sugar blend.
8. With a 2¾ oz scoop (about $^1/_3$ C), scoop dough into muffin rings. Dough should be just below the top of the rings.
9. Fill a bowl with cold water. Dip a metal spoon into water and, with quick strokes, press down dough in each ring to smooth tops.
10. Place baking sheets in oven (place oven racks on the 2nd and 4th position in oven). Let muffins rise for about 15 minutes, or until dough reaches just above the tops of the rings.
11. Raise oven temperature to 425°. Bake muffins for 40 minutes, rotating trays after 25 minutes of baking. Tops should be browned and muffins will sound hollow when you tap lightly on the tops.
12. Cool for 15 minutes on trays. Then remove muffins from rings to cool completely on wire racks.
13. Once cool, use a fork to pierce the sides of the muffins all the way around, until muffin pulls apart.
14. Enjoy freshly baked, or place in freezer-safe zip-top bags to use later. To enjoy from frozen, simply split apart and place in toaster until nicely toasted.

Makes 24 muffins

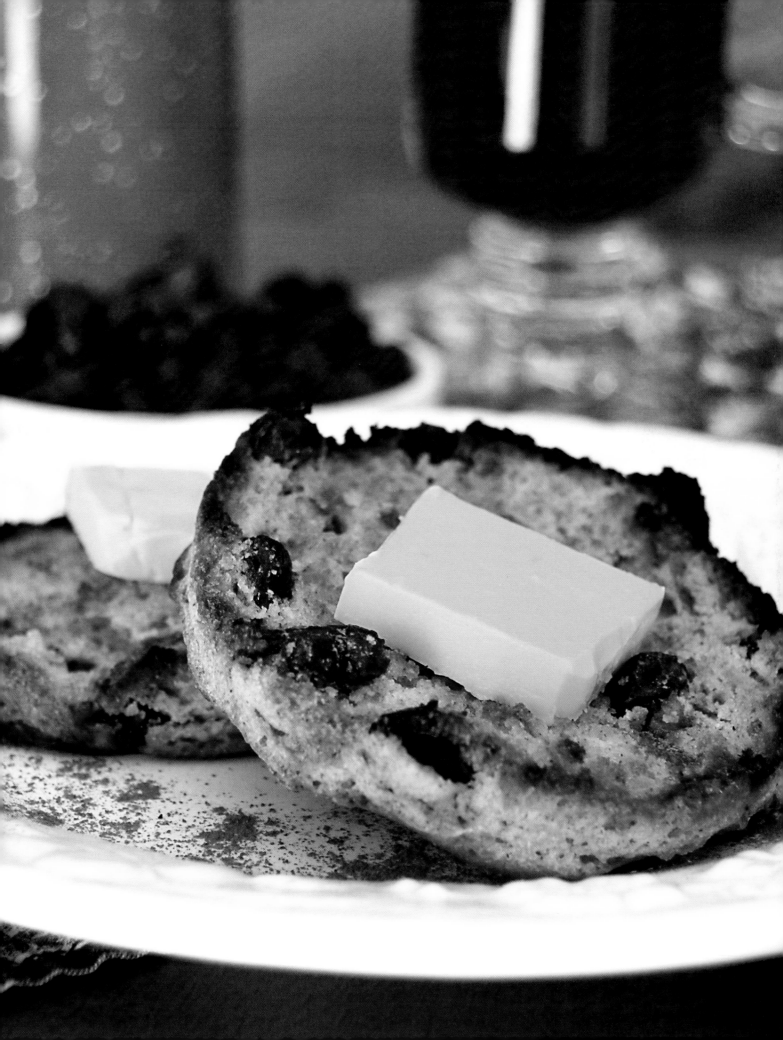

Blueberry English Muffins

Sweet wild blueberries add a touch of summer to your breakfast mornings in these English muffins! I like mine with a little honey butter (p. 270) and a fresh cup of coffee. While any frozen blueberry will work in this recipe, I really prefer the wild ones, since they are smaller and incorporate better into the batter, allowing for a higher rise and a more evenly baked muffin. With larger conventional blueberries, they can make the batter bake a little unevenly because of the temperature difference between the frozen berries and the warm dough.

Yeast Mixture:

2	C (475 mL) warm water
1	Tbsp raw organic honey
2	tsp active dry yeast

Dry Ingredients:

1	C (120 g) sorghum flour
½	C (60 g) brown rice flour
¼	C (30 g) teff flour
¾	C (90 g) potato starch
⅓	C (40 g) tapioca starch
2	tsp xanthan gum
1	tsp sea salt
½	tsp cinnamon

Wet Ingredients:

⅓	C (80 mL) coconut oil, melted
¼	C (60 mL) pure maple syrup (or raw organic honey or coconut nectar)
1	tsp apple cider vinegar
2	tsp pure vanilla extract

Add In:

2	C (300 g) frozen wild blueberries

1. Whisk together dry ingredients, set aside.
2. Preheat oven to its lowest setting, or on "warm," about 150°-170°.
3. Heat water in the microwave for about 2 minutes, or until temperature is around 100°-110°. Add honey and yeast, mix gently to combine. Set aside in a warm place, like on top of the stove or in the microwave, to proof and become frothy, for 4-5 minutes.
4. Line a half sheet pan with parchment paper. Place 12 English muffin rings on the pan. Spray rings with nonstick cooking spray.
5. In a stand mixer fit with the paddle attachment, mix dry ingredients, yeast mixture, and wet ingredients. Blend on high for 2 minutes to fully incorporate. Dough should be the consistency of a very wet bread dough. Almost like a thick muffin batter.
6. Fold in blueberries.
7. With a 2¾ oz scoop (about ⅓ C), scoop dough into muffin rings. Dough should be just below the top of the rings.
8. Fill a bowl with cold water. Dip a metal spoon into water and, with quick strokes, press down dough in each ring to smooth tops.
9. Place baking sheet in oven. Let muffins rise for about 15 minutes, or until dough reaches just above the tops of the rings.
10. Raise oven temperature to 425°. Bake muffins for 40 minutes, rotating tray after 25 minutes of baking. Tops should be browned and muffins will sound hollow when you tap lightly on the tops.
11. Cool for 15 minutes on trays. Then remove muffins from rings to cool completely on wire racks.
12. Once cool, use a fork to pierce the sides of the muffins all the way around, until muffin pulls apart.
13. Enjoy freshly baked, or place in freezer-safe zip-top bags to use later. To enjoy from frozen, simply split apart and place in toaster until nicely toasted.

Makes 12 muffins

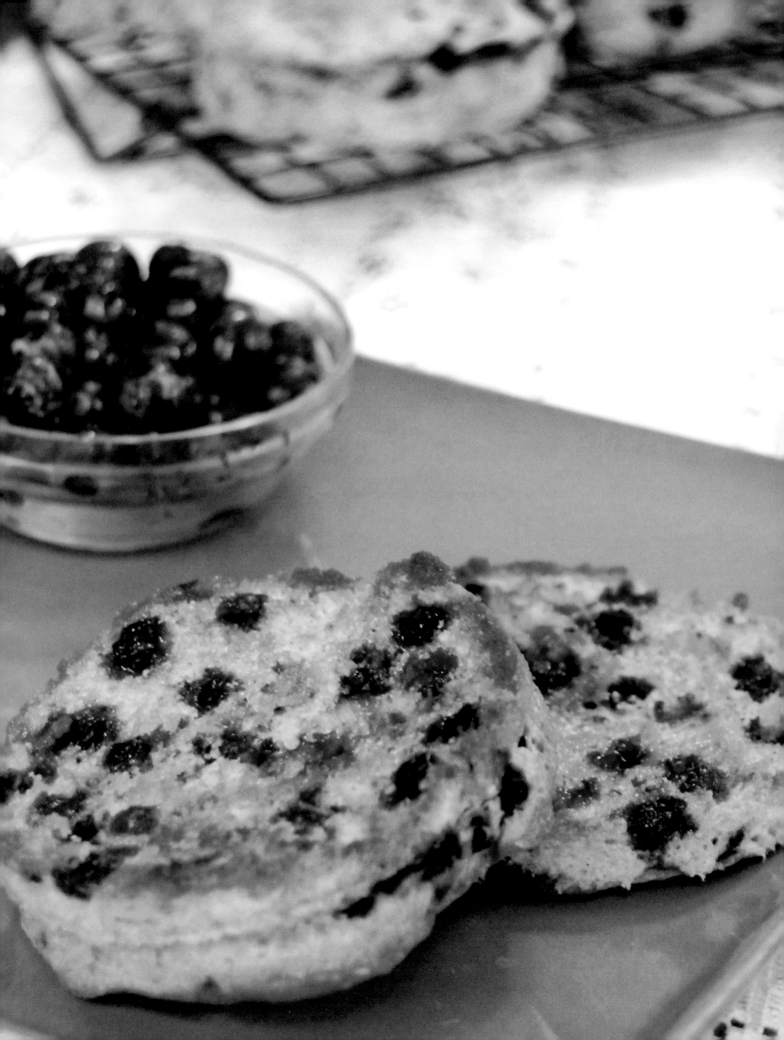

Cranberry Orange English Muffins

As you can see, the flavor combinations for my English Muffins are endless, so feel free to be creative! This flavor with the tart cranberries paired with sweet orange is a winter favorite of mine. I love making large batches in the fall and freezing them so we can enjoy them all season long. The wonderful aroma and bright flavors will cheer up any dreary winter morning!

Yeast Mixture:

2	C (475 mL) warm water
1	Tbsp raw organic honey
2	tsp active dry yeast

Dry Ingredients:

1	C (240 g) sorghum flour
½	C (60 g) brown rice flour
¼	C (30 g) teff flour
¾	C (90 g) potato starch
⅓	C (40 g) tapioca starch
2	tsp xanthan gum
1	tsp sea salt
¼	C (50 g) Sucanat/organic evaporated cane juice

Wet Ingredients:

⅓	C (80 mL) coconut oil, melted
¼	C (60 mL) pure maple syrup (or raw organic honey or coconut nectar)
½	tsp pure orange extract
¼	tsp pure vanilla extract
1	tsp orange zest
1	tsp raw apple cider vinegar

Add In:

⅔	C (100 g) organic cranberries, coarsely chopped

1. Whisk together dry ingredients, set aside.
2. Preheat oven to its lowest setting, or on "warm," about 150°-170°.
3. Heat water in the microwave for about 1 minute, or until temperature is around 100°-110°. Add honey and yeast, mix gently to combine. Set aside in a warm place, like on top of the stove or in the microwave, to proof and become frothy, for 4-5 minutes.
4. Line a half sheet pan with parchment paper. Place 12 English muffin rings on the pan. Spray rings with nonstick cooking spray.
5. In a stand mixer fit with the paddle attachment, mix dry ingredients, yeast mixture, and wet ingredients. Blend on high for 2 minutes to fully incorporate. Dough should be the consistency of a very wet bread dough. Almost like a thick muffin batter.
6. Fold in cranberries.
7. With a 2¾ oz scoop (about ⅓ C), scoop dough into muffin rings. Dough should be just below the top of the rings.
8. Fill a bowl with cold water. Dip a metal spoon into water and, with quick strokes, press down dough in each ring to smooth tops.
9. Place baking sheet in oven. Let muffins rise for about 15 minutes, or until dough reaches just above the tops of the rings.
10. Raise oven temperature to 425°. Bake muffins for 40 minutes, rotating tray after 25 minutes of baking. Tops should be browned and muffins will sound hollow when you tap lightly on the tops.
11. Cool for 15 minutes on trays. Then remove muffins from rings to cool completely on wire racks.
12. Once cool, use a fork to pierce the sides of the muffins all the way around, until muffin pulls apart.
13. Enjoy freshly baked, or place in freezer-safe zip-top bags to use later. To enjoy from frozen, simply split apart and place in toaster until nicely toasted.

Makes 12 muffins

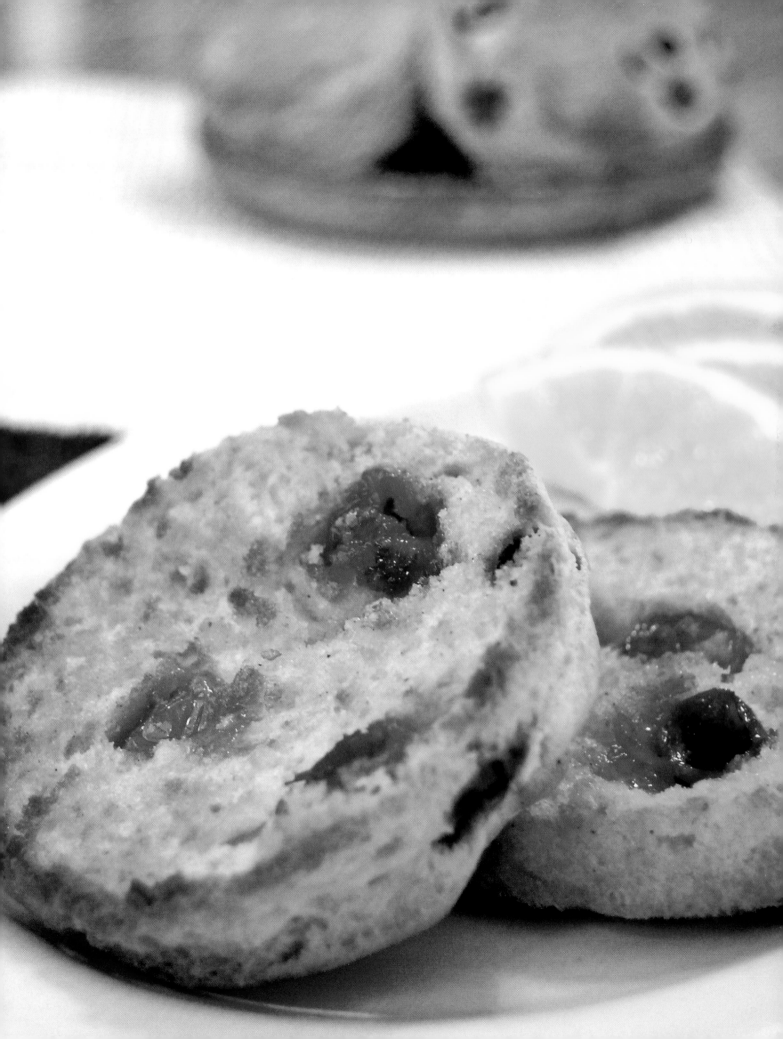

Breakfast PB & F

This is a kid favorite, and you can probably see why. My girls love to decorate their own breakfast "pies" and devour their creations. I love that they are getting a balance of whole grains, protein-packed peanut butter, and vitamin-loaded fruit, without the sugar-laden jam that usually accompanies this combo. This one makes a great after-school snack too!

1	**GF English Muffin (recipe p. 88)**
2	**tsp nondairy butter (I like Earth Balance Soy Free Spread)**
1	**Tbsp organic natural peanut butter (or almond butter or sunbutter)**
~	**Fresh organic fruit such as sliced strawberries, blackberries, raspberries, or sliced peaches**

1. Toast English muffin to desired doneness.
2. Spread nondairy butter on each side of muffin.
3. Spread nut or seed butter evenly on both sides of muffin.
4. Top with fruit and enjoy your healthy GF breakfast!

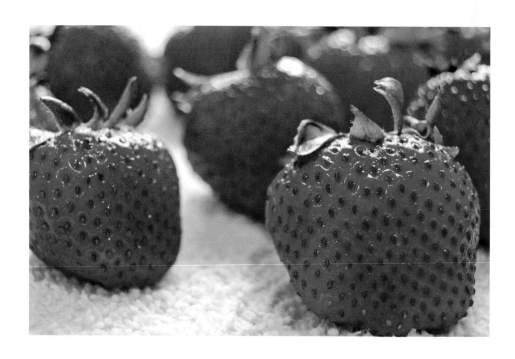

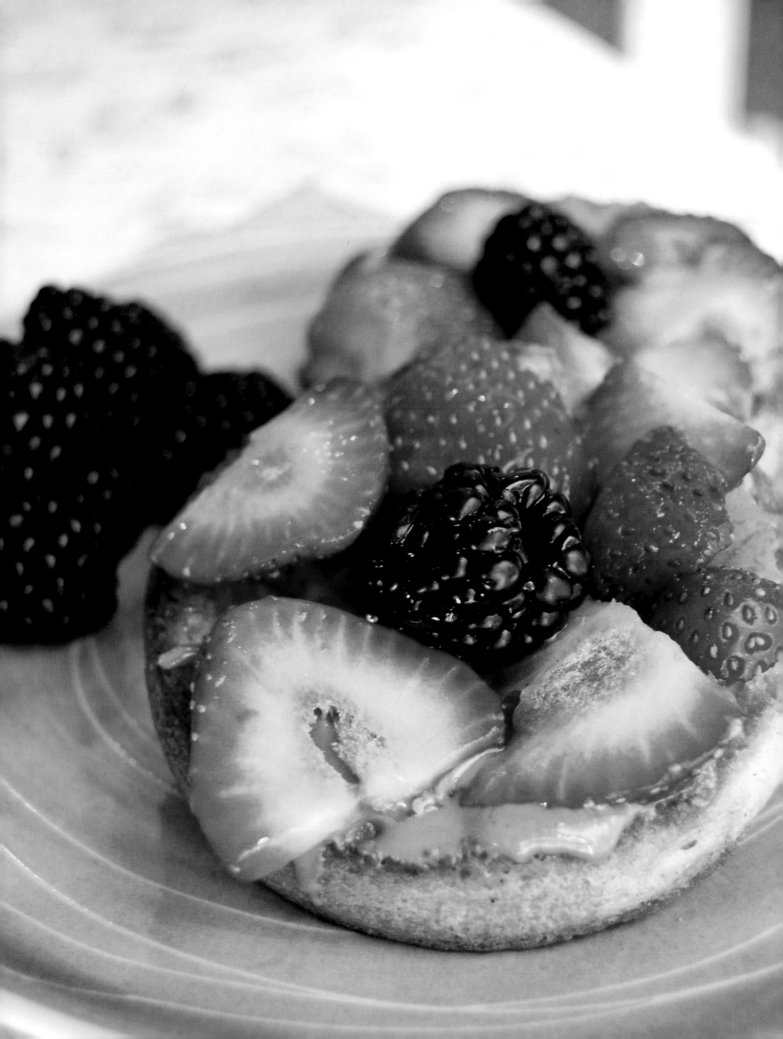

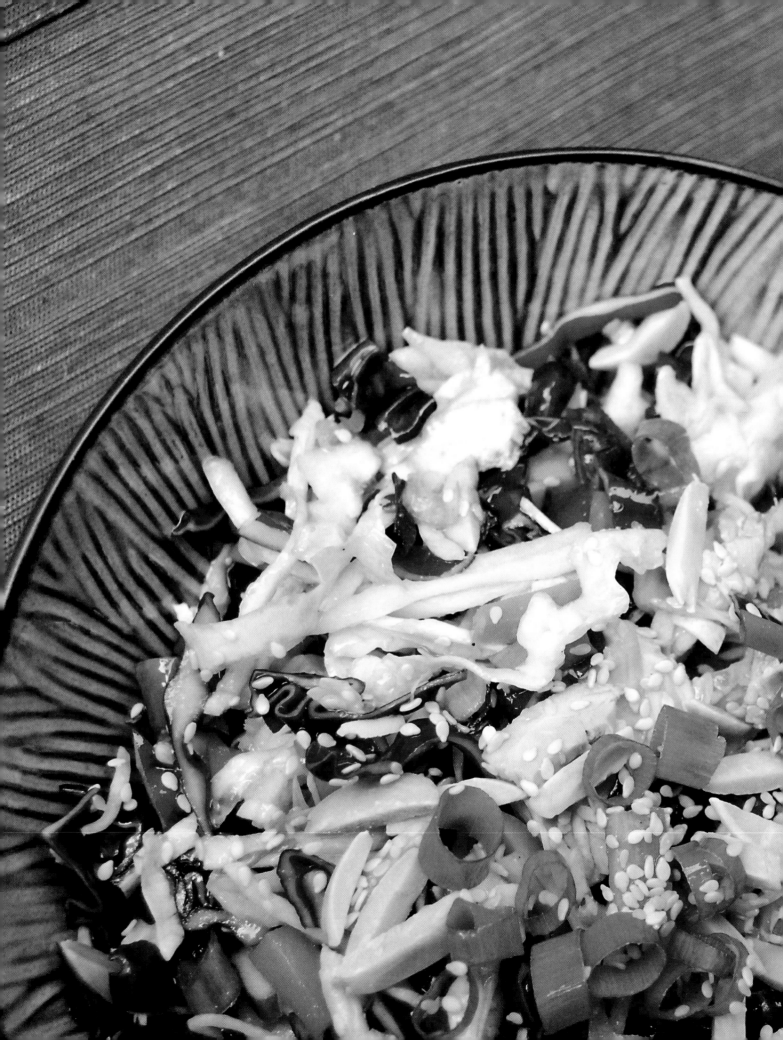

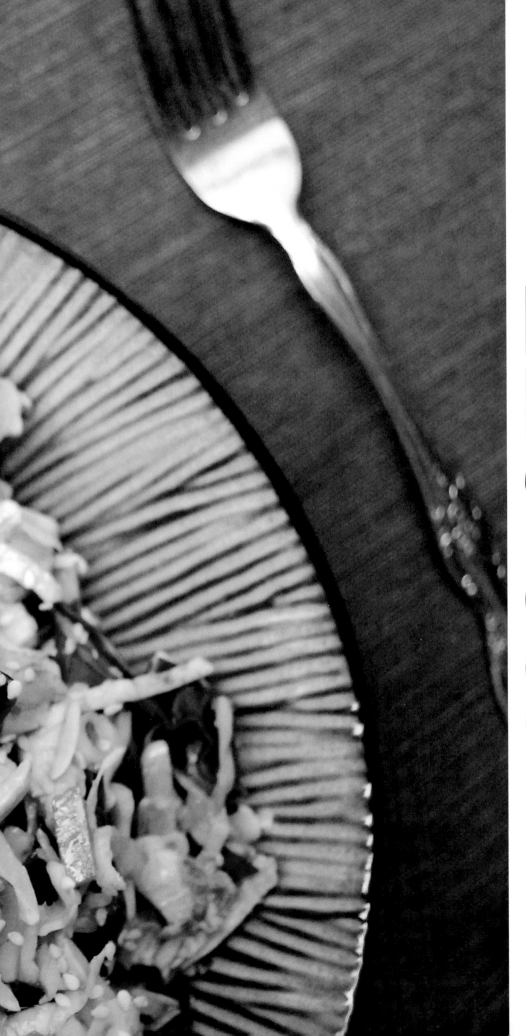

Entrées

Balsamic Chicken

This quick chicken recipe has been a go-to meal for my family for years. Inspired by those nice but allergy-pro-voking and quite expensive make-ahead meal places, this tasty chicken will become a family favorite for you too! Because let's face it, on a Tuesday "what's for dinner mom?" kind of night, even liver and onions, if it was ready to go straight from your freezer, might be a favorite recipe. Thank goodness this is way better than liver and onions!

Chicken:

~   Sea salt

~   Pepper

4   boneless skinless organic chicken breasts

Sauce:

½   cup (120 mL) organic chicken broth

¼   cup (60 mL) balsamic vinegar

1   Tbsp Dijon mustard

2   Tbsp lemon juice

2   garlic cloves, crushed

2   Tbsp olive oil (plus more for pan)

Option 1: Dinner Right Now

1. In a bowl mix together broth, vinegar, Dijon, lemon juice, garlic, and olive oil until well blended.
2. Heat about 2 Tbsp olive oil in a large skillet over medium-high heat.
3. Sprinkle salt and pepper on both sides of chicken.
4. Add chicken to hot skillet and brown chicken on both sides.
5. Add sauce to pan and over the chicken, being careful since the pan is very hot and sauce could splatter a bit. Stir up the yummy bits of goodness on the bottom of the pan as it bubbles.
6. Bring to a slight boil. Turn heat down to medium-low.
7. Simmer for about 6 minutes or until chicken is done and juices run clear.
8. To serve, spoon the delicious, slightly reduced sauce over the chicken.

Option 2: Make Ahead and Freeze Meal

1. In a freezer-safe zip-top bag (quart size) add broth, vinegar, Dijon, lemon juice, garlic, and olive oil. Close the top and squish around a bit until blended.
2. Place 4 chicken breasts and the sauce bag inside a large (gallon-size) zip-top freezer bag. Place in your freezer until ready to use. Keeps about 4 months.
3. When ready to use, remove bag from freezer and let thaw in refrigerator overnight. Follow cooking instructions above.

Tip:

When using this make-ahead method, why not make 3 or 4 at a time so you have a few meals prepared for later in the month? You're welcome.

Serves 4

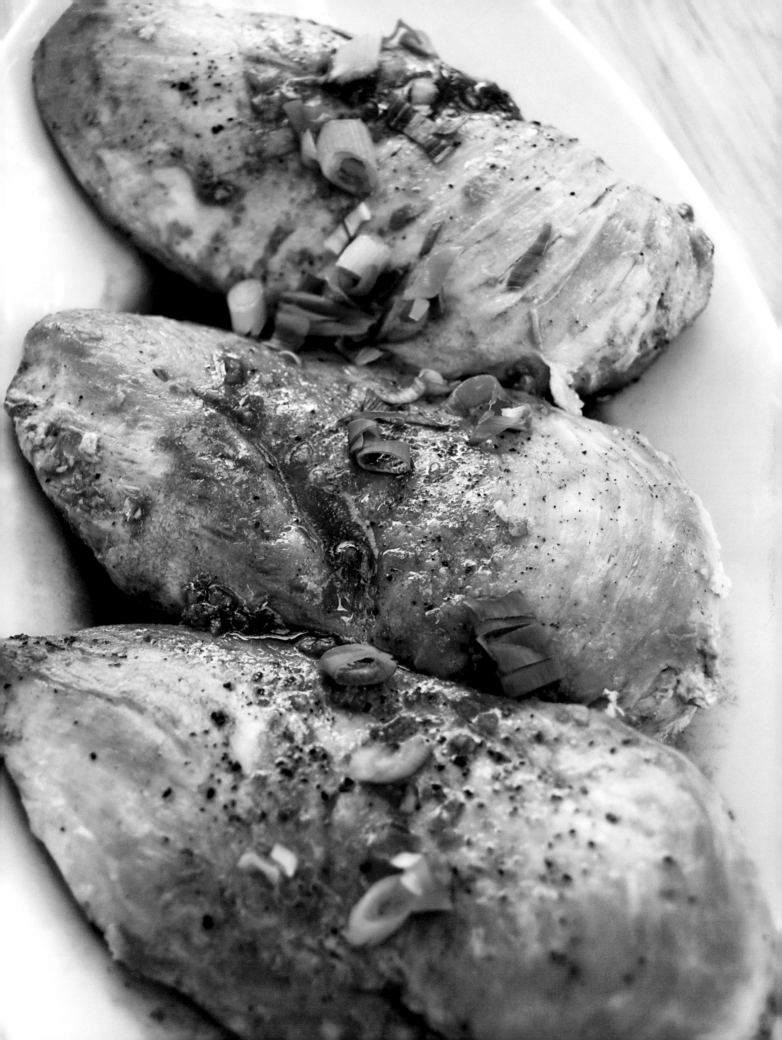

Ginger Lime Chicken Bites

These little chicken bites cook up quickly, which makes for a nice last-minute meal or a speedy school lunch for the kiddos. Make sure to heat up your wide-mouth thermos with hot water (then empty and wipe out) first, then add chicken bites and sauce, close the lid tightly, and your little ones will have a nice, warm, and healthy lunch at school! I also like to use this sauce for sautéed shrimp for another quick and tasty dinner option.

Chicken:

1   Tbsp coconut oil

3   boneless skinless organic chicken breasts, cut into bite-size pieces

Sauce:

~   Juice of 1 organic lime

2   Tbsp Bragg liquid aminos (or wheat-free tamari soy sauce or coconut aminos)

1   Tbsp olive oil

1   tsp freshly grated ginger

1   garlic clove, minced

1   Tbsp raw organic honey

1   tsp granulated onion

Topping:

~   Chopped green onions

~   Sesame seeds

1. Mix sauce ingredients in a small bowl. Set aside.
2. Heat oil in a large skillet over medium-high heat. Add chicken. Cook chicken, stirring occasionally, until browned and almost done. About 5 minutes.
3. Add sauce to skillet, turn heat to low and simmer, uncovered for another 5 minutes, or until chicken pieces are cooked through.
4. Serve with rice, or rice noodles, if desired. Top chicken bites with chopped green onions and sesame seeds. Enjoy!

Serves 2

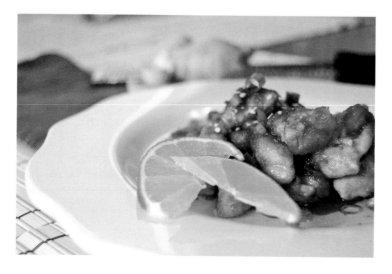

Entrées

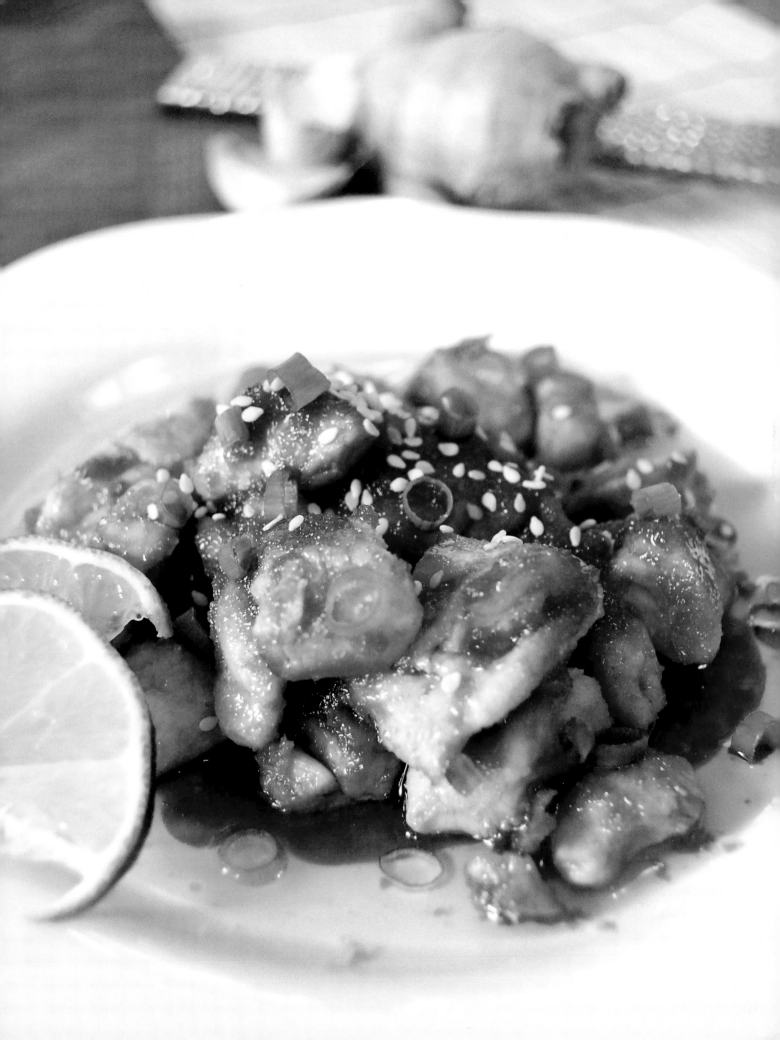

Oriental Chicken Salad

I think just about everyone has had a version of an Oriental chicken salad in their recipe box at some point. I know one of the first I tried used instant ramen noodles and the seasoning packet for the dressing. Nothing like a little sodium, MSG, BHT, and corn syrup to make a great meal! So I got to playing with a few dressings and my family unanimously agreed, this was the winner. We love this one-bowl meal in the summer because there isn't a lot of cooking (none if you use leftover cooked chicken) and it's cool but satisfying. And while this combo is our favorite, we change the veggies depending on what's in season and what we have in the fridge at that moment. Don't hesitate to put whatever veggies you love into the mix!

Salad:

3	cooked organic chicken breasts, cubed
1	small head organic green cabbage, sliced thin
½	small head organic purple cabbage, sliced thin
2	medium organic carrots, diced
1	C (150 g) organic sugar snap peas, cut in half
4	organic green onions, chopped
3	Tbsp toasted sesame seeds
1	C (150 g) toasted slivered almonds

Dressing:

1	shallot, minced
1	tsp grated fresh ginger root
¾	C (180 mL) olive oil
½	C (120 mL) rice vinegar
¼	C (60 mL) Bragg liquid aminos (or GF Tamari soy sauce or coconut aminos)
¼	C (60 mL) organic raw honey
1	tsp sesame oil
¼	tsp xanthan gum
~	Freshly ground pepper

1. In a jar with a tight fitting lid, combine dressing ingredients and shake vigorously to combine.
2. In a large bowl combine all ingredients and dressing. Toss to coat and serve.

Serves 4-6

Entrées

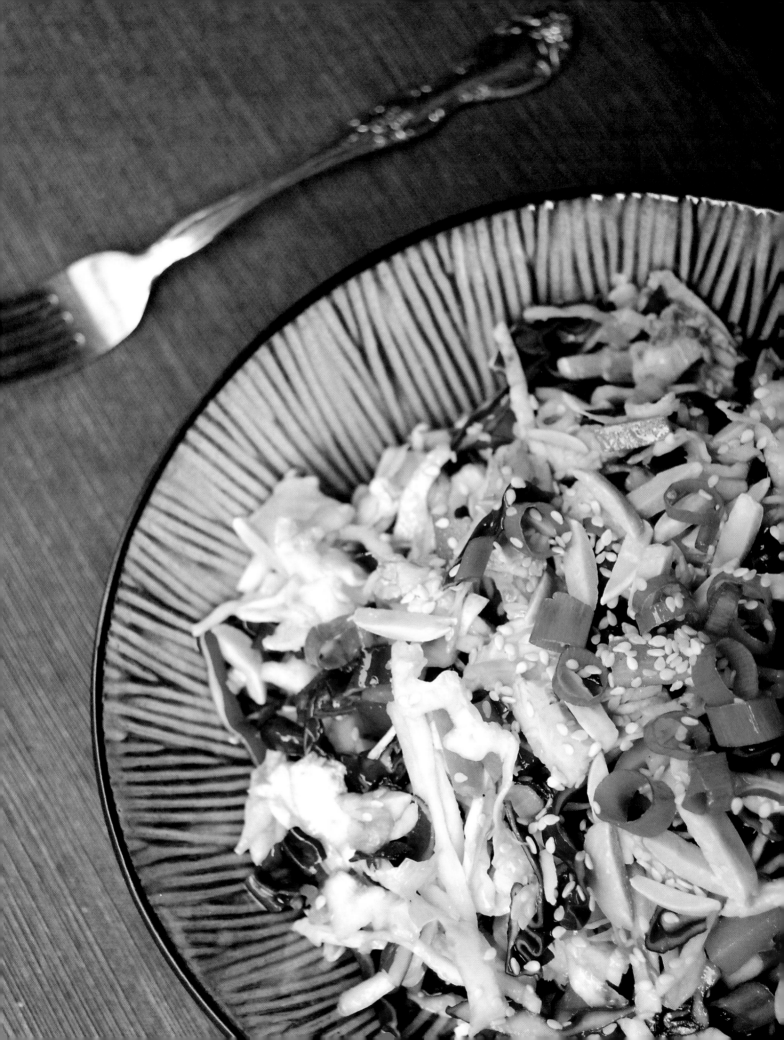

Coconut Chicken Strips

If your family is missing those weeknight drive-thru dinners, you're going to love this recipe! These crispy, tasty chicken strips are incredibly easy to make, and because they are baked, not fried, you can also feel good about serving them to your family, without the typical "post-drive-thru guilt." I love making extras for school lunches the next day. Just reheat in a frying pan with a tiny bit of oil to re-crisp the crust, then place strips in a heated wide-mouth thermos. Don't forget to include a dipping sauce like the Honey Mustard Sauce (p. 250) or the quick BBQ Sauce (p. 251)!

For the Chicken:

4	organic boneless skinless chicken breasts, cut into strips
¼	C (60 mL) coconut oil, melted

For the Breading:

1	C (150 g) finely shredded organic unsweetened coconut
¼	C (30 g) coconut flour
½	tsp sea salt
½	tsp freshly ground pepper
½	tsp granulated onion
½	tsp granulated garlic
½	tsp paprika

1. In a shallow dish, combine breading ingredients. Set aside.
2. Drizzle half of the coconut oil over chicken strips. Dredge strips in breading, covering all of the chicken.
3. Place breaded chicken in a greased 9" by 13" in glass baking dish. Pour remaining oil over strips.
4. Bake in a 375° oven for 20 minutes.
5. Change oven to Broil and broil chicken about 5 minutes, or until golden brown on top.

Serves 4

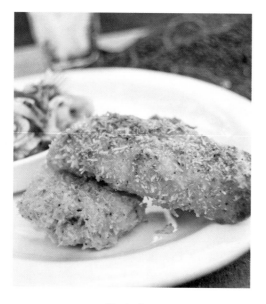

Entrées

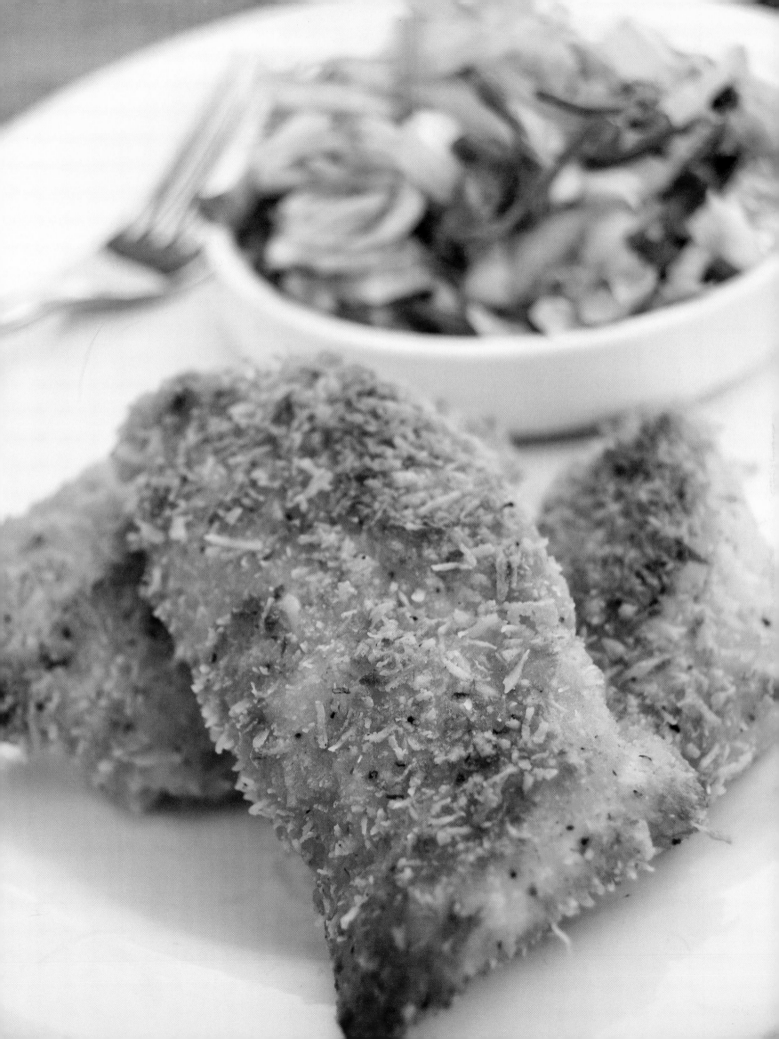

Raspberry-Glazed Chicken

Here's another great recipe inspired by those make-and-take dinner places. My sister and I tried one of those places a couple of times, but it dawned on us one day that the recipes were beyond simple and the prices were beyond reasonable! So we (OK, mostly she) proceeded to adapt a few of the recipes to our own family's tastes and budgets. This was one of our first attempts, and we were very happy with the results, not to mention the low cost! Easily made for tonight's dinner or prepared ahead and frozen for later use, this raspberry chicken makes weeknight dinner a breeze!

Chicken:

4	boneless skinless organic chicken breasts
2	Tbsp coconut oil

Sauce:

2	Tbsp balsamic vinegar
2	Tbsp olive oil
2	Tbsp lemon juice
2	tsp Dijon mustard
⅓	C organic raspberry jam
1	Tbsp raw organic honey
1	Tbsp minced red onion
½	tsp sea salt
~	Freshly ground pepper

1. In a medium bowl, combine sauce ingredients.
2. Heat oil in a large skillet over medium heat. Add chicken breasts and brown on both sides.
3. Turn heat to low and add sauce.
4. Cover and cook until chicken is cooked through, about 20 minutes.
5. Spoon extra sauce over chicken breasts to serve.

Make Ahead and Freeze!

1. In a gallon-size zip-top bag, combine sauce ingredients. Squish around to combine.
2. Add fresh boneless skinless chicken breasts to the bag, making sure they all get coated in sauce.
3. Seal bag and place in the freezer until needed.
4. To prepare, cooked thawed chicken with sauce in a baking dish at 350° until chicken is cooked, about 30 minutes.

Tip:

For a quick lunch or dinner, cut up chicken into bite-size pieces, brown in a skillet, add sauce, and simmer until done, about 10 minutes.

Option:

Try replacing the raspberry jam with apricot jelly!

Serves 4

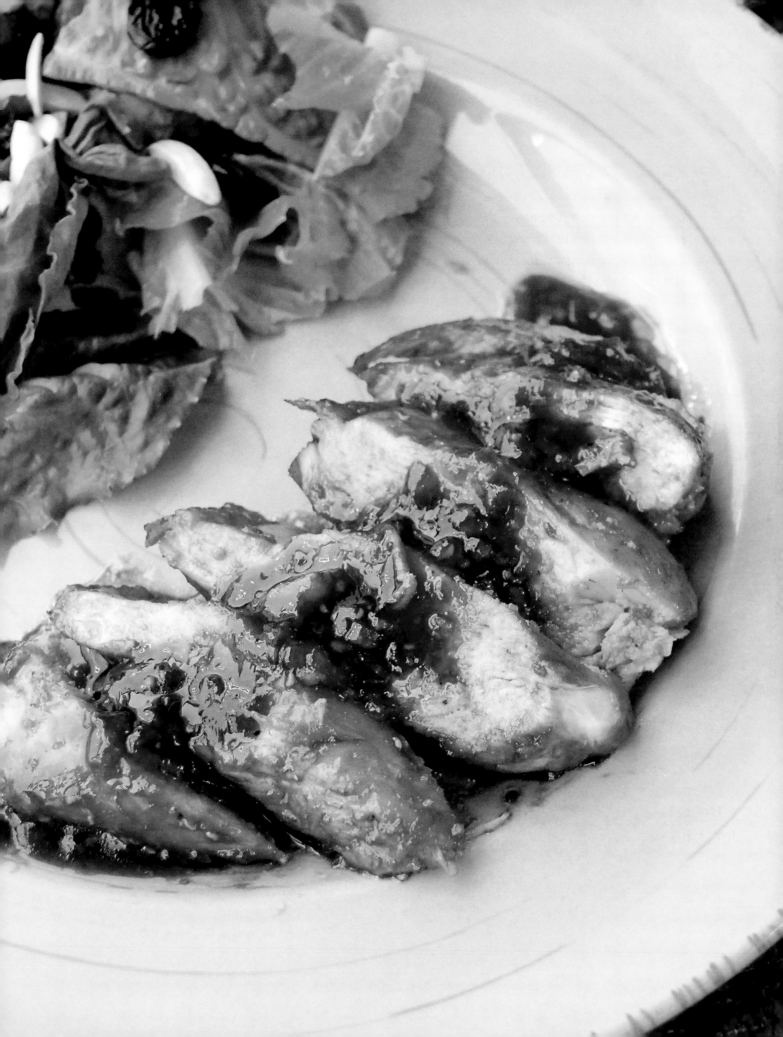

Skillet Rosemary Chicken

If you don't already have one, a great cast-iron skillet is really a kitchen essential. I love my large Lodge cast-iron skillet because it lasts forever, it's easy to clean, and I can pop it from the stovetop into the oven without thinking twice. And if you've ever hesitated getting one because you were intimidated by having to season it—guess what? Lodge seasons them for you, so you're ready to go the moment you bring it home! For this recipe you can use a good-quality, oven-proof skillet, but there's something so homey and rustic about cast-iron that I'm pretty sure it makes this dish taste even better. And to keep things easy—I love easy—this meal makes its own delicious sauce as it cooks, so make sure to spoon plenty of it over your chicken before serving!

1	tsp sea salt
~	Freshly ground pepper
2	tsp granulated onion
¼	tsp turmeric
4	bone-in organic chicken breast halves (or 4 chicken leg quarters) (US Wellness Meats)
1	Tbsp coconut oil
1	organic lemon, cut into quarters
4	sprigs fresh rosemary
2	garlic cloves, minced
8	oz (230 g) white button mushrooms, sliced
1	C (240 mL) organic chicken broth

1. Preheat oven to 400°.
2. Sprinkle salt, pepper, onion, and turmeric over chicken pieces.
3. Heat oil in a large, oven-proof skillet, over medium-high heat. Add chicken to pan and brown on both sides. Remove pan from heat.
4. Squeeze lemon over chicken and place lemon rinds and rosemary sprigs around chicken pieces.
5. Add garlic, mushrooms, and broth to pan.
6. Place skillet, uncovered, into hot oven. Bake for 30–40 minutes, or until no longer pink and juices run clear.

Serves 4

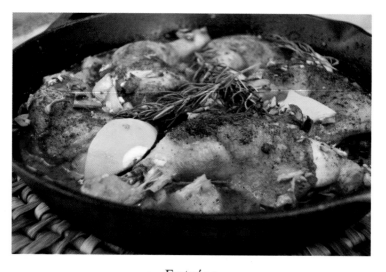

Entrées

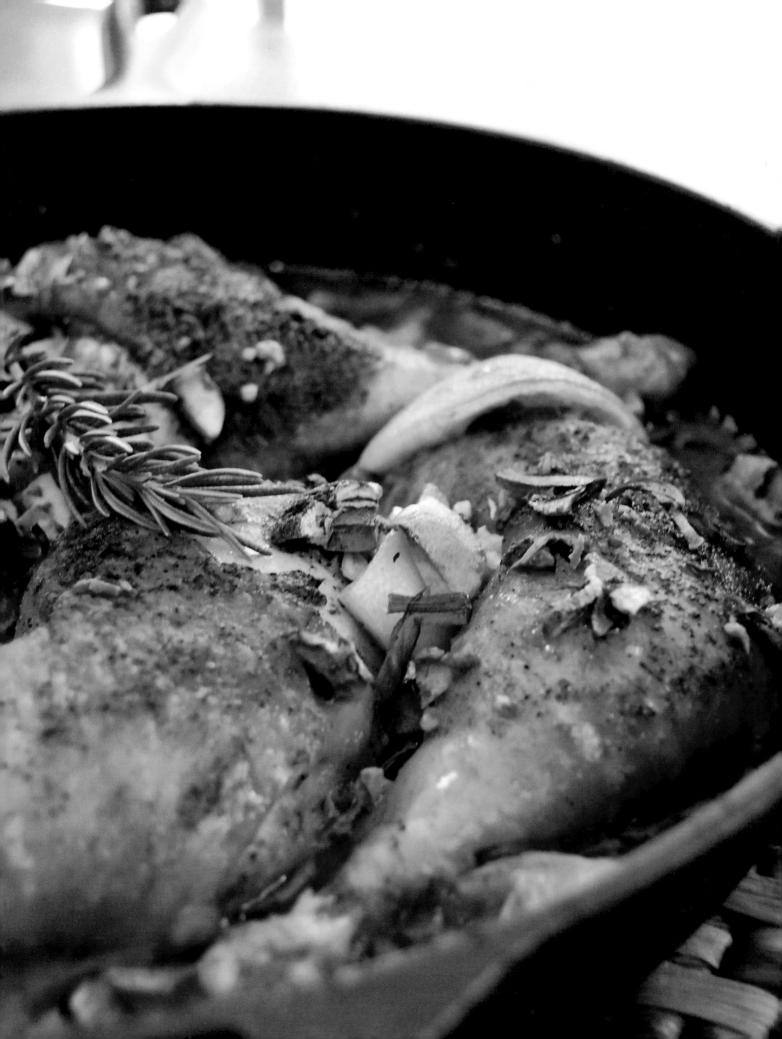

Citrus Ginger Chicken

The combination of citrus juices and ginger make this one yummy chicken dish! This recipe is another easy make-ahead meal, so feel free to make 3 or 4 at a time and freeze for another day. The next time you work late or the kids have sports until 7 PM, and everyone wants dinner in thirty minutes, you'll be glad you did!

Chicken:

4	boneless skinless organic chicken breasts, cut into 1-inch chunks
1	Tbsp Coconut oil

Sauce:

½	C (120 mL) organic orange juice
⅓	C (80 mL) fresh organic lemon juice
1	tsp yellow mustard
1	Tbsp raw organic honey
1	tsp freshly grated ginger
1	Tbsp GF tamari soy sauce (or Bragg liquid aminos or coconut aminos)
2	cloves garlic, minced
~	Freshly ground pepper
½	C (120 mL) organic chicken broth

1. Heat oil in a large skillet over medium-high heat. Add chicken and brown on both sides.
2. In a medium bowl, whisk together sauce ingredients.
3. Add sauce to the pan, making sure to scrape the pan and get all of the yumminess off of the bottom! Cover, reduce heat to low, and simmer for 15 minutes or until chicken is cooked through. Turn chicken once during cooking and baste with sauce occasionally.
4. Remove lid during the last 5 minutes of cooking to help thicken the sauce a bit.

Options:

1. For a make-ahead meal, in a large zip-top bag combine sauce ingredients.
2. Add chicken breasts to the sauce bag and seal.
3. Freeze until needed.
4. To use, thaw in the fridge overnight, place in a glass baking dish, and bake in a 375° oven for about 30 minutes or until chicken is cooked through. Baste chicken with sauce a few times while baking.

Tip:

For a speedy meal, cut chicken into bite-size pieces prior to browning and reduce cooking time to about 6 minutes.

Serves 4

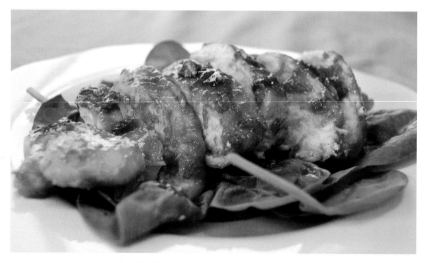

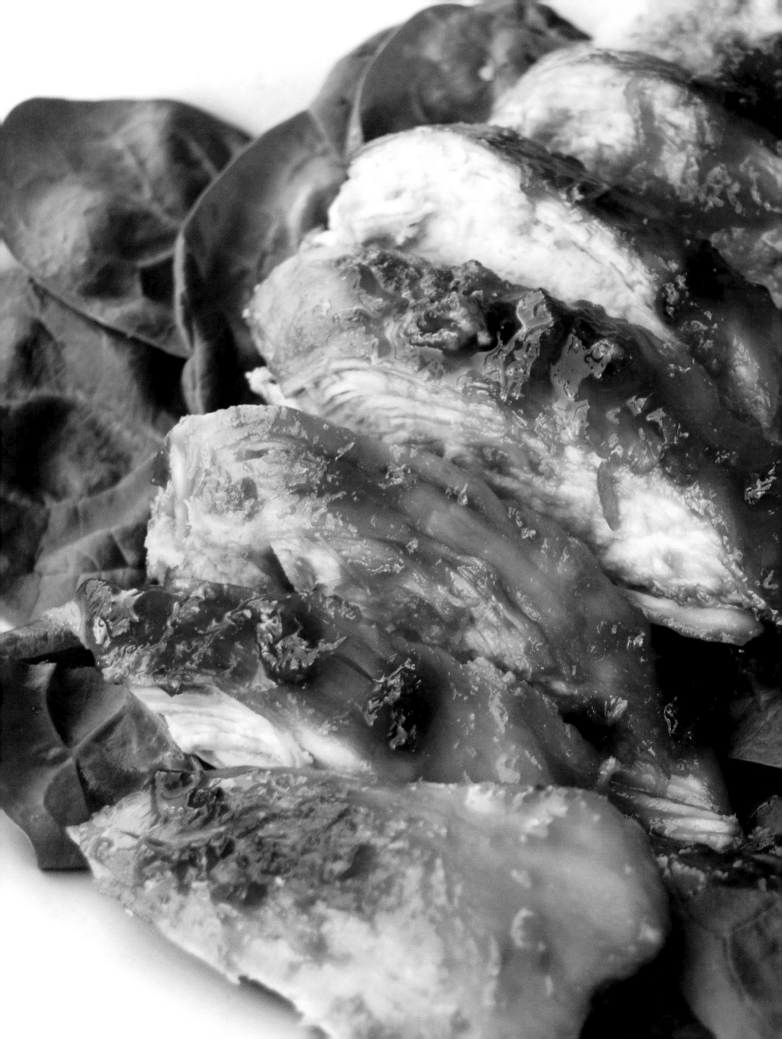

Grilled Lime Chicken

In our house, we don't even utter the word "summer" until this delicious chicken has been grilled up and served. The flavors are perfect on a hot summer day or out at the lake BBQ-ing. Just mix up a bowl of the Cherry Tomato Salad on page 202 and a heaping helping of the Cucumber Salad on page 226 and you've got yourself a satisfying summer picnic that just happens to be gluten-free! I love this recipe for how easy it is to throw together in a pinch, and that you can make it ahead of time for even more convenience. Yay summer!

4	Boneless skinless organic chicken breasts
~	Juice of 2 organic limes (about ½ C)
⅓	C (80 mL) olive oil
3	green onions, chopped
4	garlic cloves, minced
1	Tbsp dried dill (or about 3 Tbsp chopped fresh dill)
~	Freshly ground pepper (to taste)

1. Pound chicken breasts to flatten.
2. In a small bowl, combine remaining ingredients.
3. In a large zip-top bag, add chicken breasts and marinade. Seal and refrigerate for a few hours or overnight.
4. To prepare, grill chicken (discard remaining marinade) until browned and cooked through, about 3–4 minutes per side. Garnish with chopped green onions or chopped cilantro if desired.

Options:

~To make ahead, combine marinade ingredients in a quart-size zip-top bag and seal. Place marinade bag and 4 chicken breasts in a gallon-size zip-top bag. Seal and freeze until needed. To prepare, thaw in refrigerator overnight then proceed with step #3.

~Try this marinade with shrimp instead of chicken and grill on skewers until no longer pink. Another tasty summer meal!

Serves 4

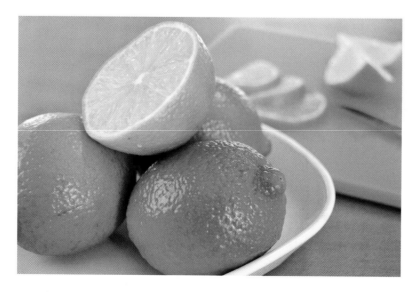

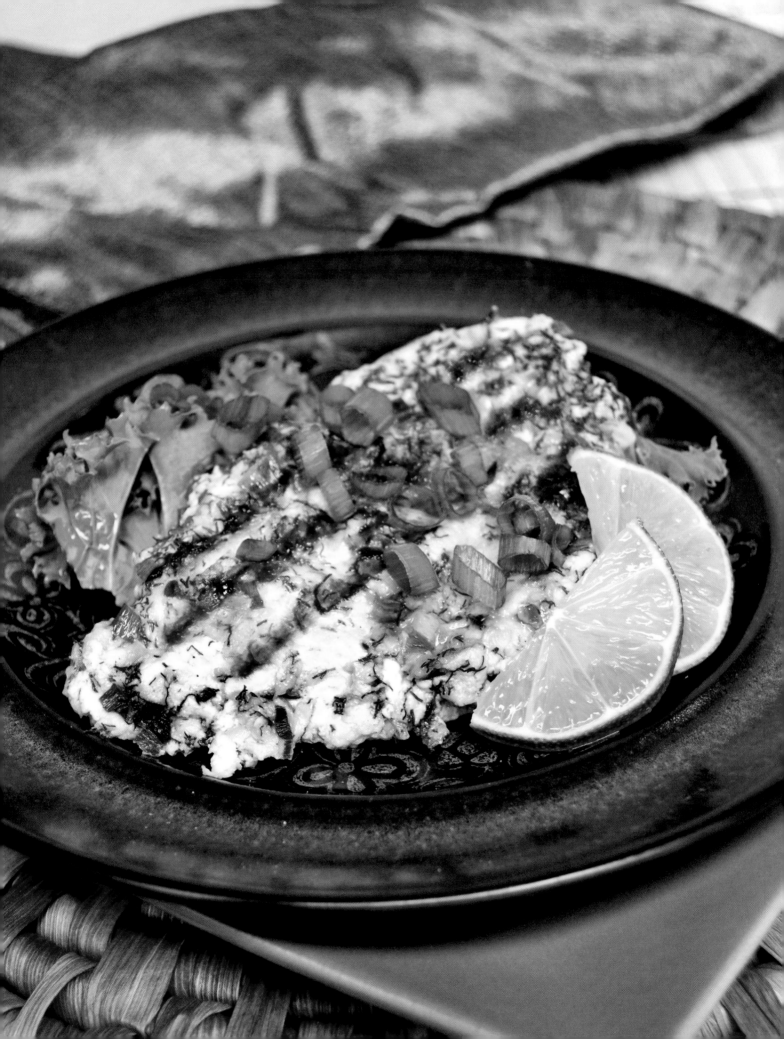

P.F. Chicken Lettuce Cups
(as in Pretty Fantastic!)

So we all know about a famous and delicious Chinese Food restaurant chain that also happens to be very gluten aware for their customers. The downside? I have to drive 3 hours to get to the nearest restaurant! Sometimes, a person needs the PF Lettuce Cups and nothing else will do. And so these chicken lettuce cups were born! Delivering the same fresh lettuce crunch and tangy, bursting-with-flavor chicken filling, but without the 3-hour drive or hour-long wait for a table. Enjoy these lettuce cups as a light summer dinner or as an elegant appetizer.

Sauce:

⅓   C (80 mL) Bragg liquid aminos or wheat-free tamari soy sauce (or coconut aminos)

2   Tbsp fish sauce (Thai Kitchen has a great one)

¼   C (60 mL) rice vinegar

1   tsp GF Worcestershire sauce

Filling:

2   Tbsp olive oil

1   lb (450 g) boneless skinless organic chicken breast, cut into small pieces (or you can use 1 lb ground turkey or chicken)

8   oz (230 g) white mushrooms, finely chopped

1   tsp freshly grated ginger (or ½ tsp dried ground ginger)

2   garlic cloves, minced

Shells:

1   head organic romaine lettuce, washed and leaves separated

Toppings:

~   Diced carrots

~   Diced cucumbers

~   Chopped green onions

~   Sesame seeds

~   Toasted almonds

~   Diced radishes

1. In a small bowl, mix together liquid aminos/soy sauce, fish sauce, rice vinegar, and Worcestershire sauce. Set aside.
2. Heat oil in a large skillet over medium-high heat. Add chicken. Cook for 1 minute.
3. Stir in mushrooms, ginger, and garlic. Cook and stir for about 4 minutes, or until some of the liquid has evaporated.
4. Stir in liquid amino sauce mixture. Reduce heat and simmer for about 4–5 minutes, or until chicken is cooked through.
5. To serve, spoon chicken mixture into lettuce cups. Add your favorite toppings and enjoy!

Serves 4

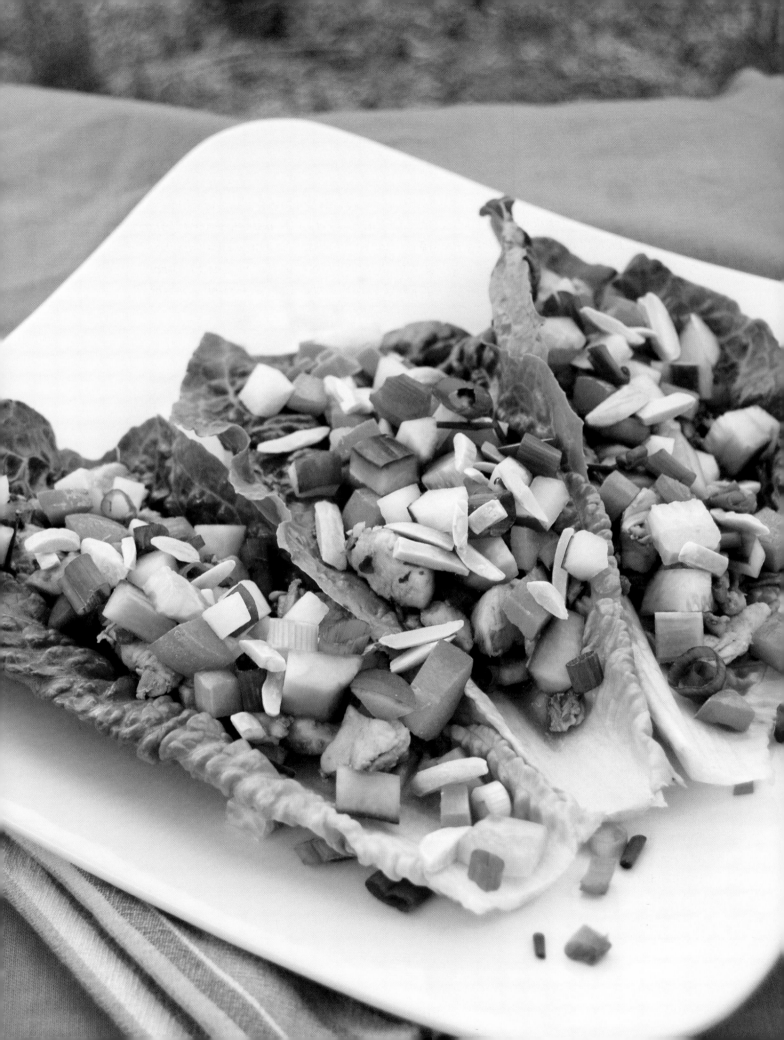

Crock Pot Chicken

There is nothing like walking into your home at the end of a long day and being greeted by a wonderful aroma and the realization that dinner is all done! Crock Pot Chicken is the much healthier and GF equivalent to fast food, without the drive-thru, the high sodium, the cost, the mistaken order, the stomach ache, the 5 lbs on your thighs... shall I go on? Sometimes being gluten-free forces us to do the right thing by our bodies, even though we should have been doing it all along. This is fast food you can feel good about feeding yourself and your family. And leftovers make a great lunch the next day too!

Chicken:

1	whole organic chicken (size depends on what will fit into your crock pot—I have a 6-quart crock pot so I get the biggest bird I can find)
1	large organic yellow onion, sliced
2	medium organic sweet potatoes, diced into bite-size chunks
6	large organic carrots, diced in to bite-size chunks

Seasoning Blend:

1	tsp granulated onion
1	tsp granulated garlic
¼	tsp turmeric
½	tsp paprika
¼	tsp poultry seasoning
1	tsp Italian seasoning
~	Salt and pepper

1. Wash your bird and take out the unmentionables in the cavity.
2. In a small bowl, combine seasoning blend. Rub seasoning mixture all over the bird and make sure to tuck some in under the skin where you can. Wash hands thoroughly.
3. Layer onions, then potatoes, then some carrots in the crock Pot. Place bird on top. Wash hands again.
4. Place the remaining carrots around the bird, tucking them in nicely.
5. Cook for 6–8 hrs on low or 4–5 hours on high.
6. Serve sliced chicken over potatoes and carrots with sliced onions on top and a little of the juices spooned over! Yummerific and not a lot of work!

Serves 4–6

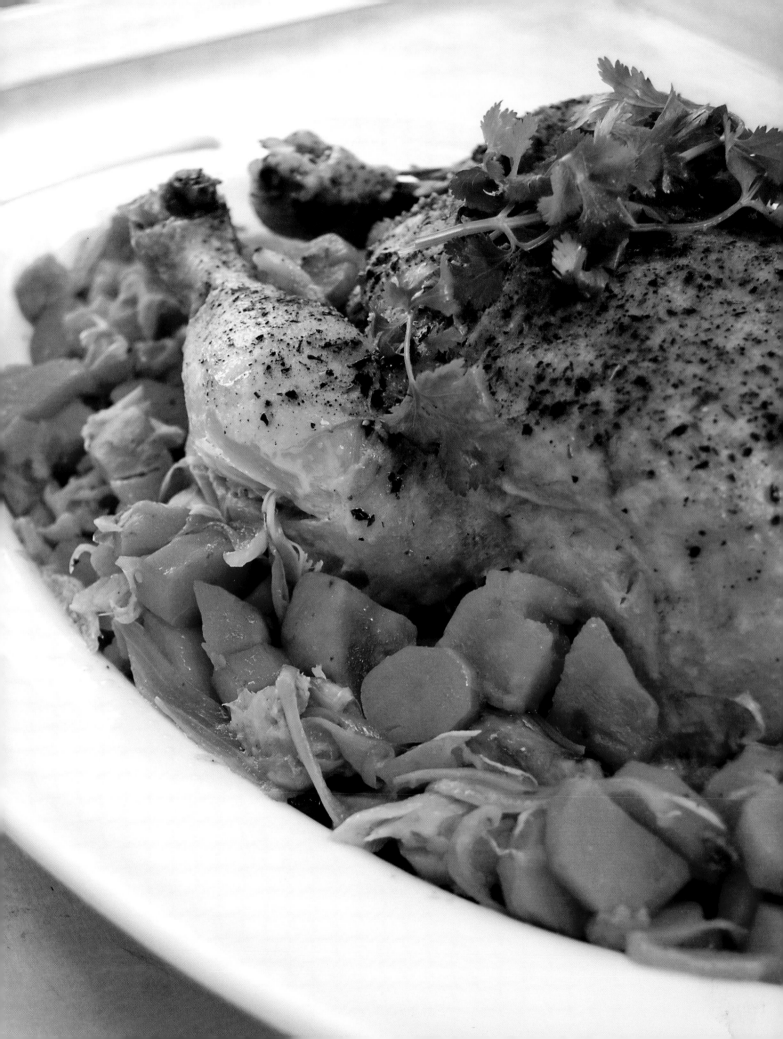

Sweet and Sour Chicken Stir Fry

For the first 5 years of our marriage, when The Maniac said he would cook, I knew what I was in for. Stir-fry chicken with veggies and some soy sauce. And while that was really sweet and wonderful the first, oh, ten times he made it, after a few years it was time to up his game a little. So I taught him how to make an actual sauce for the stir fry. It went over so well, I'm hoping to graduate him to a real cooked chicken breast or maybe a steak someday. A girl can dream.

Sauce:

3	Tbsp GF tamari soy sauce (or Bragg liquid aminos or coconut aminos)
3	Tbsp raw apple cider vinegar
2	Tbsp raw organic honey
¼	tsp red pepper flakes
2	Tbsp GF ketchup
½	tsp freshly grated ginger
1	tsp arrowroot starch

Stir Fry:

3	Tbsp coconut oil
3	boneless skinless organic chicken breasts, cubed
3	C (450 g) stir-fry veggies of choice

1. Mix sauce ingredients in a medium bowl, set aside.
2. Heat a wok (or large skillet) over high heat. Add oil to pan. When hot, add chicken and cook until browned, about 4 minutes.
3. Add in veggies, stirring until chicken is done and veggies are cooked, about 4 minutes.
4. Add sauce to pan, stir to coat. Enjoy!

Serves 4

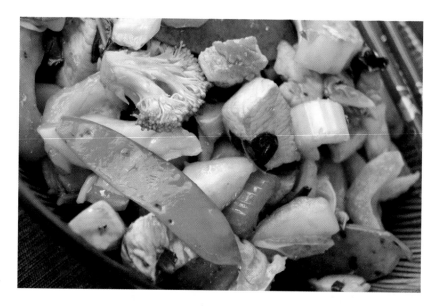

Entrées

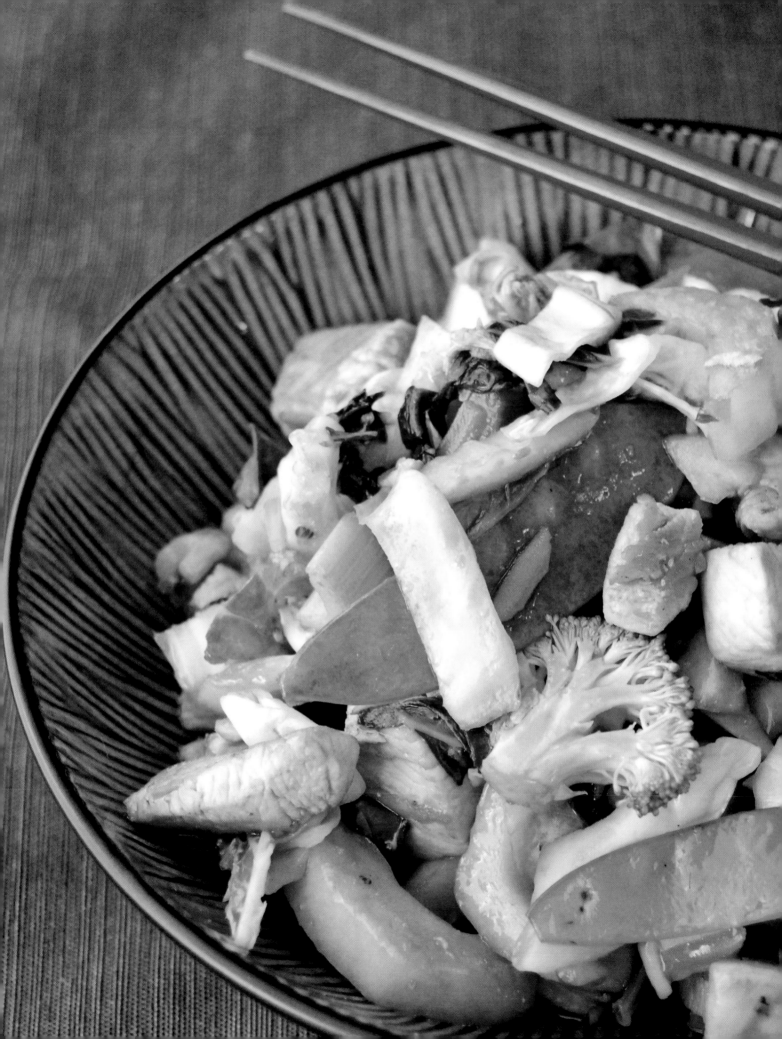

Walnut Basil Chicken

My kids call this "ugly chicken." It's not the prettiest meal we make at our house, but it's so full of flavor and goodness from the fresh basil and walnuts, we just ignore that fact and dig in! You should do the same. Trust me.

1	C (40 g) organic basil leaves, loosely packed
¾	C (110 g) raw walnuts
3	garlic cloves, coarsely chopped
½	tsp sea salt
~	Freshly ground pepper
4	boneless skinless organic chicken breasts

1. Add basil, walnuts, garlic, salt, and pepper to a food processor. Pulse until a meal forms.
2. Place chicken onto a greased baking sheet. Pat basil mixture evenly over each chicken breast.
3. Bake in a 375° oven until chicken is done and top is browned, about 20–25 minutes.

Serves 4

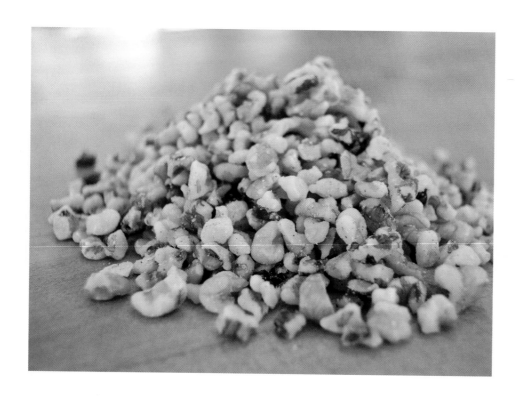

Entrées

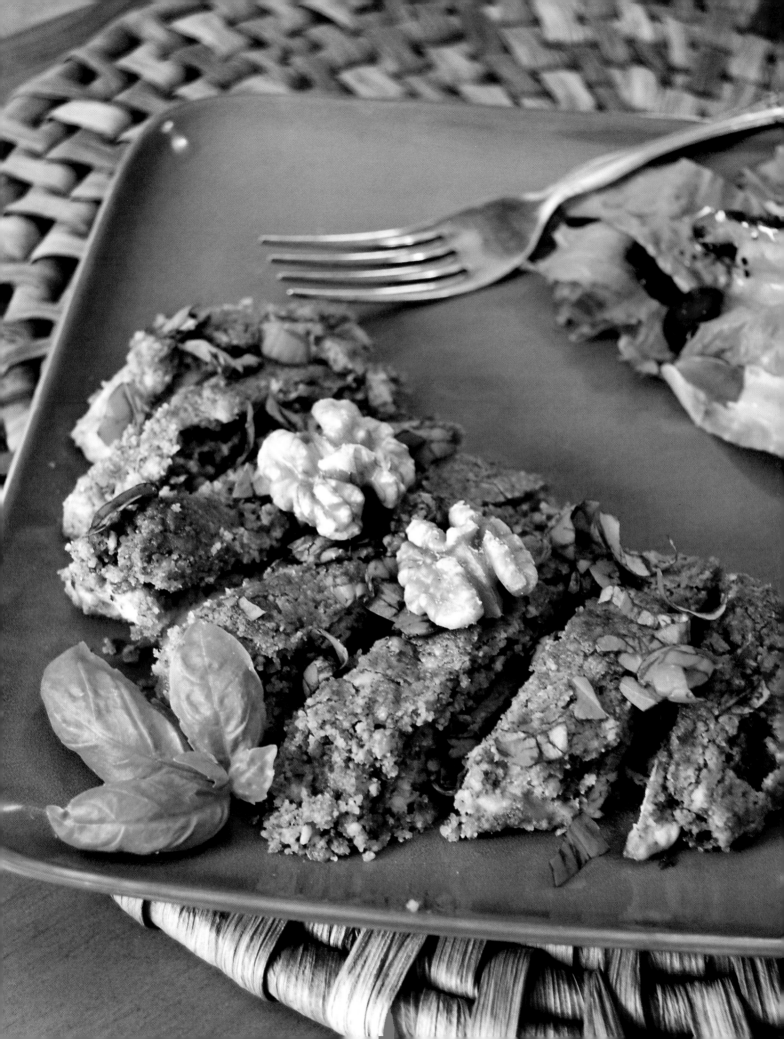

Baked Chicken Legs

Chicken legs are a great, kid-approved dinner in our house. They are inexpensive and full of great flavor and more iron than a dry chicken breast, plus the kids love that they don't have to use a fork! Who doesn't love food that is also a handle? Anyone? Just make sure to make plenty so you have leftovers for lunches the next day!

Seasoning:

1	tsp granulated onion
½	tsp granulated garlic
½	tsp rosemary
1	tsp dried parsley
¼	tsp turmeric
½	tsp paprika
½	tsp basil
1	tsp sea salt
~	Freshly ground pepper
3	lbs (1,350 g) organic chicken legs

1. Mix seasonings in a small bowl.
2. In a large bowl, place chicken legs and sprinkle and rub seasoning all over each leg.
3. Place chicken legs in a greased 9" by 13" baking dish.
4. Bake legs in a 375° oven for about 40 minutes, or until chicken is browned and juices run clear.

Serves 4

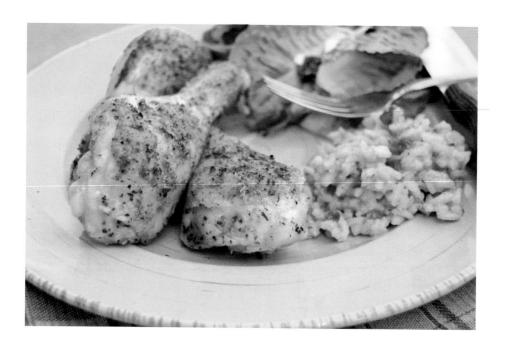

Entrées

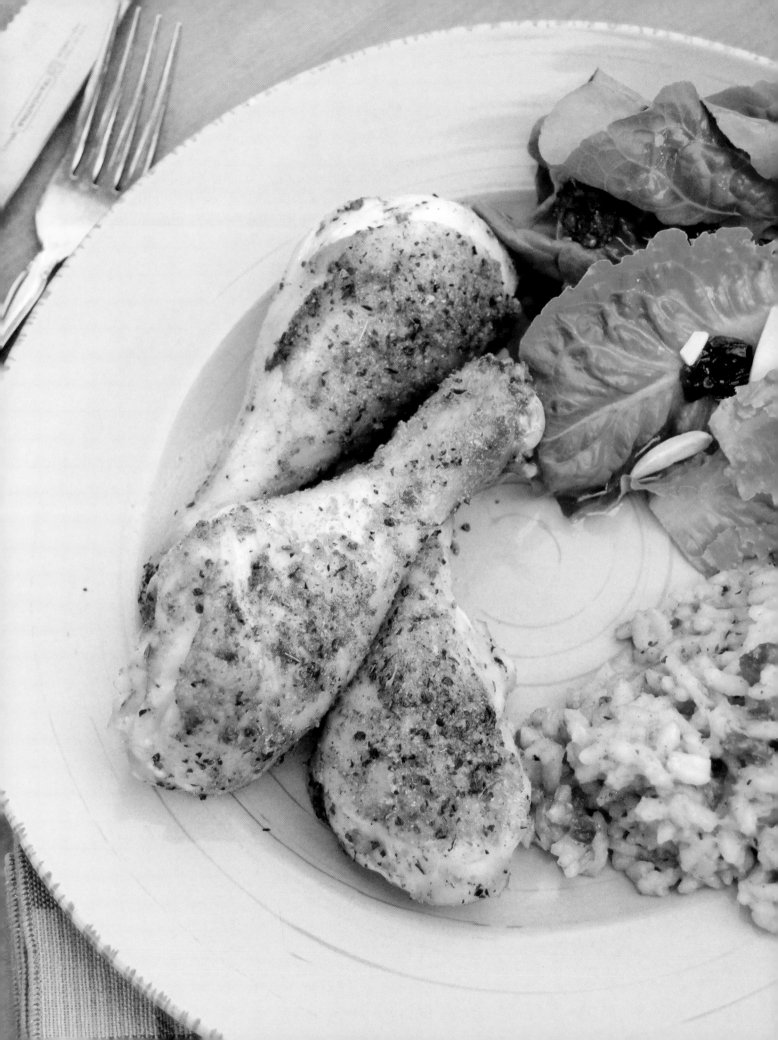

Chippy Chicken Thighs

There are a lot of great, gluten-free potato chips on the market without a lot of disgusting ingredients. Many of the higher-quality brands like Kettle simple use potatoes, oil, and salt. Also check out Trader Joe's. Many of their chips are gluten-free and contain minimal ingredients. Occasionally, it's nice to utilize something that's not too bad for us to help boost the flavor of a meal. My kids love the flavor, but mostly the lovely crunchy coating on this chicken. If you're missing a great crispy piece of chicken that isn't fried or coated in nuts or even coconut, this one will be a nice change!

4	C (240 g) GF potato chips of your choice
1½	lbs (675 g) boneless skinless organic chicken thighs
⅓	C (80 mL) melted nondairy butter or coconut oil
~	Sea salt to taste
~	Freshly ground pepper to taste

1. Place chips in a large zip-top bag and seal, making sure to let all of the air out so the bag doesn't pop. Roll a rolling pin over the bag to create crumbs.

2. Dip chicken thighs in butter/coconut oil and then in chip crumbs. Place in a greased 9" by 13" glass baking dish. Season chicken with salt and pepper.

3. Bake chicken in a 350° oven for 25–30 minutes, or until chicken is done and no longer pink.

4. Turn on broiler. Broil chicken, watching carefully so it doesn't burn, for about 4 minutes to brown the top.

Serves 4

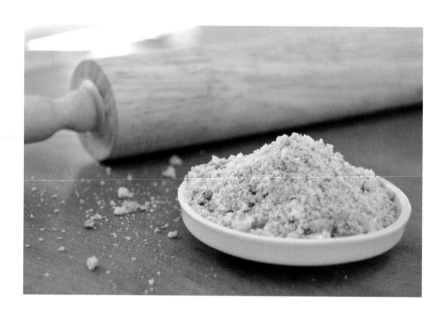

Entrées

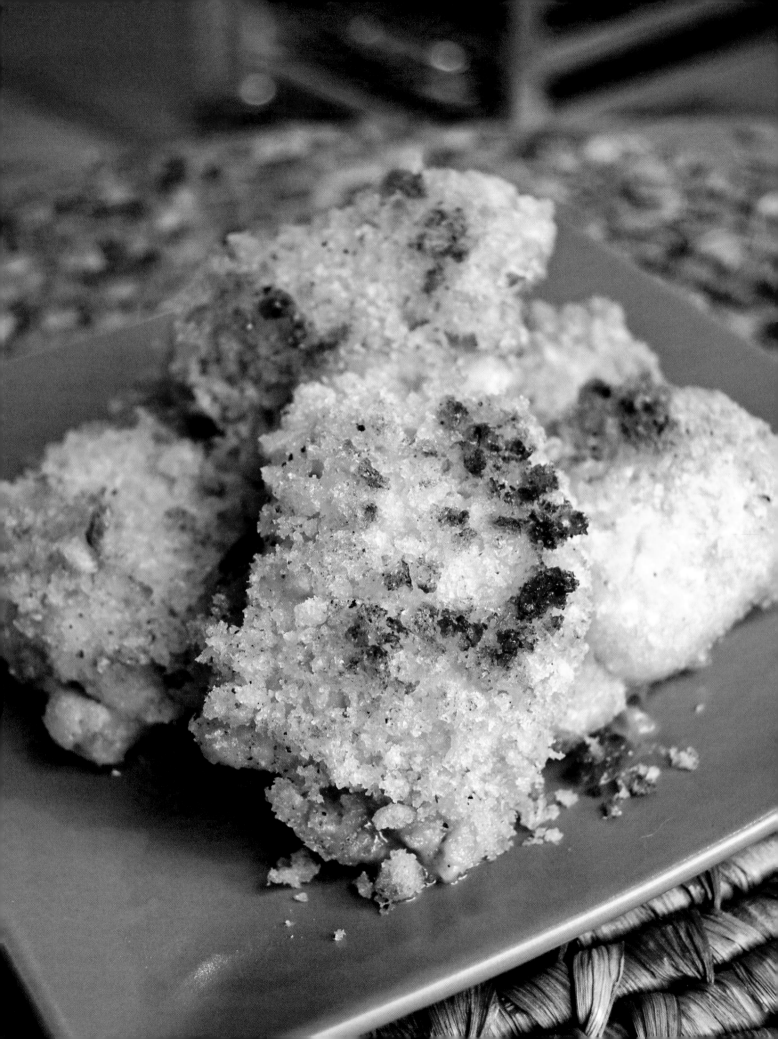

Lemon Artichoke Chicken Piccata

I love meals I can make ahead without a lot of time or ingredients. This flavorful chicken is all that in a freezer bag! Make it quickly for tonight's dinner, or prepare a few packages ahead and freeze until needed. Either way, this dish will be appreciated and devoured! It's even fancy enough to serve to guests, without spending your whole night in the kitchen.

~ **Salt and pepper to taste**

4 **boneless skinless organic chicken breasts**

½ **C (120 mL) organic lemon juice**

½ **C (120 mL) white wine (Always double-check your brand to make sure it's gluten-free. Most are. You can omit the wine and still have a great dinner, but the flavor is enhanced with the wine).**

1 **C (240 mL) organic GF chicken broth**

2 **garlic cloves, crushed**

2 **Tbsp olive oil**

2 **Tbsp capers**

2 **C (300 g) artichoke hearts (You can do frozen or canned. I like Trader Joe's brand canned artichoke hearts in water. Takes about 2 [14 oz] cans.)**

Dinner Tonight:

1. Sprinkle salt and pepper on both sides of chicken.
2. In a medium bowl, mix together lemon juice, white wine, chicken broth, garlic, and capers. Set aside.
3. Heat 2 Tbsp olive oil in a large skillet over medium-high heat. Place chicken in pan and cook until browned, about 3 minutes.
4. Flip chicken breast, turn heat to medium-low.
5. Pour sauce into pan, over chicken, scraping up the yummies on the bottom of the pan as you go.
6. Add artichoke hearts to the pan.
7. Bring to a simmer and cook, uncovered, for about 7 minutes, or until chicken is done and juices run clear.

Make Ahead and Freeze:

1. In a quart-size zip-top bag, combine lemon juice, white wine, chicken broth, garlic, capers, and artichoke hearts. Squish around to combine ingredients. Make sure the top is closed first . . . I should have mentioned that earlier.
2. In a large, gallon-sized, zip-top freezer bag, place bag of sauce and 4 boneless chicken breasts.
3. Place in freezer until ready to use. Lasts about 4 months.
4. When ready, remove bag from freezer and allow to thaw in refrigerator overnight.
5. To prepare, follow steps 1–7 above.
6. Enjoy a great meal and give thanks that someone told you to do this so you didn't have to cook dinner from square-one tonight!

Tip:

To speed up cooking time, pound chicken breasts (placed in a large zip-top bag with air removed) to about ½-inch thickness. Reduce cooking time to 3–4 minutes in step 7.

Serves 4

Entrées

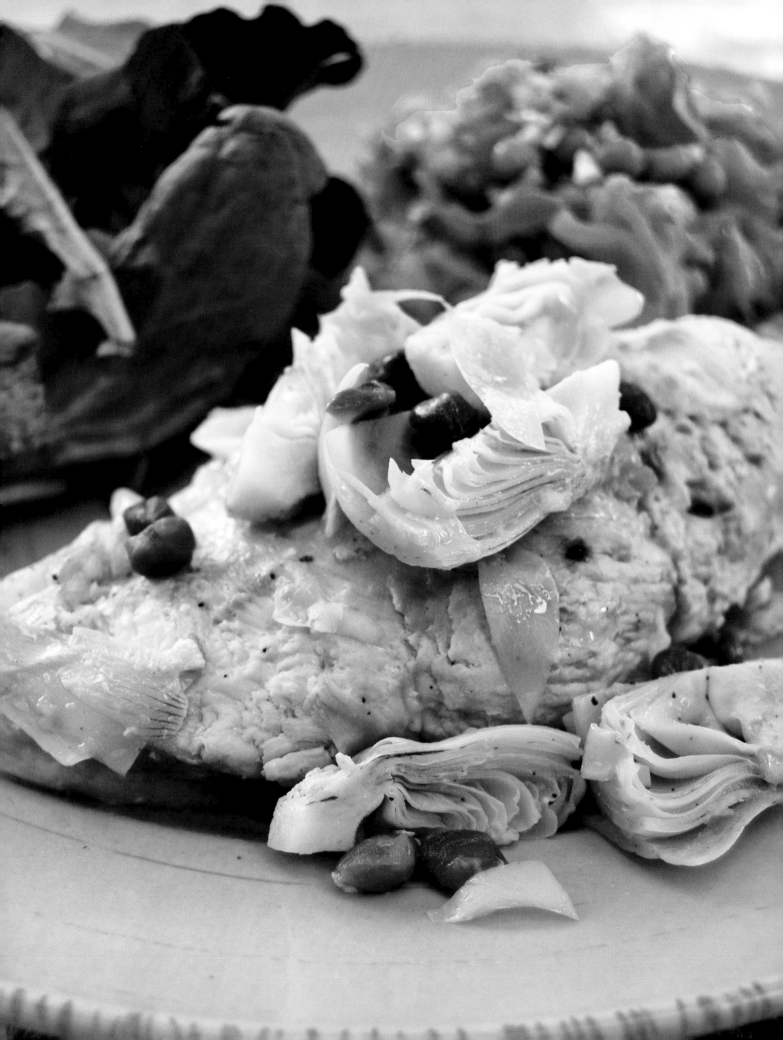

Garlic Rosemary Chicken Bites

I love making this chicken for a weeknight meal because it's oh so easy, yet still packs a lot of flavor. When I can, I make 3 or 4 of these meals ahead of time and pop them in the freezer. Nothing better than a freezer full of meals you don't have to think about and can grab when you need them!

Bites:

2	boneless skinless organic chicken breasts, cut into 1-inch chunks
1	Tbsp coconut oil

Sauce:

2	Tbsp balsamic vinegar
2	Tbsp olive oil
1	tsp fresh chopped rosemary
2	garlic cloves, minced
~	Sea salt to taste
~	Freshly ground pepper to taste

1. Heat oil in a large skillet over medium-high heat. Add chicken and brown on all sides.
2. In a medium bowl, whisk together sauce ingredients.
3. Add sauce to the pan, reduce heat to low, and simmer for 5 minutes or until chicken is cooked through.
4. To serve, spoon chicken pieces onto a platter and fill a small bowl with the juices from the pan for dipping!

Option:

1. For a make-ahead meal, use 4 chicken breasts and leave whole.
2. In a large zip-top bag combine sauce ingredients.
3. Add chicken breasts to the sauce bag and seal.
4. Freeze until needed.
5. To use, thaw in the fridge overnight, place in a glass baking dish and bake in a 375° oven for about 30 minutes or until chicken is cooked through. Baste chicken with sauce a few times while baking.

Serves 2

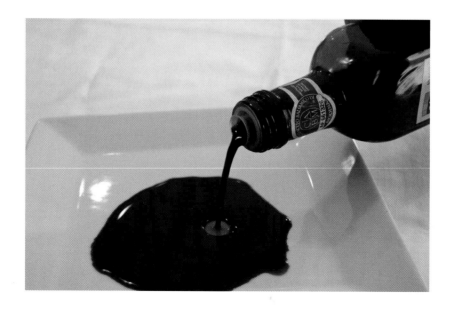

Entrées

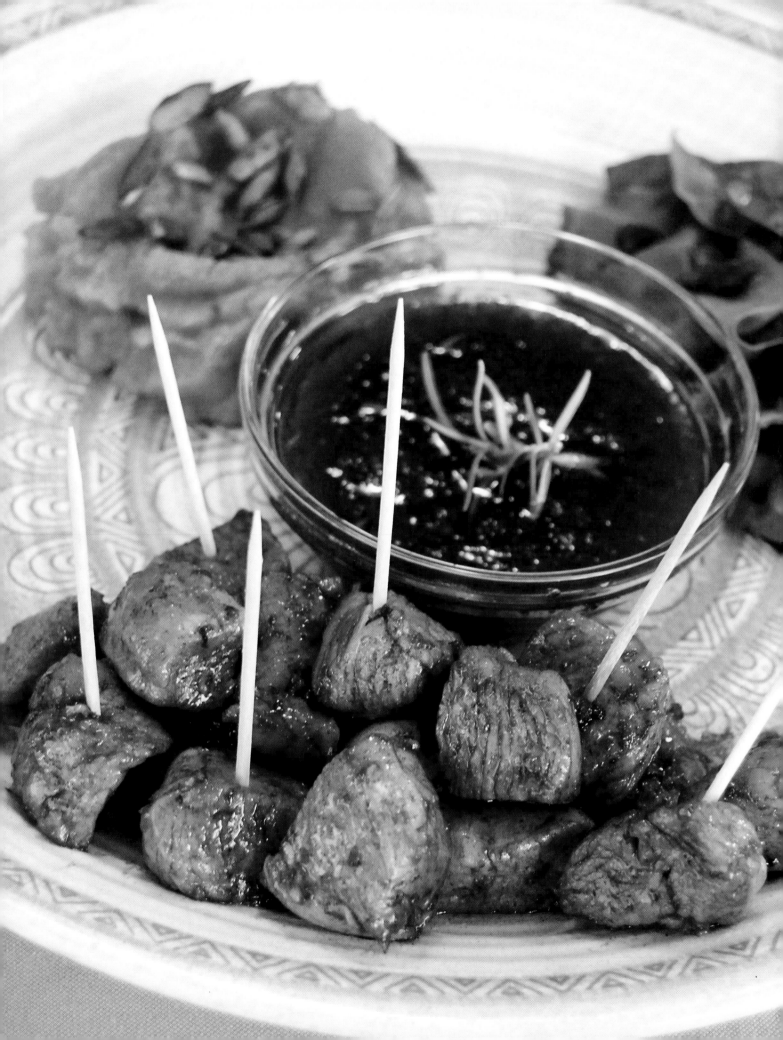

Classic Chicken Noodle Soup

I believe every person needs to be able to make a version of chicken noodle soup, especially in those long winter months when colds and flu are prevalent. Studies have shown that homemade chicken soup really does have immune-boosting properties, plus it's just plain yummy. It also serves as a great base for any variety of soup you'd like. Feel like sweet potatoes? Add some chunks! In the mood for turnips? Toss those babies in! Go crazy! Well—as crazy as you can get with soup.

2	C (280 g) gluten-free spiral noodles
2	qts (2 L) homemade chicken broth (or store bought GF organic chicken broth)
½	medium organic yellow onion, diced
3	large organic carrots, chopped
3	stalks organic celery, chopped
¼	C chopped fresh organic parsley
2	C (300 g) cubed cooked organic chicken
~	Sea salt to taste
~	Freshly ground pepper to taste

1. Cook pasta according to package directions. Drain.
2. Meanwhile, place remaining ingredients in a large pot over medium-high heat. Bring to a boil.
3. Turn heat to low and simmer, covered, until veggies are tender, about 45 minutes.
4. Add sea salt and pepper to taste.

Tip:

Cooking the noodles separately and adding to your soup as needed ensures that any leftover soup can be stored and used at a later date with no soggy noodles.

Options:

Try adding roasted garlic cloves and peas to this soup for a little flavor variety.

Serves 4-6

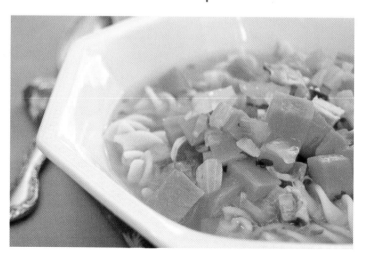

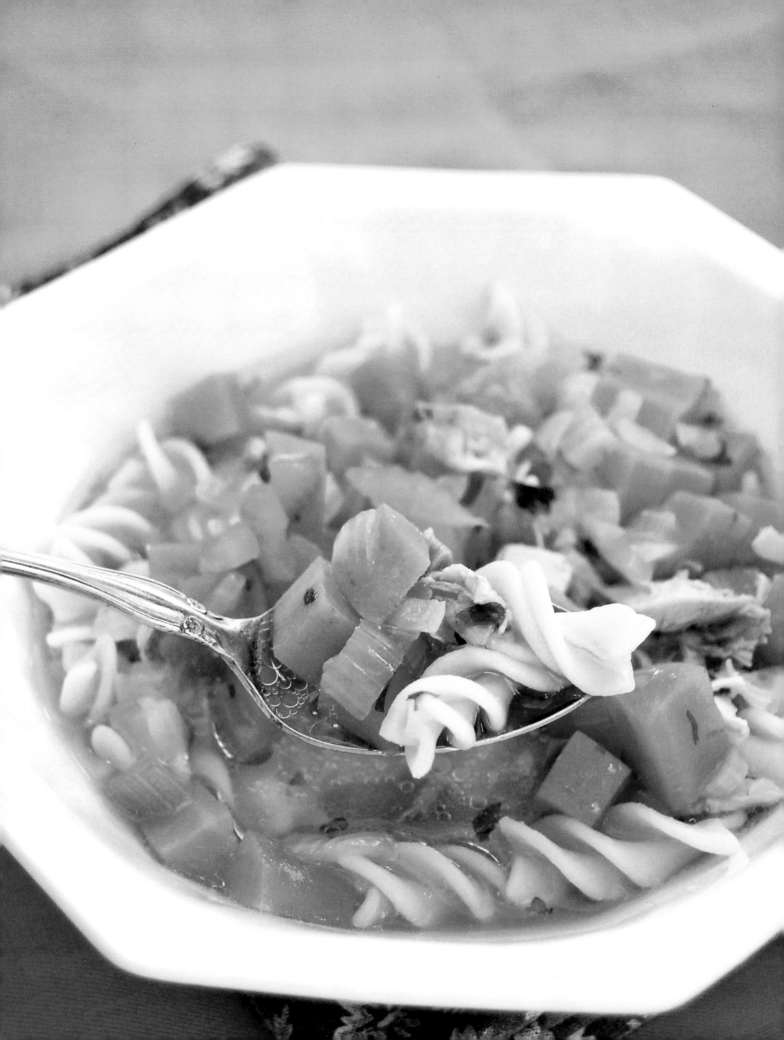

Chicken Wings

Please do not underestimate the deliciousness of the mighty chicken wing! Flavorful and such a nice size for little hands, wings make a great Family Fun Night dinner and are fantastic in the Thermos for school lunch the next day. This recipe makes lots of sauce, which is good because it's so versatile. Plus, it can be refrigerated or frozen so you always have some ready to go when that wing craving hits!

Seasoning:

1	Tbsp paprika
2	tsp granulated onion
½	tsp granulated garlic
¼	tsp smoked paprika
1	tsp sea salt
~	Freshly ground pepper to taste

Wings:

24	chicken organic wings, washed and patted dry
2	Tbsp coconut oil, melted

Wing Sauce:

1	(15 oz) can (about 475 mL) organic tomato sauce
1	(6 oz) can (180 mL) organic tomato paste
3	Tbsp raw organic honey or pure maple syrup
3	Tbsp organic raw apple cider vinegar
2	tsp sea salt
1	Tbsp granulated onion
1	tsp paprika
½	tsp smoked paprika
2	tsp granulated garlic
1	Tbsp coconut aminos (or GF tamari soy sauce or Bragg liquid aminos)

1. Mix wing seasoning together in a small bowl.
2. Coat wings with oil. Sprinkle all of the seasoning over wings and rub in evenly with your hands. Don't forget to wash your hands now!
3. Cover a large baking sheet with foil. Grease or spray foil. Place seasoned wings evenly on pan, trying to not let them touch so they bake evenly and get crispy.
4. Cook wings in a 450° oven for about 35 minutes, or until wings are browned, crispy, and cooked through.
5. Meanwhile, combine all sauce ingredients in a large saucepan. Heat over medium-low until heated through.
6. Place cooked wings in a large bowl, add enough sauce to make yourself happy, and toss lightly to coat wings evenly. Serve and devour . . . remember the napkins!
7. Refrigerate extra sauce to use with coconut chicken strips (p. 106), steak bites (p. 160), or to top mini meatloaf (p. 150).

Options:

Like it hot? Add as much of your favorite GF hot sauce to the sauce mixture as you like! Mmmm, spicy!

Serves 4

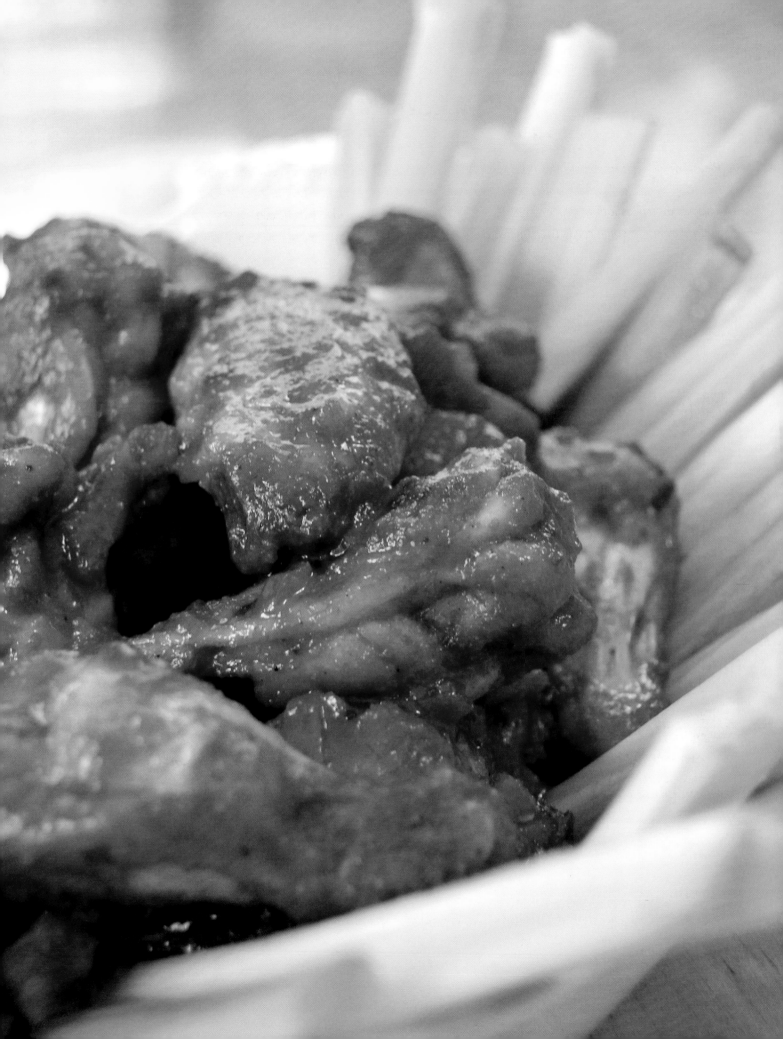

Cranberry Chicken Fingers

I love using cranberries any way I can when they're in season, and these quick-cooking tenders are a great way to utilize such an antioxidant rich food. I especially make this post-Turkey Day to use up that leftover sugar-free cranberry sauce (p. 252).

Chicken:

1	Tbsp coconut oil
1–1½	lbs (450–675 g) organic chicken tenders
~	Sea salt to taste
~	Freshly ground pepper to taste

Sauce:

1	C (240 mL) Cranberry Sauce (p. 252)
2	Tbsp GF tamari (or Bragg liquid aminos or coconut aminos)
1	Tbsp raw organic honey
½	tsp tarragon
½	tsp granulated onion
~	Freshly ground pepper

1. Sprinkle chicken with sea salt and pepper.
2. In a medium bowl, whisk together sauce ingredients until combined.
3. Heat oil in a large skillet over medium-high heat. Add chicken tenders and brown on both sides. Turn heat to low.
4. Add sauce (carefully) to the pan, scraping up any yummy bits off the pan. Simmer on low for 5 minutes, or until chicken is cooked through.

Serves 4

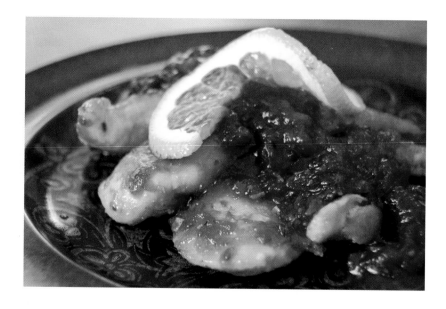

Entrées

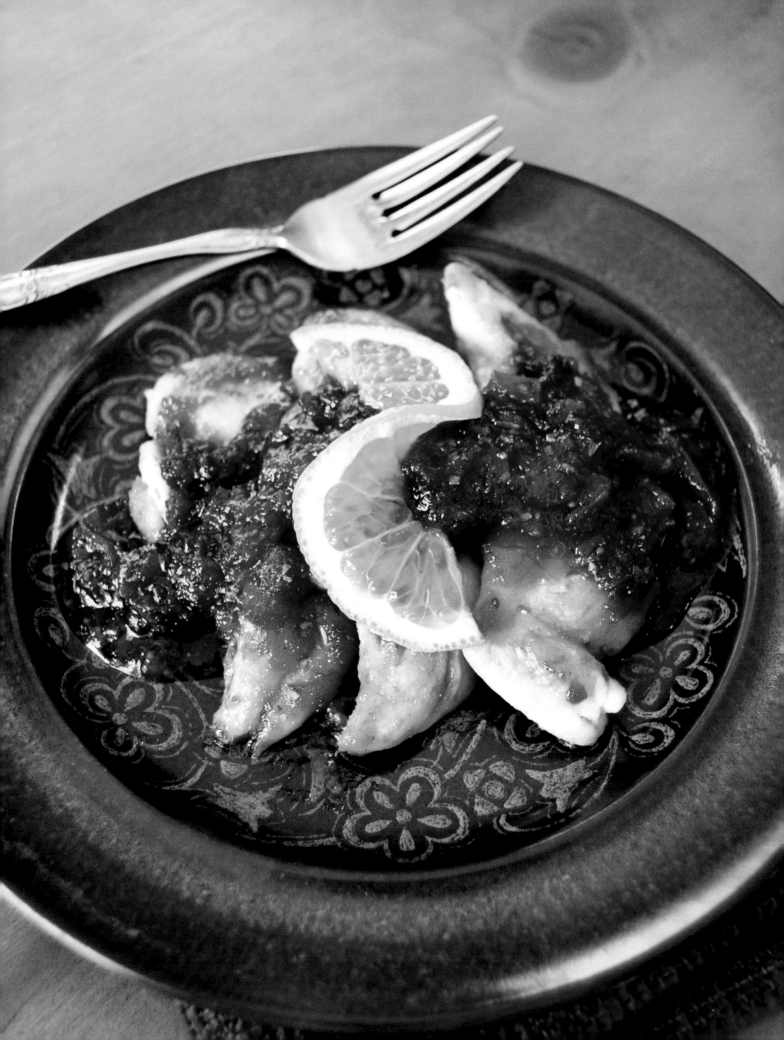

My Favorite Chicken Salad

The first "Wow!" chicken salad I ever had was at a small deli in the city where I went to college. There's something about those neighborhood, hole-in-the-wall places that seem to serve the best food. I had never ordered chicken salad out because it never seemed special enough, but that day I was in a mood, so I tried it. And wow! I've come close to its wonderfulness here, but only close. That chicken salad will always be untouchable it seems, but for now, this is my favorite... at home.

2	C (300 g) cooked boneless skinless orgainic chicken breast, diced
1	small stalk organic celery, diced
1	small organic green onion, chopped
1	Tbsp chopped fresh organic Italian parsley
½	tsp dill
½	tsp Dijon mustard
2	Tbsp vegan mayo (I like Spectrum)
~	Squeeze of fresh lemon juice
⅛	tsp granulated onion
~	Sea salt to taste
~	Freshly ground pepper to taste

Optional Add ins:

2	Tbsp chopped walnuts
¼	C (40 g) organic grapes, sliced in half

1. In a medium bowl, mix all ingredients gently until combined. Add in walnuts and/or grapes if desired.
2. To serve, pile up chicken salad on a lightly toasted English Muffin (recipe p. 88), on a bed of lettuce with sliced tomatoes, or perhaps in half of an avocado.

Serves 2

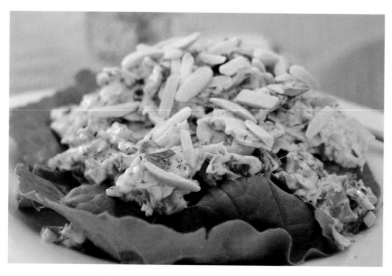

Entrées

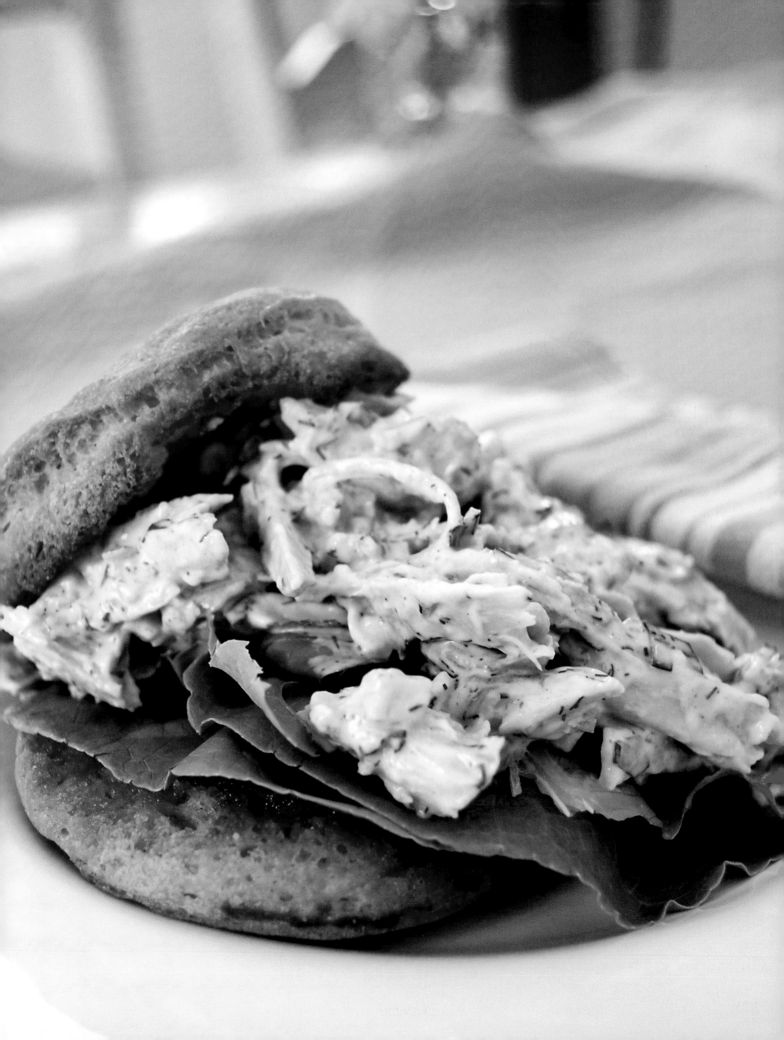

Bacon-Wrapped Chicken Bites

This recipe originated as "wrapped water chestnuts." I'm sure you know it. It made an appearance at just about every party over the last ten years. But I was over the water chestnuts as well as the insane amount of sugar in the sauce. I needed an appetizer that actually had substance without sending me to the dentist. So in honor of my husband's bottomless stomach, I changed things up a bit and made bacon-wrapped chicken. Filling, but not too heavy, these little bites of heaven will get you rave reviews at your next party!

Sauce:

1   C (240 mL) GF ketchup

½   C (90 g) organic brown sugar

⅓   C (80 mL) raw honey

2–3 Tbsp Worcestershire sauce (You decide how much you like!)

Bites:

1   lb (450 g) uncured bacon

3   boneless skinless organic chicken breasts, cut into bite-size pieces

1. Preheat oven to 375°.
2. In a small saucepan, combine sauce ingredients, stir, and heat just to boiling. Set aside.
3. Meanwhile, cut bacon slices into thirds.
4. Wrap each piece of chicken with a piece of bacon and secure with a toothpick. Place in a greased 9" by 13" baking dish.
5. Bake until bacon is almost done, about 40 minutes.
6. Pour warmed sauce over bacon-wrapped chicken pieces and put back into oven.
7. Bake an additional 15 minutes or until bacon is completely cooked and sauce is bubbly.

Serves 4-6

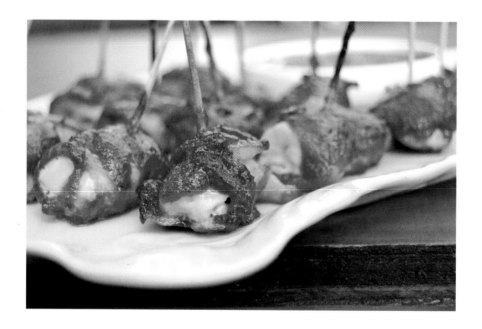

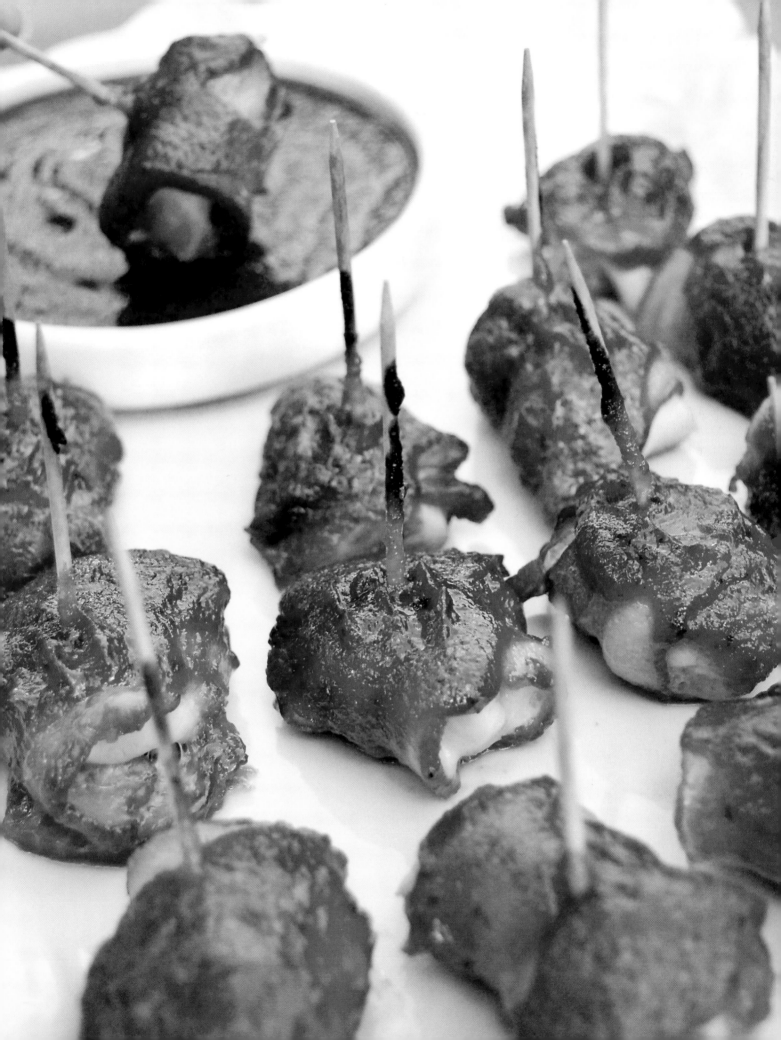

Citrus Chicken Pasta Salad

I found inspiration for this dish in a free Warehouse Store cookbook that was being given away one Thanksgiving weekend. It reminds me to look around my kitchen, TV, magazines—whatever—for inspiration to create great tasting, healthy, gluten-free meals. Remember to look beyond the initial ingredients in a recipe. Is there a sauce that would work well or can one ingredient be replaced or eliminated? Just because the recipe isn't allergy friendly to start with doesn't mean it's not a good jumping-off point to create your own masterpiece!

Salad:

1	C (150 g) chopped walnuts
2	C (280 g) gluten-free spiral pasta
2	C (300 g) cooked, diced organic chicken
½	C (75 g) chopped organic celery
⅓	C (50 g) finely chopped organic red onion
2	Tbsp chopped fresh organic parsley
¼	C (40 g) chopped green onions

Dressing:

½	C (120 mL) fresh orange juice
¼	C (60 mL) fresh lemon juice
¼	C (60 mL) olive oil
2	tsp Dijon mustard
1	Tbsp raw organic honey
1	tsp sea salt
~	Freshly ground pepper
2	Tbsp rice vinegar

1. Toast walnuts until lightly browned.
2. Cook pasta according to package directions, drain and rinse with cold water (to prevent sticking).
3. Combine dressing ingredients in a jar with a tight fitting lid and shake until combined.
4. In a large bowl, combine pasta, chicken, walnuts, celery, red onions, and parsley. Toss to combine. Top with green onions and, if desired, a sprinkle of nondairy cheese.

Serves 4–6

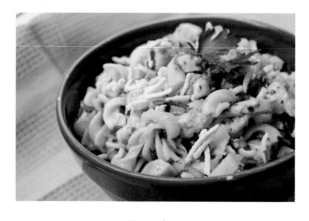

Entrées

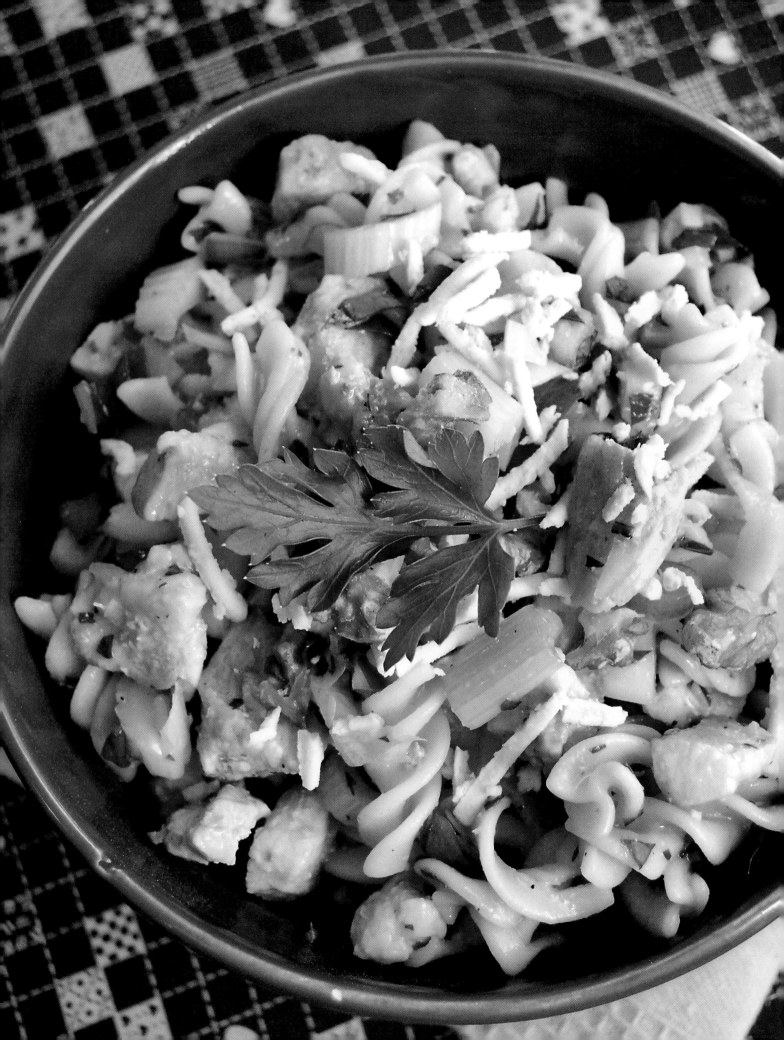

Rosemary Kale Chicken Soup

When cold snowy days hit our area, soup is the one thing we all crave at my house. It's warm, comforting, and filling—everything you want on a cold January day. I love making super-large batches of this soup and freezing leftovers in quart glass jars. Then for months I have a quick and healthy lunch available when we need it. This soup is also the one way I can guarantee my kids will eat nutrient-packed kale! But let's keep that one between us, OK?

2	qts (2 L) homemade chicken broth
1	garlic clove, minced
½	medium organic yellow onion, diced
2	organic celery stalks, chopped
2	C (85 g) chopped organic kale
1	small sprig rosemary, stem removed, leaved finely chopped
1	C (150 g) cubed cooked organic chicken breast
~	Sea salt to taste
~	Freshly ground pepper to taste

1. Place all ingredients in a large pot over medium-high heat. Bring to a boil.
2. Turn heat to low and simmer, covered, until veggies are tender, about 30 minutes.
3. Add sea salt and pepper to taste.

Serves 4

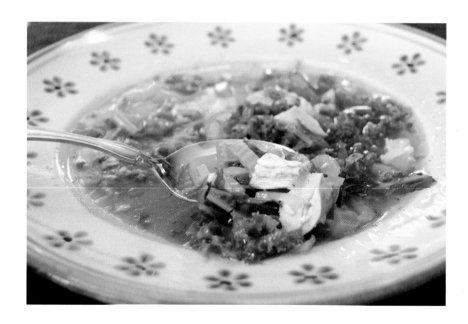

Entrées

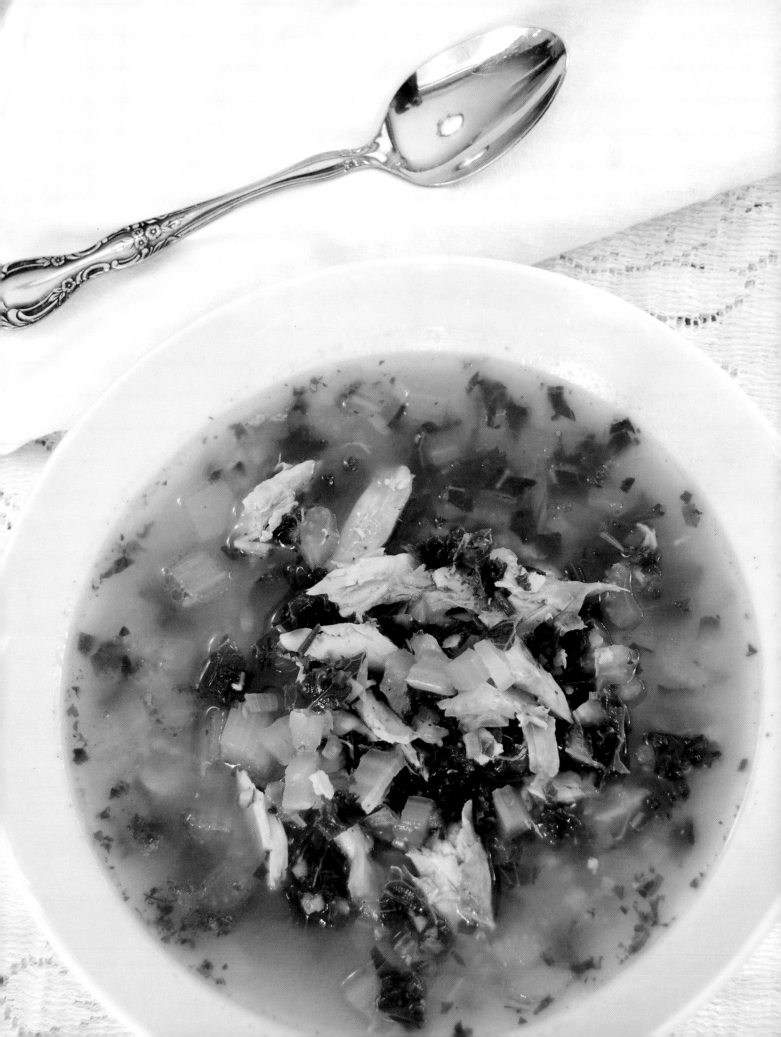

Favorite Turkey Burgers

Super-easy, economical, healthy, and oh, so tasty. What more could you ask for in a gluten-free dinner? Oh, and did I mention there's spinach hidden in these beauties, but the kids love them and ask for them each and every week? Don't worry, I won't tell... it'll be our little secret!

1–1½	lbs (675 g) organic ground turkey
2	C (85 g) fresh organic spinach, chopped
1	shallot, finely chopped
1	clove garlic, minced
12	large basil leaves, finely chopped
3	Tbsp finely chopped parsley
1	Tbsp Dijon mustard
~	Sea salt
~	Freshly ground pepper
~	Olive oil

1. Put all ingredients together in a large mixing bowl. Add a pinch of sea salt and some freshly ground pepper.
2. Mix meat mixture with hands, gently, until everything is incorporated.
3. Divide meat into quarters in the bowl. Take ¼ of the meat and shape into round patties. Repeat for other patties.
4. Grill about 3 minutes per side until no longer pink.
5. Serve with quick dinner rolls (p.386) or English muffins (p.88) and favorite toppings like sautéed mushrooms and avocado.

Make Ahead and Freeze:

Make patties as directed, place on a platter lined with wax paper. If needed, place wax paper between patties to stack. Freeze until solid. Place patties, with wax paper between each, in a freezer bag and freeze until needed, up to 4 months. When ready, let patties thaw in refrigerator and grill as usual. Don't forget to double or triple recipe and make enough patties for a month!

Serves 4

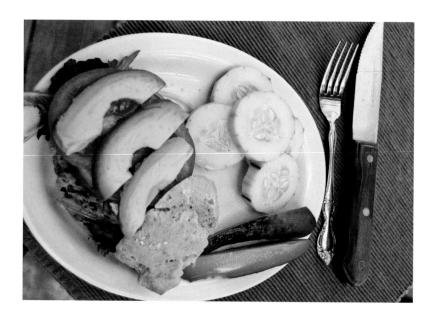

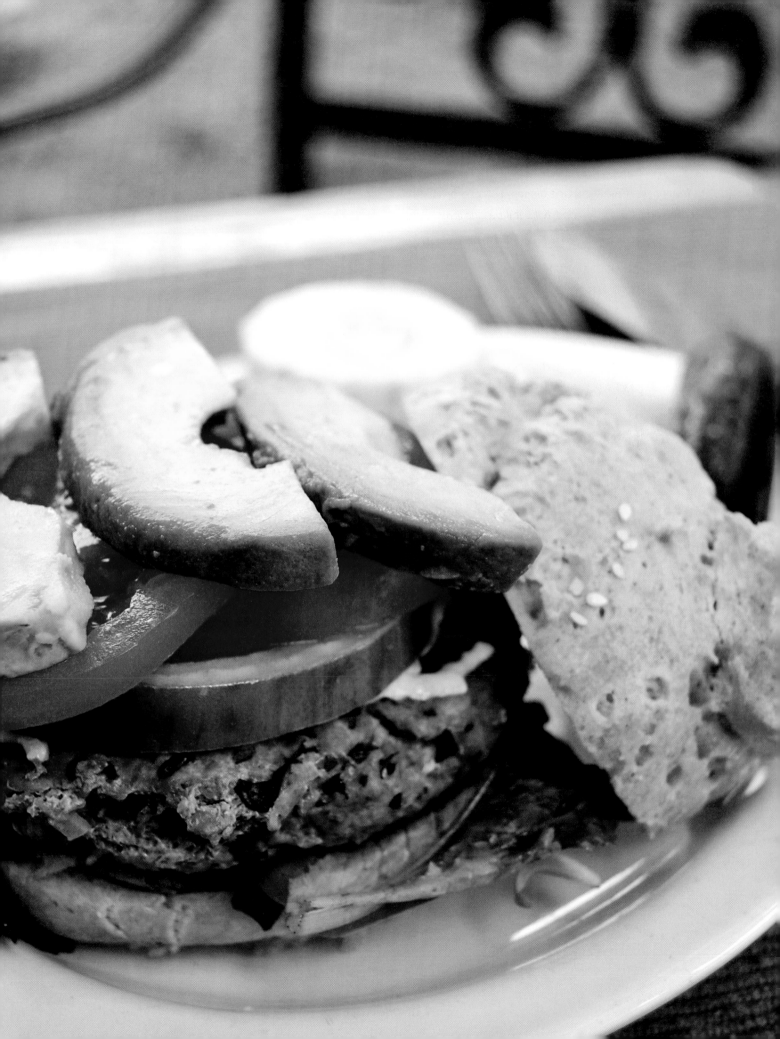

Flank Steak Rub

Another recipe from my sis! If there's one thing I've learned from being the youngest, it's to let big sis be the guinea pig. So I let her search, shop, try, and tweak a recipe. Then and only then will I try them, love them, and keep them for my own. Hey, I occasionally give her credit, so I figure we're good.

Rub:

½	tsp freshly ground black pepper
2	tsp sea salt
1	Tbsp paprika
½	tsp cumin
1	Tbsp organic brown sugar
¼	tsp cayenne pepper
1	tsp allspice
2	tsp freshly grated ginger
1	Tbsp chopped fresh Italian parsley

Steak:

2	lbs grass fed flank steak (US Wellness Meats)

1. In a plastic zip-top bag, combine all of the rub ingredients.
2. Add flank steak and squish around the bag to coat steak on all sides.
3. Seal bag and refrigerate for 2-plus hours or overnight.
4. Grill steak over high heat about 4 minutes per side. Allow meat to rest for 10 minutes.
5. Slice against the grain and serve!

Serves 4

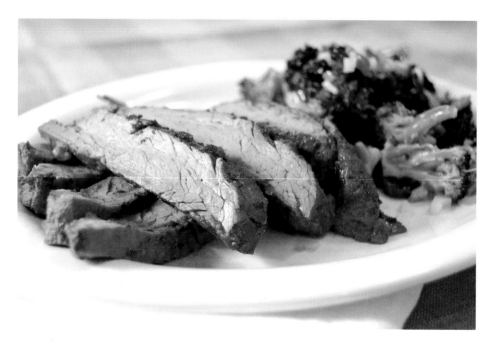

Entrées

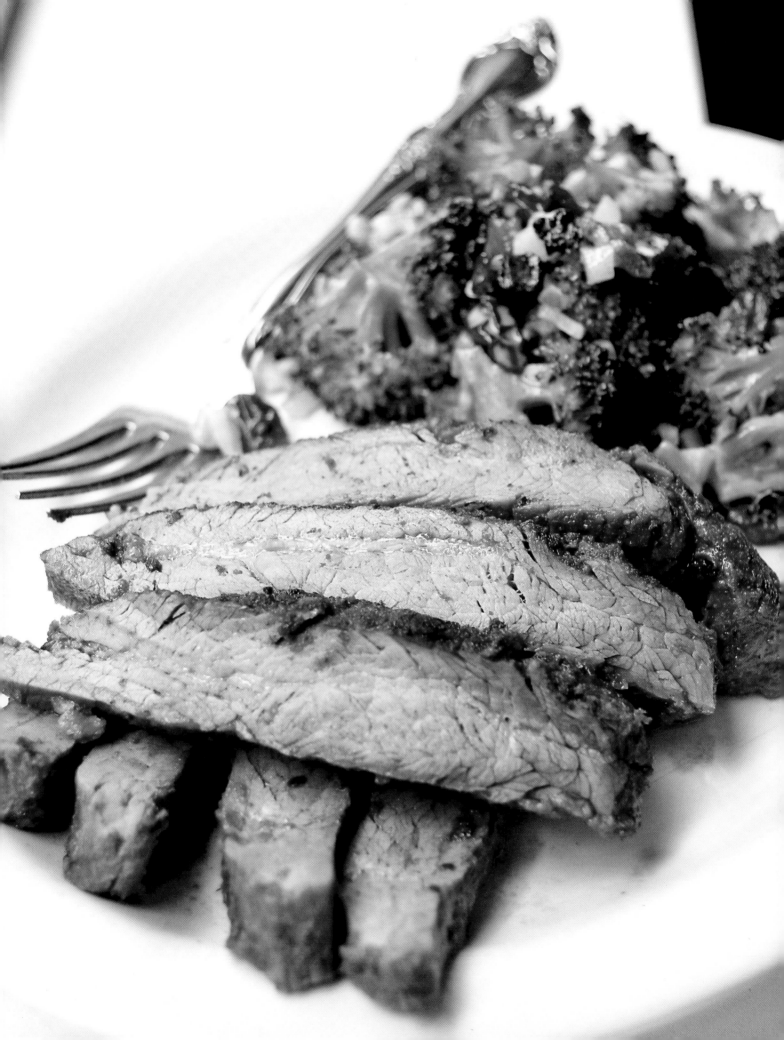

Mini Meatloaves

I distinctly remember my mom making meatloaf often when I was a kid. And while having it for dinner was a take-it-or-leave-it thing for me, I definitely remember craving it the next day for lunch. There is nothing better than a little leftover meatloaf for a satisfying lunch. Unlike some meatloaves that bake into one large loaf that can become mushy and greasy while cooking, these minis stay moist with a nice caramelized top for each and every one! And the leftovers? Yep, just like you remember. And with this recipe making 18 minis, you are almost guaranteed to have a few leftover. Of course, that depends on if your husband sneaks downstairs after you've gone to bed and eats them as a late-night snack. Sadly, I know this from experience. Good luck.

For the Loaves:

½	medium organic yellow onion, diced
2	cloves garlic, minced
2	lbs (900 g) organic ground beef (US Wellness Meats)
1½	tsp sea salt
½	tsp freshly ground pepper
1	Tbsp GF Worcestershire sauce
1	C (240 mL) organic tomato sauce (about ½ of a 15 oz can)
1	tsp granulated onion
1	tsp marjoram
½	tsp dried basil
¾	C (90 g) almond meal (if you happen to have some GF bread crumbs on hand, you can use those instead)
¼	C (20 g) fresh Italian parsley, chopped (or 1 Tbsp dried parsley)
2	Tbsp flax meal mixed with ⅓ C hot water

Sauce:

3	Tbsp organic tomato paste
~	Remaining can of tomato sauce (about ¾ C/180 mL)
3	Tbsp raw organic honey
1	Tbsp raw apple cider vinegar
1	tsp granulated onion
½	tsp granulated garlic
1	tsp sea salt
~	Freshly ground pepper to taste

1. In a medium skillet over medium-high heat, sauté onions and garlic until soft. About 5 minutes.
2. Meanwhile, in a large bowl, add beef, and remaining meat ingredients. Add cooked onions/garlic. Carefully (onions will be hot) stir and combine meat mixture until all ingredients are incorporated.
3. Spray muffin pans with nonstick spray. Fill muffin pans, just to the tops, with the meat mixture. Press down slightly to level tops.
4. In a small bowl, combine sauce ingredients.
5. Place a small spoonful of sauce on top of each mini meatloaf. With the back of the spoon, spread the sauce evenly over each loaf.
6. Fill any empty muffin cups halfway with water so meat bakes evenly. Bake in a 375° oven for about 30 minutes, rotating trays halfway through. Meat should be cooked through and top edges just turning brown.

Option: Pizza Mini Meatloaf

~Replace 1 lb of the burger with 1 lb (450 g) Italian sausage

Add:

~1 tsp Italian seasoning

~1 garlic clove, minced

~½ C (75 g) chopped olives

~¼ C (22 g) shredded nondairy cheese (Daiya)

~Replace sauce with about 1½ C (350 mL) of your favorite GF spaghetti sauce

Makes 18 Minis

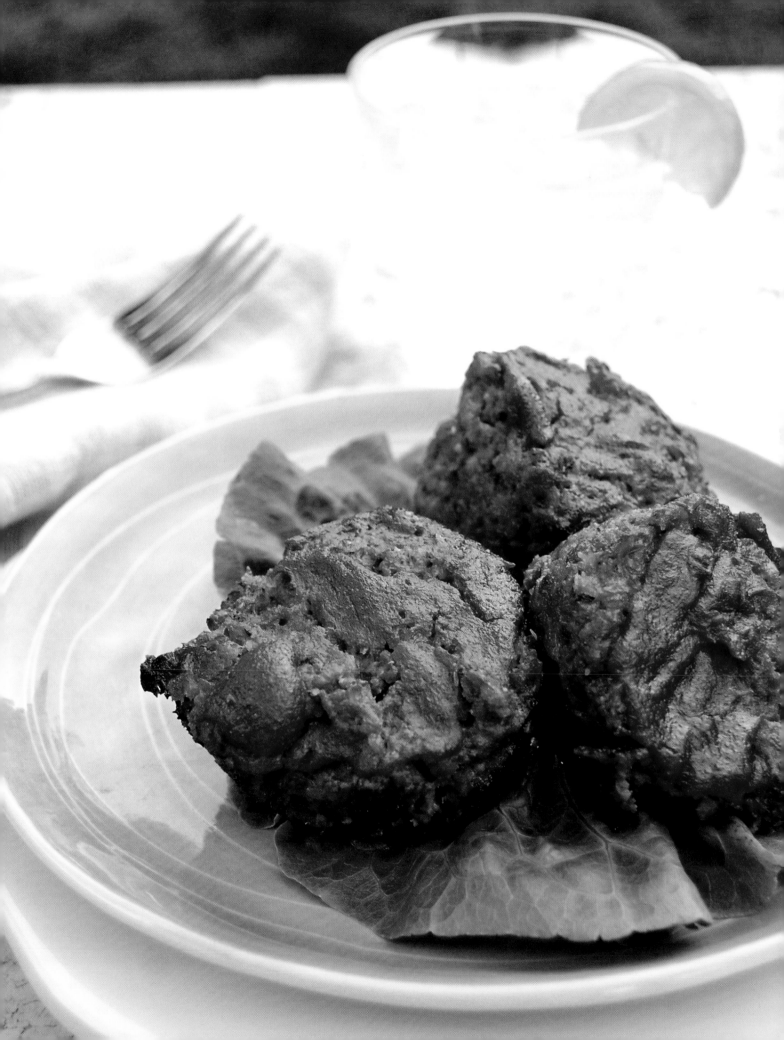

Holy Cow! Short Ribs

Oh short ribs... where have you been all my life? For some reason—we will call it a lapse of common sense—I avoided these guys for years, not sure what to do with them. What a mistake! Reasonably priced and packed with delicious meaty goodness, short ribs are so flavorful they really should be a part of everyone's Sunday supper repertoire. And please don't be afraid of the long cook time. The prep is actually very quick and the three hours they are in the oven give you plenty of time to take a walk with the kids, fold some laundry, or lock yourself in the bedroom with a glass of wine and a gossip magazine—I'm just offering options here, not that I've ever done the latter. Really. Either way, at the end, you can sit down to a satisfying, amazingly flavorful dinner that everyone will think you slaved over. And you won't be lying when you tell them it took you "three long hours" to prepare this meal. Wink, wink. Nudge, nudge.

For the Ribs:

3	lbs (1,350 g) short ribs (US Wellness Meats)
~	Granulated garlic
~	Granulated onion
~	Sea salt
~	Freshly ground pepper
1	Tbsp oil

For the Sauce:

5	organic celery stalks, chopped
8	large organic carrots, chopped
1	large organic yellow onion, chopped
1	qt (1 L) organic beef (or chicken) broth
1	sprig fresh rosemary

1. Season ribs liberally with garlic, onion, salt, and pepper on all sides.
2. Heat oil over medium-high heat in a large Dutch oven. Brown ribs on all sides, about 8 minutes. Remove ribs to a plate; cover to keep warm.
3. Add chopped veggies to Dutch oven and cook, stirring occasionally, for 3 minutes. Add broth, rosemary, and ribs back to pot. Cover and place in a 300° oven for about 3 hours. The meat should be very tender and falling off of the bone.
4. If desired, take about 1 cup of the veggies and liquid and carefully puree it in a food processor or blender until semi-smooth. Serve sauce over ribs.

Optional:

~Try adding 1 can diced tomatoes to the sauce for a little tomato-y flavor.

~Add ½ C (120 mL) red wine to the sauce for an amazing Burgundy-type rib.

Serves 4

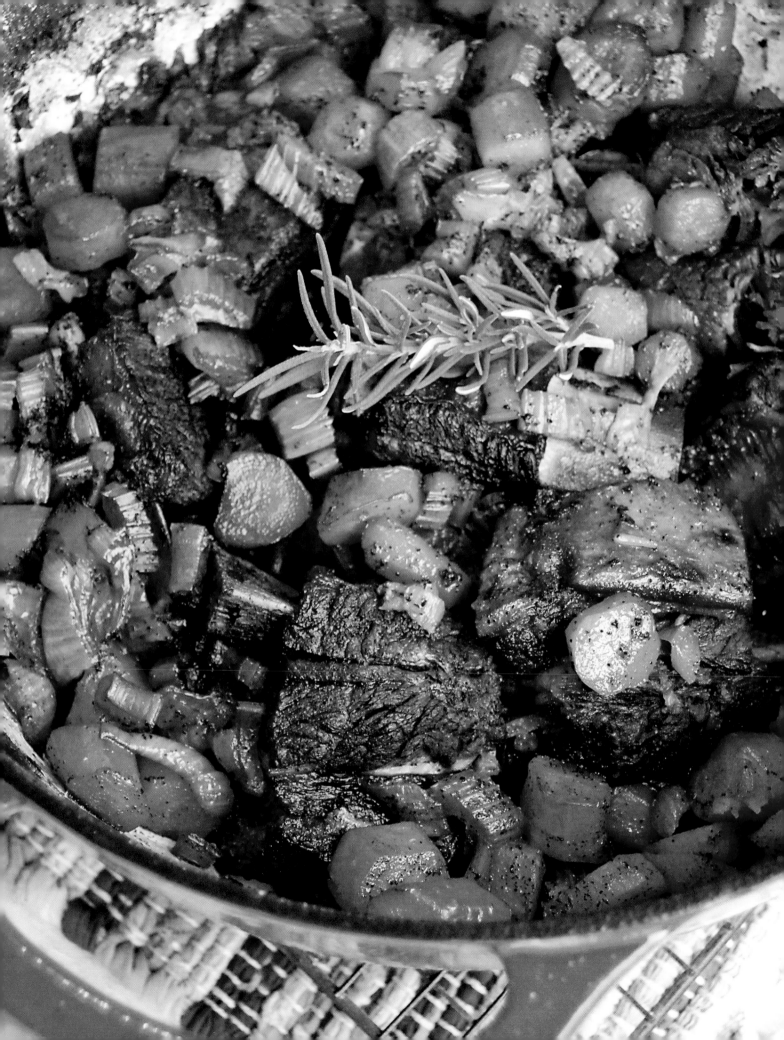

Grilled Marinated Tri-Tip

My family loves to grill and these tri-tip steaks have become a staple at our summer BBQ's. Perfectly tender, super flavorful, and just the right amount of sweet and savory in the marinade make these steaks disappear quickly! I like to use the tri-tip steaks from US Wellness Meats because they are grass-fed and come in convenient sizes that cook quickly, but this marinade will work well with a large tri-tip roast too!

Marinade:

½	C (120 mL) GF ketchup
2	Tbsp tamari wheat-free soy sauce (or coconut aminos)
3	cloves garlic, minced
1	Tbsp sesame seeds
2	Tbsp raw organic honey
5	large basil leaves, torn into pieces

Steak:

2	lb (450 g) tri-tip steaks (US Wellness Meats)
~	Sea salt to taste
~	Freshly ground pepper to taste

1. Combine marinade ingredients in a 9" by 13" glass baking dish.
2. Season tri tip with a little salt and pepper. Add tri-tip steaks to marinade, turning to coat.
3. Cover pan and refrigerate 5 hours, or overnight. Turn meat once part way through.
4. Bring meat to room temperature. Grill steaks, about 5 minutes per side. Let rest 10 minutes before slicing and serving.

Serves 4

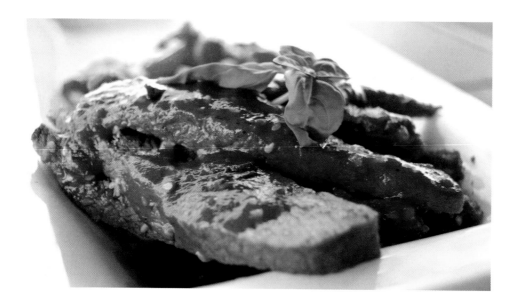

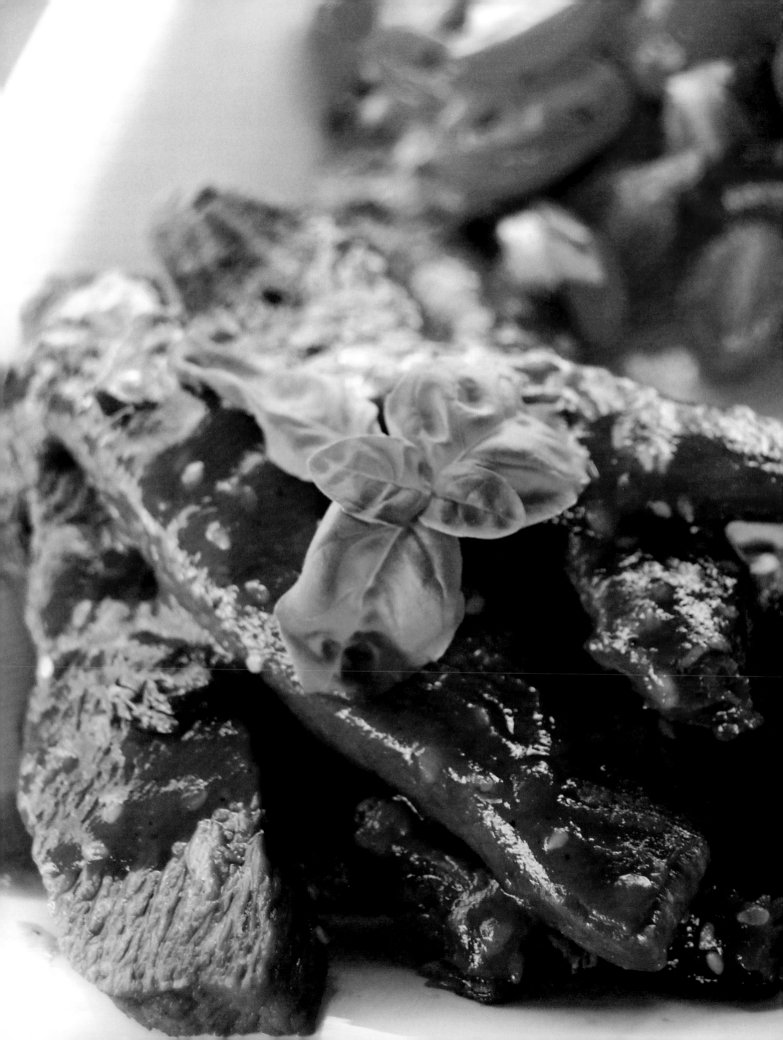

Sloppy Joes

Darn you, Adam Sandler! I can't make this dish or look at this recipe without singing his silly spoof of a song about a lunch lady making "sloppy joes, sloppy, sloppy joes!" Of course the voice he uses is what makes the song. Now I have to go and sing it until my head explodes because I can't get it out of my head once it's in there. Sigh. In the meantime, make these—they are delicious and nutritious. Way better than any pseudo-food sauce that comes in a can. Freeze any leftovers for later. Oh, and the kiddos love these for school lunches! Just heat the filling and put in a heated wide-mouth thermos. Give them some Cornbread (p.218) or a slice of Sandwich Bread (p. 384) and they'll be singing a happy tune as well!

Filling:

1	Tbsp olive oil
1	small organic yellow onion, diced
1	large organic orange bell pepper, diced
1	lb (450 g) grass-fed ground beef (US Wellness Meats)
3	Tbsp raw organic honey
1	tsp sea salt
~	Freshly ground pepper to taste
1	tsp granulated garlic
1	tsp granulated onion
1	tsp Italian seasoning
1	tsp caraway seeds

Sauce:

1	Tbsp red wine vinegar
1	Tbsp GF Worcestershire sauce
1	(15 oz) can (about 475 mL) organic tomato sauce
2	Tbsp organic tomato paste

1. Heat oil in a large skillet with high sides. Add onions and sauté 2 minutes.
2. Add bell pepper and sauté 1 minute.
3. Add ground beef, honey, and spices. Stir.
4. When meat has browned but isn't quite cooked through, reduce heat to low. Add red wine vinegar and Worcestershire sauce, stirring to combine.
5. Add tomato sauce and tomato paste. Stir well and cook for about 6 minutes, stirring occasionally.
6. Serve in a bowl or as a sandwich with a toasted English Muffin (p. 88) or on top of a slice of Cornbread (p. 218).

Make Ahead and Freeze:

Follow all steps to the end. Cool meat and store in airtight containers in the freezer until needed. To use, thaw and reheat over medium heat in a saucepan.

Serves 4

Entrées

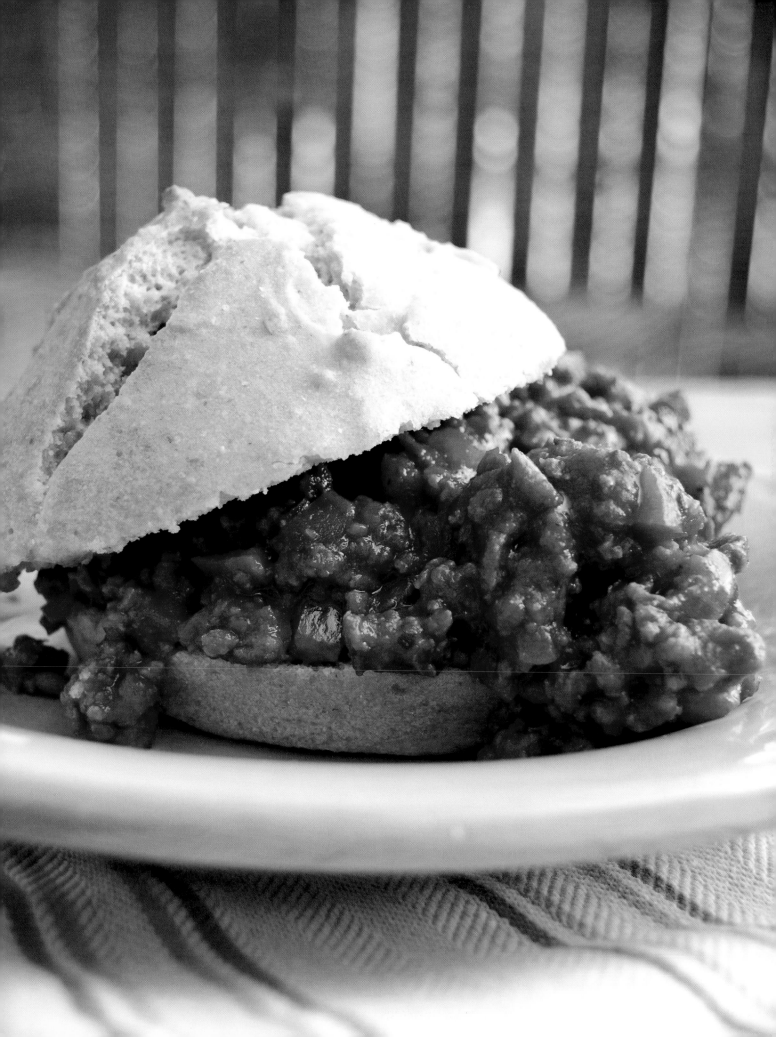

Quick Beef Burgundy
with Caramelized Onions

Traditional beef Burgundy can be a lengthy and labor-intensive process. And while it is very delicious, sometimes (OK all the time) I don't want to be in the kitchen that long. My motto is quick, easy, and delicious for all meals in my kitchen, no three-hour prep times and endless chopping! So if you love the flavor of beef Burgundy, but without the tornado-struck kitchen look and achy back, give this recipe a whirl. All the great taste of traditional beef Burgundy in a fraction of the time.

Sauce:

- ½   C (120 mL) organic red wine
- 2   Tbsp coconut aminos or Bragg liquid aminos
- 2   cloves garlic, minced
- ~   Freshly ground pepper to taste
- 1   Tbsp olive oil
- ~   Pinch of sea salt
- ½   tsp dried basil

Beef:

- 2   lb (900 g) flank steak (US Wellness Meats), slice thin across the grain
- 1   large organic red onion, slice into thin rings
- 3   Tbsp Coconut oil

1. Mix sauce ingredients in a medium bowl. Set aside.
2. In a large skillet, heat 2 Tbsp coconut oil over high heat. Sauté onions until softened, browned, and caramelized. Set aside.
3. Meanwhile, heat additional 1 Tbsp coconut oil in another large skillet over medium-high heat. Add steak strips. Sear steak on both sides, about 1–2 minutes per side.
4. Add sauce to steak pan, turn down heat to medium and simmer, uncovered, until meat is done but still pink and sauce has reduced a bit. About 2–3 minutes.
5. To serve, place steak strips on a plate, cover with caramelized onions, and top with a little sauce.

Serves 4

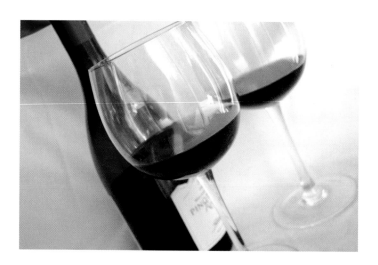

Entrées

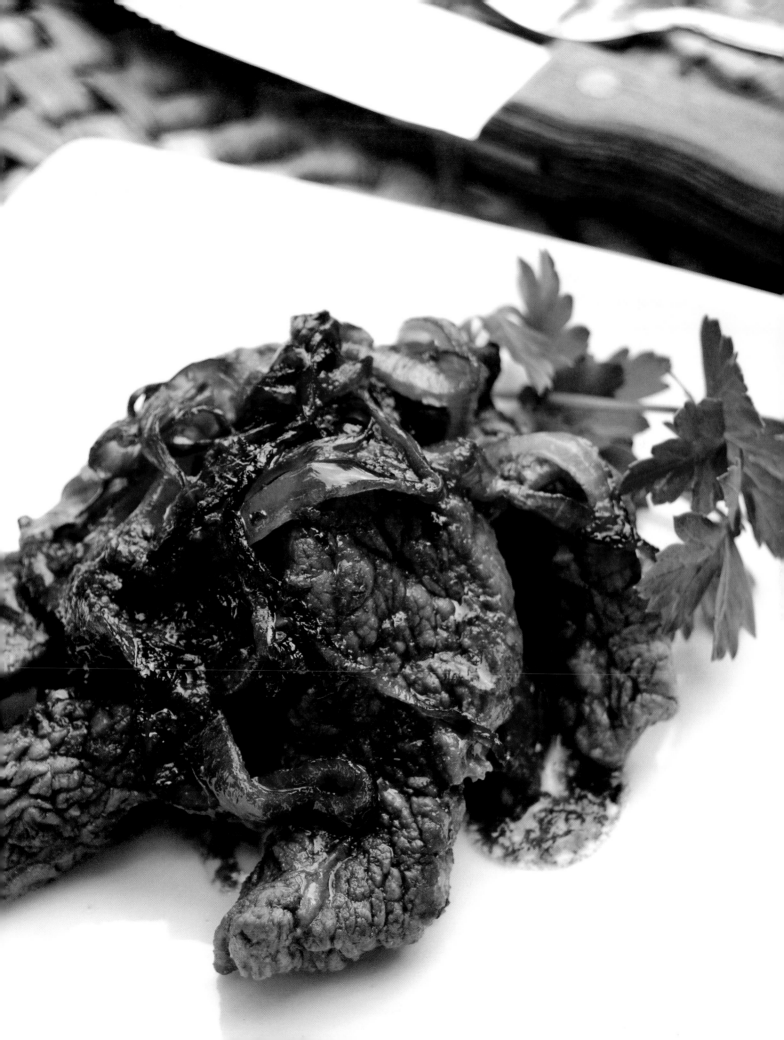

Steak Bites

These quick-cooking steak bites make a great midweek meal or a fun lunch for the kiddos. For school lunches, just preheat a wide-mouth thermos and fill with cooked steak and warmed sauce. It will be warm and yummy at lunchtime!

Bites:

2	lb (900 g) grass-fed sirloin steak (US Wellness Meats), cut into bite-size pieces
~	Granulated garlic
~	Granulated onion
~	Sea salt
~	Freshly ground pepper
1	Tbsp coconut oil

Sauce:

1	(15 oz) can (about 475 mL) organic tomato sauce
1	(6 oz) can (180 mL) organic tomato paste
3	Tbsp raw honey or maple syrup
3	Tbsp organic apple cider vinegar
2	tsp sea salt
1	Tbsp granulated onion
1	tsp paprika
½	tsp smoked paprika
2	tsp granulated garlic
1	Tbsp coconut aminos or GF tamari soy sauce or Bragg liquid aminos

1. Season meat with garlic, onion, salt, and pepper to taste.
2. In a small saucepan, combine sauce ingredients. Stir to combine and heat over medium until very warm. Set aside.
3. Heat coconut oil in a large skillet over medium-high heat. Add seasoned steak pieces, and don't stir! Let them sit for a few minutes to caramelize.
4. Stir and let steaks cook until just pink inside, about 6 minutes. Serve steak bites alongside sauce for dipping.

Serves 4

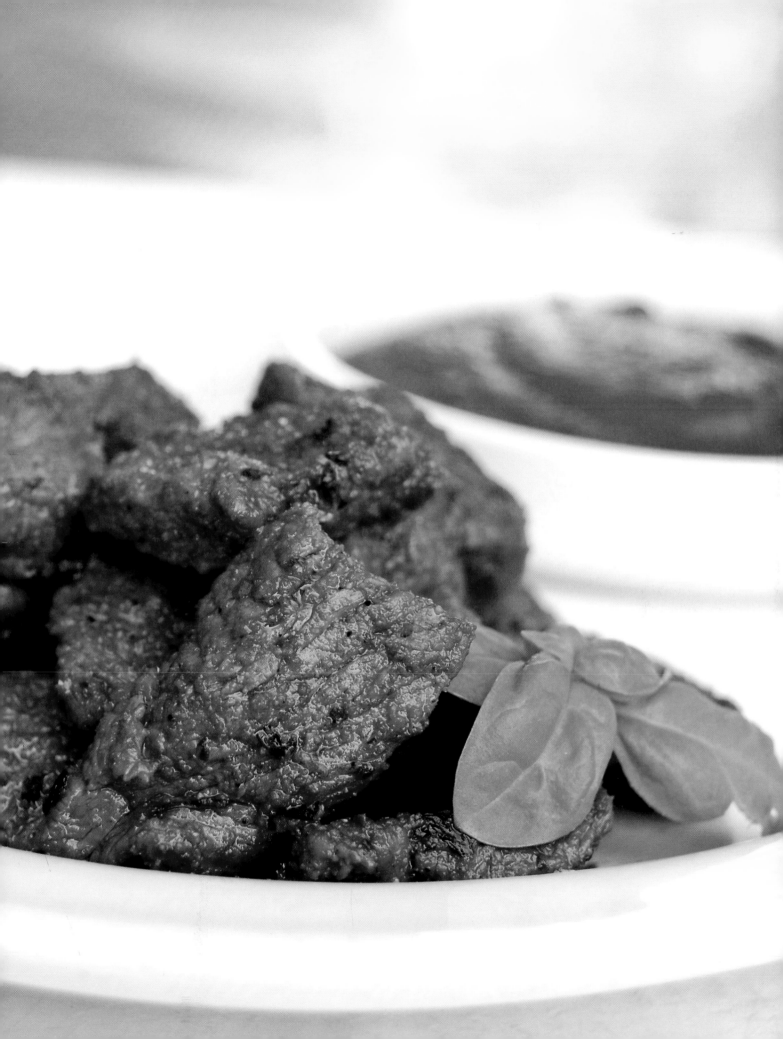

Salisbury Steak with Mushroom Gravy

Sometimes after being diagnosed with multiple food intolerances, folks feel like their favorite comfort foods will be off limits . . . bread, lasagna, spaghetti, gravy. But most of these meals can be recreated with a little imagination—and a good craving! Because let's face it, sometimes nothing satisfies a grumbly tummy like a hearty, tasty, filling meal like yummy Salisbury Steak with Mushroom Gravy. I guarantee you will love this way more than any TV dinner you've had in the past! Serve alongside some creamy mashed potatoes and cooked carrots for comfort food at its best.

For the Steaks:

1½	lbs (675 g) organic grass-fed ground beef (US Wellness Meats)
½	medium yellow onion, finely chopped
1	tsp granulated garlic
2	tsp granulated onion
½	tsp dried rosemary
1	tsp paprika
1	tsp fennel seed
1	tsp sea salt
~	Freshly ground pepper to taste
2	Tbsp coconut oil, for the pan

For the Gravy:

8	oz (230 g) white mushrooms, chopped
~	Sea salt and pepper to taste
2	C (475 mL) organic beef broth
½	C (120 mL) coconut milk (or your favorite nondairy milk)
1	Tbsp coconut flour
1	Tbsp arrowroot starch mixed with a tiny bit of cold water to make a slurry

1. Mix all of the steak ingredients gently in a bowl to combine.
2. Form 4 large oval patties, about 1 inch thick.
3. Heat oil in a large nonstick skillet over medium-high heat. Add steak patties to the hot pan.
4. Cook meat until browned and caramelized, about 6 minutes per side.
5. Remove patties to a platter and keep warm by tenting with foil.
6. Add mushrooms to hot pan. Season mushrooms with salt and pepper and cook until tender, about 5 minutes.
7. Add beef broth and coconut milk to pan.
8. Add coconut flour to pan and stir. Bring to a boil.
9. Add arrowroot slurry and stir until thick, about 1 minute. Remove gravy from heat.
10. Serve Salisbury steaks with mushroom gravy poured over the top!

Serves 4

Entrées

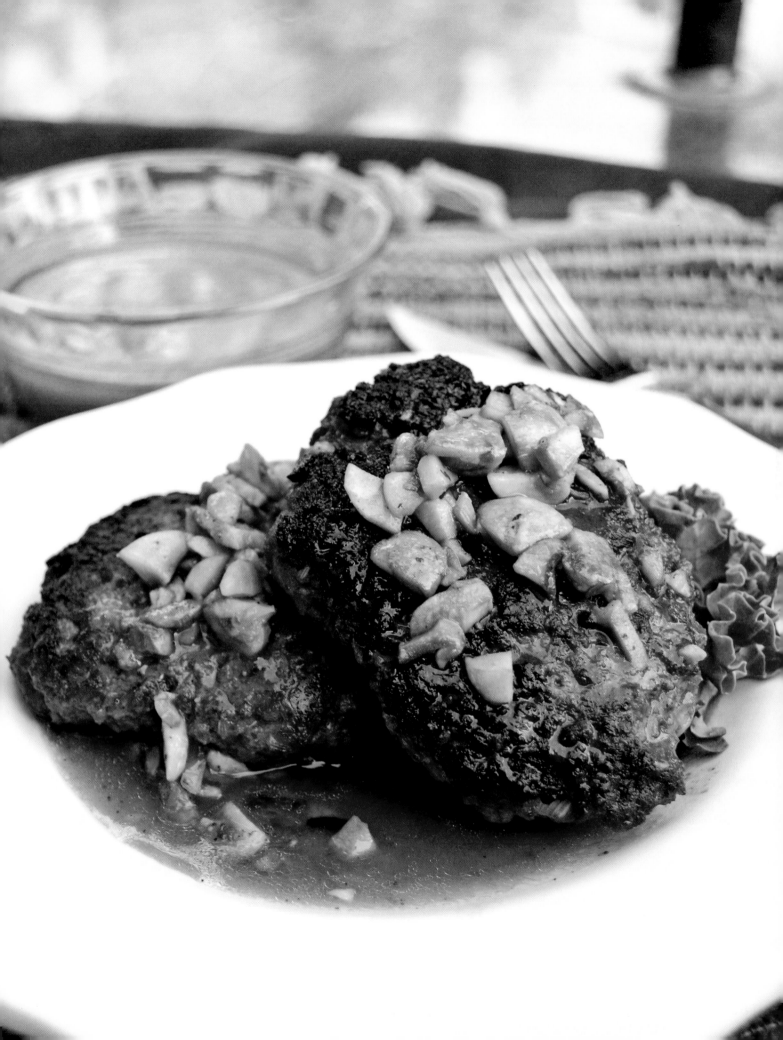

Italian Meatballs

I'm going to warn you now—these things are addicting. The sauce simmering with the meatballs creates such a delicious, satisfying meal, you'll keep coming back for more, and maybe a little more, and then just another one.... I also love how versatile the recipe is. First, I make them as is for a nice dinner. Second, I can make the meatballs ahead of time, freeze them prior to cooking, then thaw and cook as usual—a great make-ahead meal! And third, I like to bring these along to potlucks or parties, so I cook them most of the way through, place the meatballs and sauce in a slow cooker on low, and then take them to the event. People will adore you and want your autograph. Signed, The Master of Meatballs...

1	lb (450 g) grass-fed ground beef (US Wellness Meats)
1	lb (450 g) grass-fed ground pork (US Wellness Meats)
½	medium organic onion, finely chopped
3	garlic cloves, minced
¼	C (about 11 g) chopped fresh parsley
½	tsp sea salt
1	tsp oregano
½	tsp dried basil
~	Pinch of dried rosemary
½	tsp freshly ground pepper
2	Tbsp coconut flour
¼	C (30 g) almond meal
2	Tbsp olive oil
1	C homemade spaghetti sauce (p.248)

1. In a large bowl, mix all ingredients lightly with your hands until combined.
2. Roll into 1½-inch meatballs.
3. Heat oil in a large skillet over medium-high heat. Add meatballs, spacing evenly around pan. Make sure not to touch them for a few minutes and really let them brown and caramelize on the bottoms. Turn meatballs and brown on all sides, turning down heat to medium if necessary.
4. When meatballs are all browned and just about cooked through, add 1 C Spaghetti Sauce and deglaze the pan (i.e., scrape up all the yummy meatball goodness on the bottom of the pan, but be careful not to break up the balls).
5. Let sauce heat through and simmer slightly for about 5 minutes.
6. Serve and enjoy!

Option:

If you're avoiding nuts, process ½ C (75 g) raw sunflower seeds in the food processor to replace the almond meal.

Serves 4-6

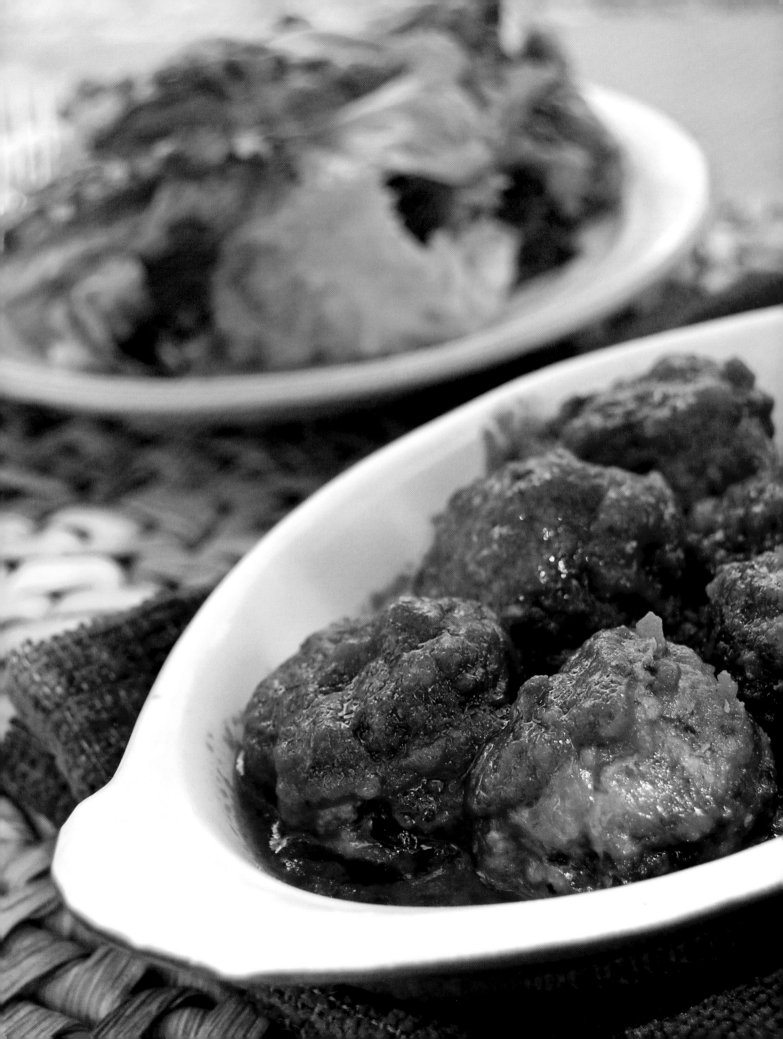

Pork Chops with Pineapple Mango Salsa

Pork chops can be a little, shall we say, plain and boring? And if there's one thing kids don't like, it's boring. So I had to come up with a quick fix one night while staring at a plate of uncooked pork chops with the kids at my heels asking, "What's for dinner, Mom?" Luckily, after rummaging through the kitchen, I was inspired to throw together, um, I mean masterfully create, a fresh salsa to help make those chops a little more exciting! The family was happy, the chops were delicious, and dinner was saved. I love a happy ending!

Chops:

4	boneless organic pork chops (US Wellness Meats)
~	Sea salt to taste
~	Freshly ground black pepper to taste
~	Granulated garlic to taste
1	Tbsp olive oil

Salsa:

1	organic mango, peeled and diced
1	C (150 g) diced organic pineapple (can use frozen, canned, or fresh)
4	basil leaves, finely chopped
½	medium organic red onion, finely chopped
~	Juice of 1 small organic lime
2	Tbsp olive oil
~	Sea salt and freshly ground pepper to taste

1. Sprinkle pork chops with salt, pepper, and garlic.
2. Heat oil in a large skillet over medium-high heat. Add pork chops and brown on each side. Cook until done and no longer pink, about 5 minutes per side.
3. Meanwhile, make the salsa. Add all salsa ingredients, except water, to a bowl and stir gently to combine.
4. To serve, place a pork chop on a plate and spoon salsa over the top.

Serves 4

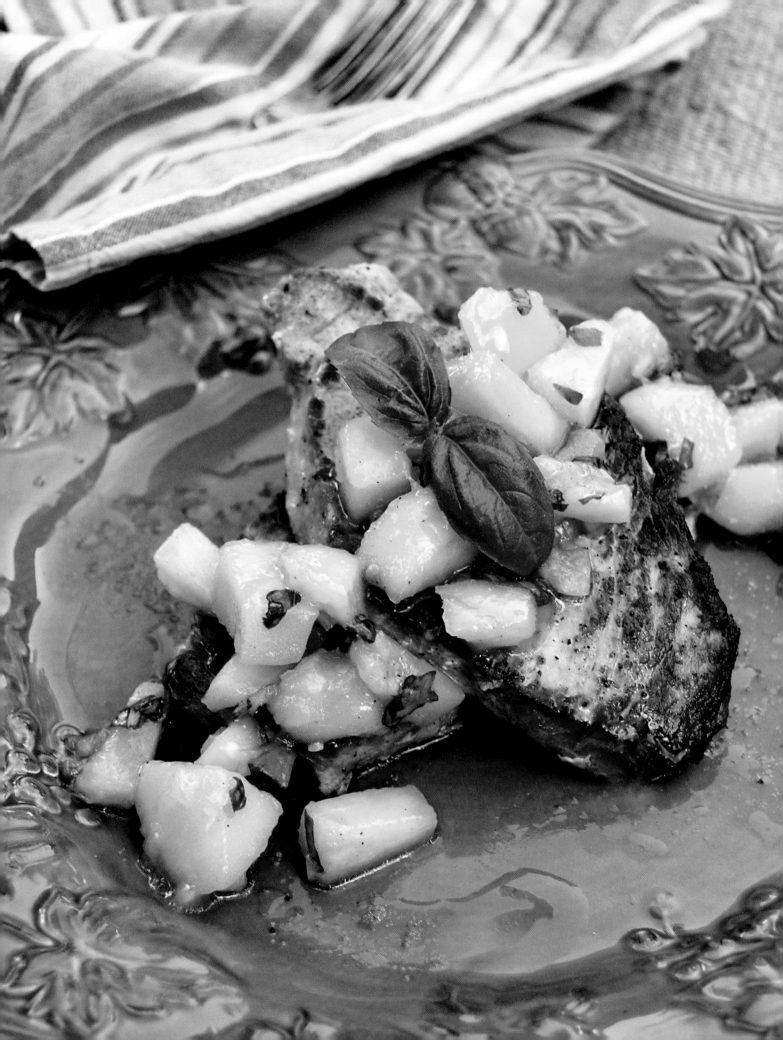

Dutch Oven Pork Roast

I love a one-pot meal, and one that can be made and forgotten about is even better! This pork roast is amazingly tender and delicious. Enjoy it thoroughly for dinner, and then use leftovers in everything from sandwiches to tacos.

Roast:

5	lb (2,250 g) organic pork roast (US Wellness Meats)
2	Tbsp coconut oil
~	Sea salt and pepper to taste

For Sauce:

1	organic yellow onion, quartered
3	garlic cloves
3	Tbsp olive oil
3	Tbsp raw apple cider vinegar
3	Tbsp raw organic honey
1	tsp oregano
1	tsp chili powder
1	tsp rosemary
2	tsp granulated onion
1	tsp cumin
2	tsp sea salt
~	Freshly ground pepper to taste
3	C (700 mL) water

1. Rub roast with salt and pepper.
2. In a food processor, puree sauce ingredients until blended but still slightly chunky.
3. In a Dutch oven, heat oil over medium-high heat. Add pork roast and brown on all sides. Remove from heat.
4. Pour sauce over roast, being careful of the hot steam.
5. Pour 3 C water around roast.
6. Cover with lid and place in 325° oven. Cook for 2½–3 hours, or until roast is done and fork tender.

Serves 4-6

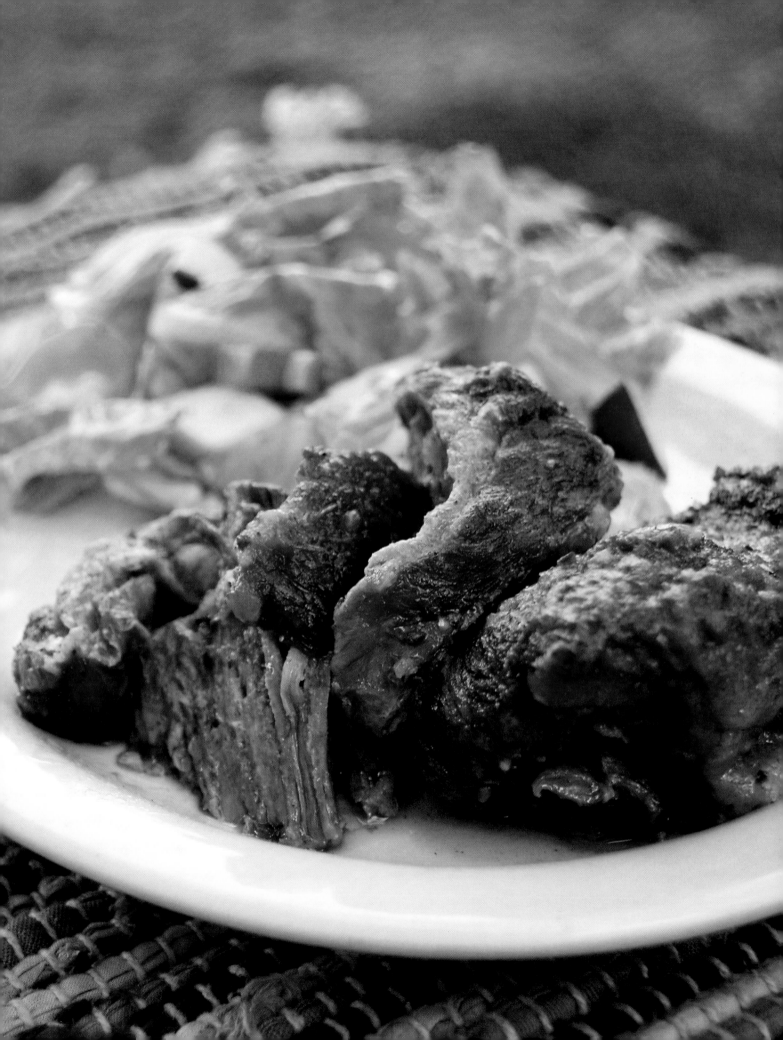

Stuffed Mushrooms

My family has a tradition of eating snacky, appetizer-type foods on Christmas Eve. Everyone is usually so excited on this special night and, as a kid, it was much more enjoyable to nibble all evening than try and sit through a big family meal. After twenty-five-plus years of doing this (I was an embryo when it began... really) there are a few key treats that always make a return appearance, including these stuffed mushrooms. And while they originally contained bread crumbs, egg, and cream cheese, the modifications I've made have not affected the taste one bit. I still hear "Where are those stuffed mushrooms?" every year when I walk in the door and the platter is still empty at the end of the night. Another happy holiday, sans gluten.

30	large white button mushroom, cleaned
1	lb (450 g) GF Italian sausage (bulk, or links with casings removed)
3	organic green onions, chopped
8	oz (230 g) room-temperature vegan cream cheese (see note below for soy free option)

1. Pop stems off of mushrooms and scoop out a small opening in each cap.
2. Cook sausage until done and browned. Add green onions, stir, and remove from heat.
3. Add cream cheese. Stir until combined.
4. With a teaspoon, scoop sausage filling into each mushroom cap. Place mushrooms on a foil-lined baking sheet.
5. Bake in a 400° oven for 15–20 minutes, or until mushrooms are cooked and top of filling starts to brown and bubble.
6. Serve immediately.

Option: *I have not found a vegan cream cheese that doesn't contain soy, but since we eat these just once a year during Christmas, we are OK with that. If you don't want the soy cream cheese, try adding just enough plain non-dairy yogurt (such as coconut milk or rice milk) to get the filling to stick together. Proceed with step 4.*

Tip: *You can make these a day ahead! Complete steps 1–4, cover baking sheet with plastic wrap and store in the fridge until ready to use. Proceed with baking in step 5, keeping in mind they may take a few extra minutes to cook since they will be starting from a colder temperature.*

Makes about 30 mushrooms

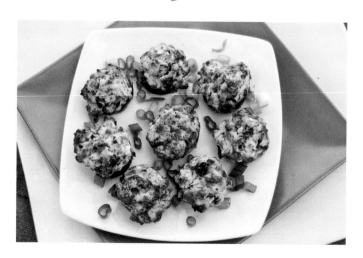

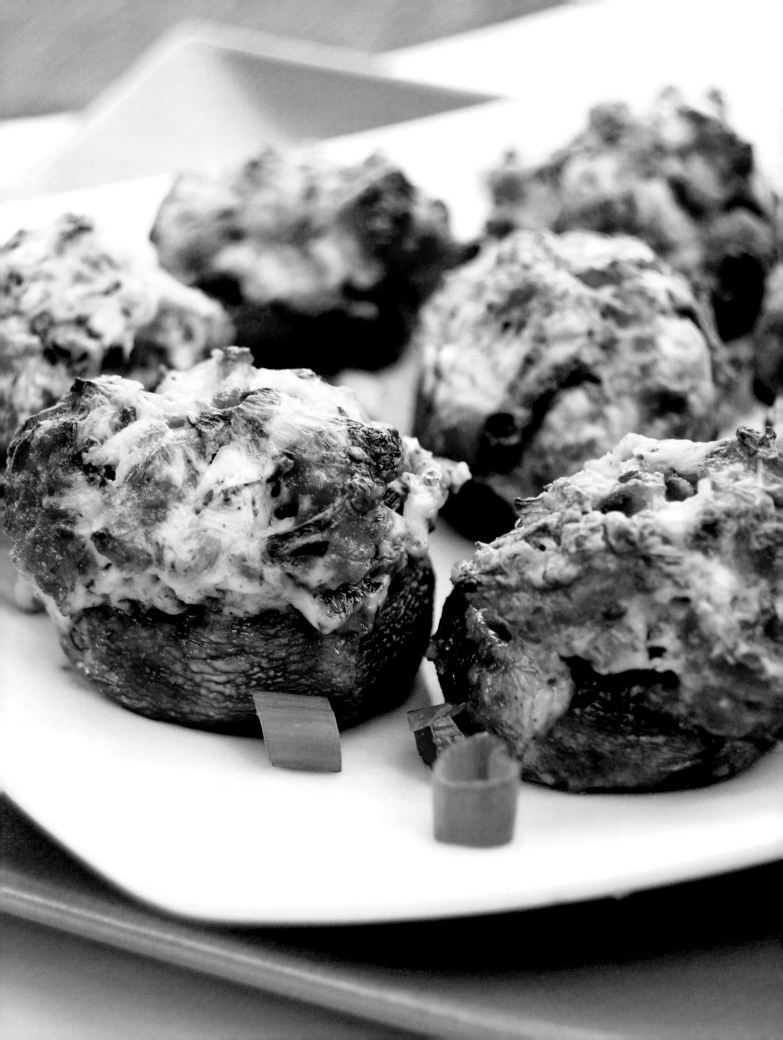

Garlicky Crock Pot Pork Roast

I absolutely love the wonderful aroma created by this exceptionally easy recipe. And the only thing better than a yummy-smelling crock pot roast is the entire yummy meal in the crock pot that's ready when you are! Homey, filling, healthy, and satisfying, pork roast with carrots and potatoes provide comfort food for the GF and non-GF alike.

Roast:

1	5 lb organic pork roast
~	Sea salt
~	Freshly ground black pepper
2	Tbsp coconut oil

Sauce:

4	cloves of garlic, minced
1	C (240 mL) organic chicken broth
1	tsp onion powder (granulated onion)
1	tsp tarragon
¼	tsp thyme
1	Tbsp raw organic honey
2	Tbsp raw apple cider vinegar
3	Tbsp organic tomato paste (or in a pinch you can use a GF ketchup)
½	tsp orange zest

Add Ins:

1	medium organic yellow onion, sliced
4	medium organic russet potatoes, peeled and cut into large chunks
6	large organic carrots, chopped into large chunks

1. Sprinkle salt and pepper over pork roast.
2. Heat oil in large skillet over medium-high heat. When pan is hot, add pork roast and brown on all sides.
3. While pork is browning, mix sauce ingredients in a medium bowl until combined.
4. Place onions over the bottom of the slow cooker, followed by the potatoes.
5. Add browned roast to slow cooker, followed by the carrots around the roast.
6. Pour all of the sauce mixture over the roast and veggies.
7. Cook on high for 4–5 hours, or low 6–8 hours.
8. Serve pork with onions and sauce over the top, with potatoes and carrots on the side.

Serves 4- 6

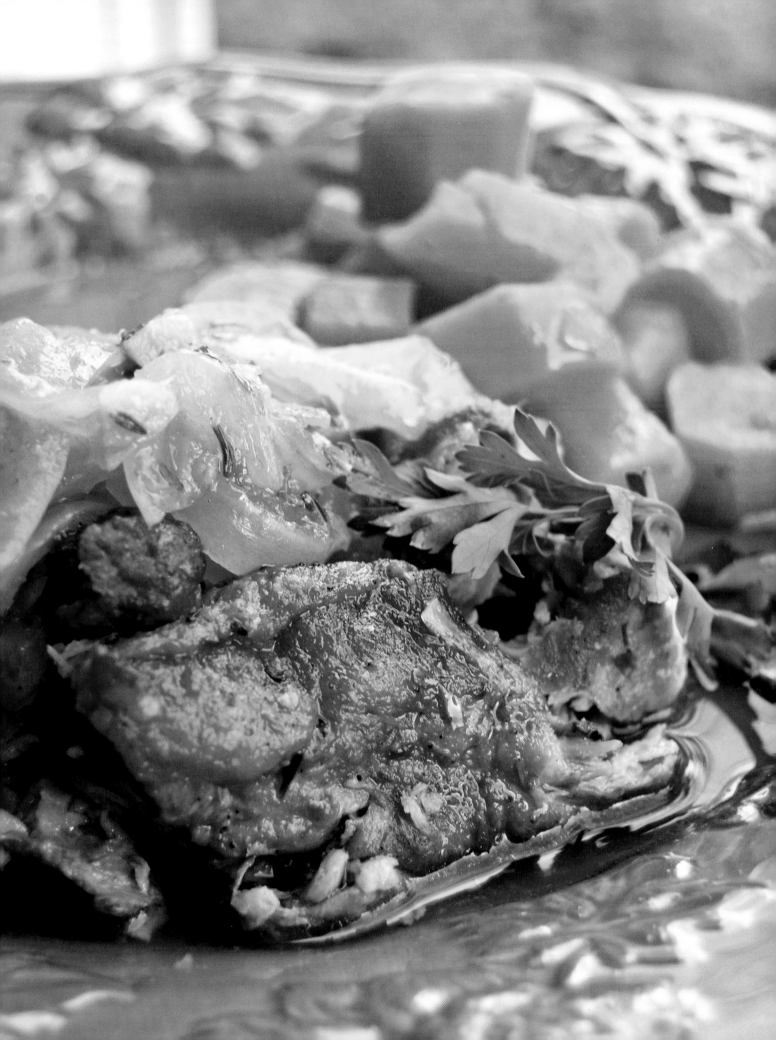

Pork Tacos with Pineapple Salsa

A little bit country, a little bit rock 'n' roll... uh, wait, I mean, a little bit smoky, a little bit sweet! These yummy tacos are a hit with the family and guests alike. So much flavor from every angle, no one you know will guess these are naturally gluten-free! Plus, you'll look like a rock star when you serve up a platter of these with the sweet pineapple salsa AND a smoky sauce. Because really, who ever makes two sauces for tacos? Rock on, Senorita, rock on.

Sauce & Salsa:

1	small organic yellow onion, cut in half
1	small jalapeño, cut in half, seeds removed and discarded
3	Tbsp raw organic honey
3	cloves of garlic, minced (or use garlic press)
1	Tbsp chili powder
1	tsp oregano
2	tsp cumin
2	tsp sea salt
~	Freshly ground pepper to taste
1	(20 oz) (about 500 mL) can organic pineapple chunks in juice
2	Tbsp chopped fresh cilantro, plus more for garnish
~	Lime wedges

Filling:

1½–2 lbs (900 g) boneless organic pork chops

Shells:

~ Organic GF Corn tortillas (Try using homemade corn tortillas on p. 232. Either microwave for a few seconds to soften, or fry lightly in oil until soft.)

Toppings:

~ Shredded lettuce
~ Diced tomatoes
~ Diced avocado
~ Dairy-free cheese

1. In food processor, puree half of onion, half of jalapeño, honey, garlic, chili powder, oregano, cumin, salt, pepper, about $^1/_3$ of the can of pineapple with ½ cup of the juice. Puree until semi-smooth.

2. Pour $^1/_3$ cup of sauce into a plate. Add pork and turn to coat pork in the sauce.

3. Grill pork 6–8 minutes (turning pork once), or until no longer pink. Let rest.

4. While pork is cooking, dice remaining ½ onion and ½ jalapeño; place in a small bowl. Add remaining $^2/_3$ can of pineapple including a Tbsp of the juice and 2 Tbsp of chopped cilantro. Squeeze in the juice of one lime wedge. Season with sea salt and pepper to taste.

5. Cut pork into bite-size chunks.

6. To serve: place pork in warmed tortillas. Top with pineapple salsa and reserved sauce and a squeeze of lime. Add any toppings you like!

7. For an even healthier twist, use lettuce leaves instead of corn tortillas.

Options:

~Use the pureed sauce over a pork roast in the crock pot. When done, shred pork and serve in warm tortillas with a squeeze of lime.

~The pureed sauce also makes a great salsa with tortilla chips!

Serves 4

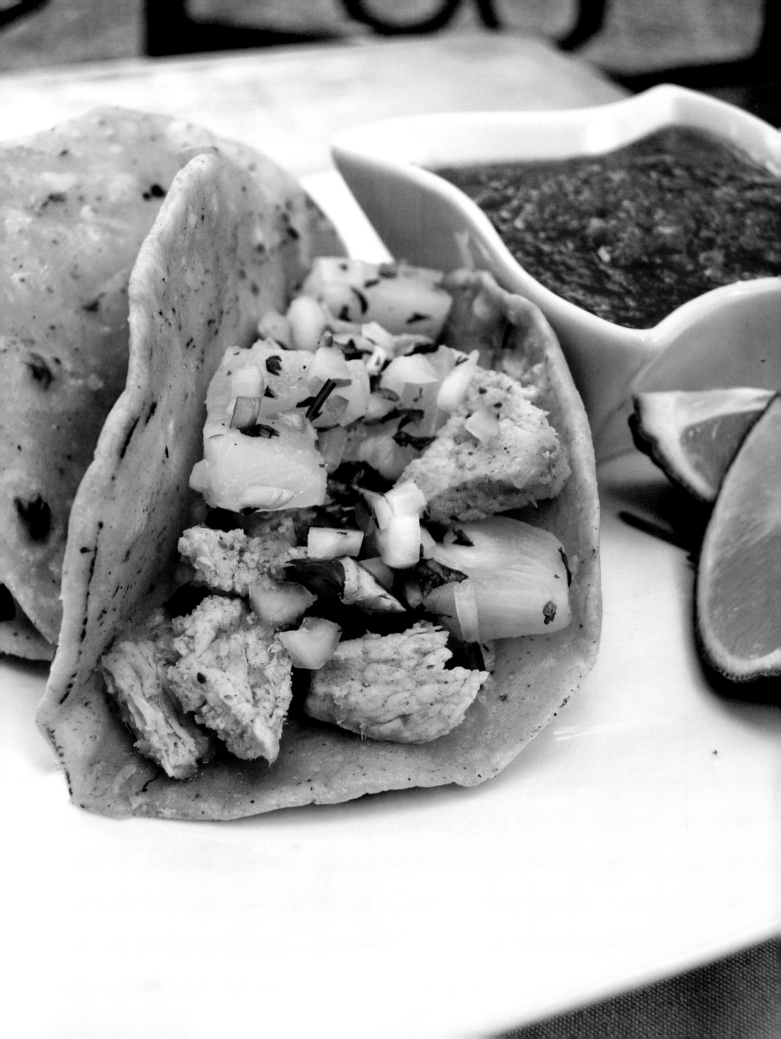

BLAT's to Go
(Bacon, Lettuce, Avocado and Tomato)

We travel a lot, especially in the summer, and you can't always find safe places to eat while on the road. Our solution is to pack an ice chest wherever we go, and this lettuce wrap has quickly become a favorite on-the-go meal for us. Tasty and filling, it really hits the spot when tummies start rumbling on the road.

8	organic romaine lettuce leaves, washed and dried
1	package of organic, uncured bacon, cooked (US Wellness Meats)
2	small organic avocados, mashed
1	pint (450 g) organic cherry tomatoes, washed and dried

1. When you're ready to eat, spread a spoonful of avocado onto each lettuce leaf.
2. Place slices of cooked bacon on top of avocado.
3. Sprinkle each lettuce cup with tomatoes.
4. Enjoy!

Option:

~Try adding diced red onions on top!

~How about a drizzle of Italian vinaigrette? (p. 258)

Makes 8

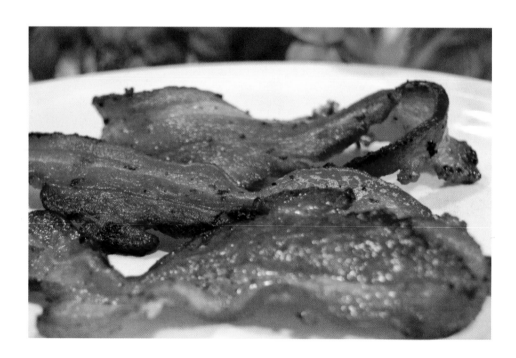

Entrées

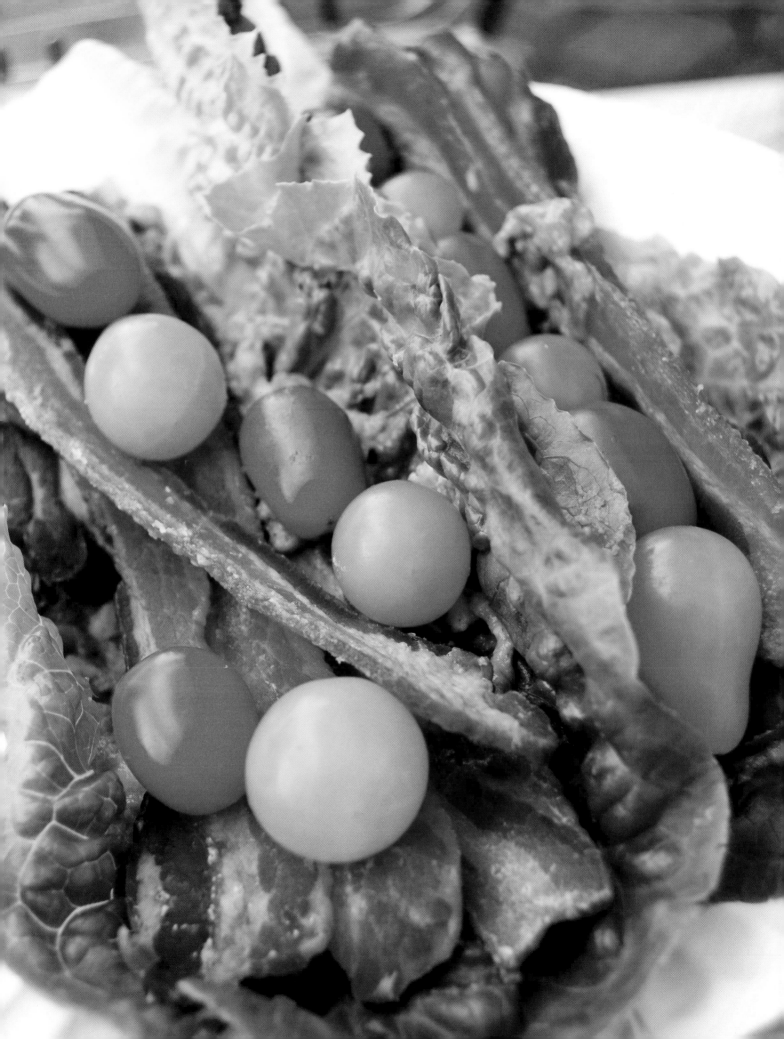

Shrimp Basil Pasta

This dish has had many makeovers over the years. It started out as a salad with tomato slices and basil. Then I turned it into a delicious side dish by chopping the tomatoes and adding pasta. Liking the idea of a one-bowl dinner, I added shrimp and, voila! A dish about twelve years in the making! No one ever said I was a fast cook. But it has turned into another family favorite, especially during the summer months. My youngest usually begs for me to make it at least once a week, so you just know it must be good! This also makes a great take-along meal for picnics and traveling since it's great served cold or heated up a bit.

Pasta:

⅓	C (80 mL) olive oil
3	cloves of garlic, minced
18	basil leaves (about 1 small herb package or ½ C [20 g] packed), finely chopped
8	ripe organic Roma tomatoes, diced
1	(16oz) pkg. (450 g) GF pasta (brown rice spirals or penne work well)

Shrimp:

1	lb (450 g) frozen raw peeled wild shrimp, thawed, tails removed
1	Tbsp olive oil
~	Sea salt and pepper
½	tsp granulated garlic
½	tsp dried basil

Optional:

3	Tbsp nondairy cheese, such as Daiya shredded mozzarella

1. Pour olive oil into a large serving bowl. Add garlic and let sit for 10 minutes.
2. Add chopped basil and tomatoes to bowl, stir gently to combine. Set aside.
3. Cook pasta according to package directions and drain.
4. Meanwhile, cook the shrimp. Heat oil in a large skillet over medium-high heat. Add shrimp.
5. Season shrimp with salt, pepper, garlic, and basil. Stir and let shrimp cook until done and no longer pink.
6. Add pasta and shrimp to tomato mixture and stir gently to combine.
7. If desired, sprinkle with nondairy cheese and enjoy!

Serves 4–6

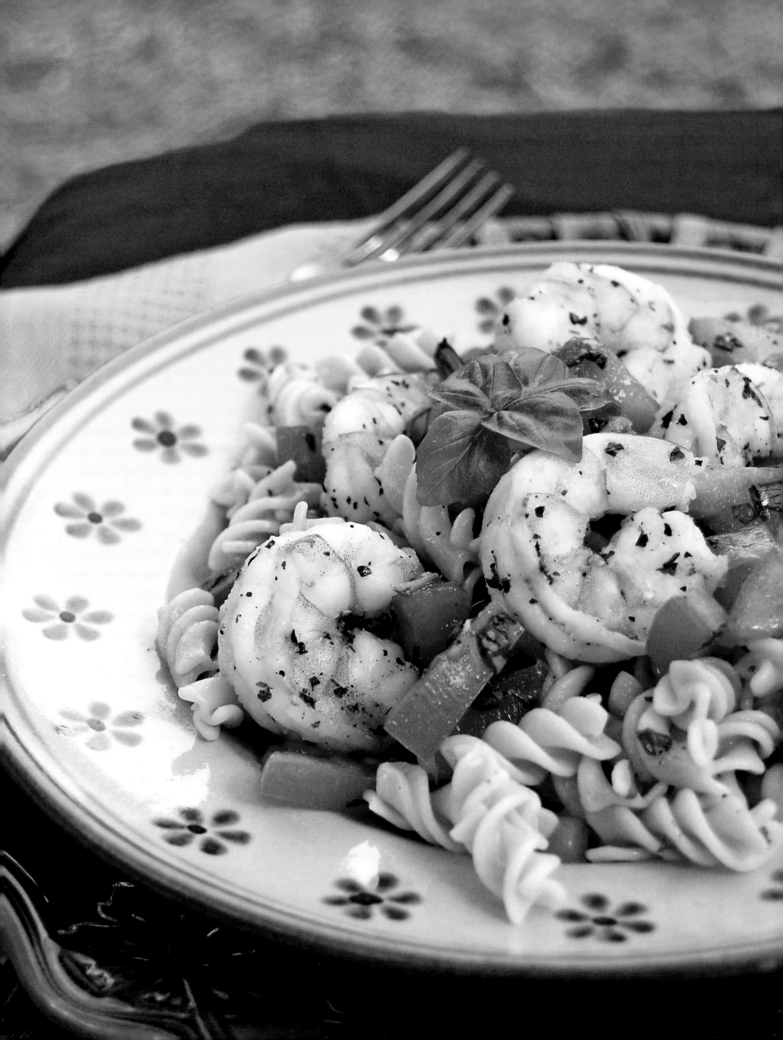

Ginger Salmon

It's hard to believe now, but I wasn't always a fan of salmon. Shhhhh... don't tell anyone! Everyone knows healthy people eat salmon, right? But, sadly, I just never loved its flavor. And then one day, determined to eat this amazingly heart-healthy fish, I created this sauce to help me along. And you know what? I love salmon now! Try this easy Ginger Salmon for anyone in your family who's a bit fish-phobic and I'll bet they'll be cleaning their plates in no time!

Sauce:

3	Tbsp GF tamari soy sauce (can substitute coconut aminos)
2	tsp grated fresh ginger
1	Tbsp lemon juice
2	Tbsp raw organic honey
½	tsp granulated onion
~	Freshly ground pepper to taste
2	Tbsp olive oil

Salmon:

4	boneless skinless wild salmon fillets

Toppings:

~	Chopped green onion
~	Sesame seeds

1. Whisk together soy sauce, ginger, lemon juice, honey, granulated onion, a little freshly ground pepper, and olive oil. Set aside.

2. Heat a large nonstick skillet over med-high heat. Spray with cooking spray or use a small amount of your favorite oil in the pan. Add salmon fillets. Cook for about 1 minute.

3. Turn salmon fillets. Reduce heat to medium-low, cover and cook for 3 minutes.

4. Pour sauce over salmon, into pan. Simmer, uncovered, for about 2 minutes, or until salmon is cooked through and flakes with a fork. If sauce starts thickening too much, reduce heat to low.

5. To serve, place salmon on plates and spoon some of the sauce on top. Garnish with chopped green onions and/or sesame seeds.

Serves 4

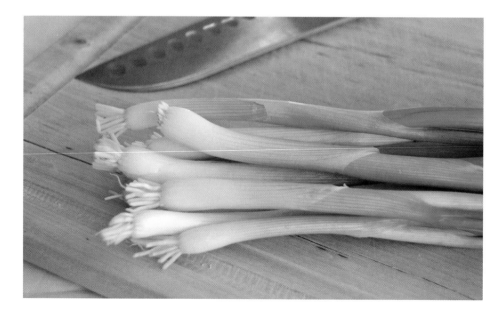

Entrées

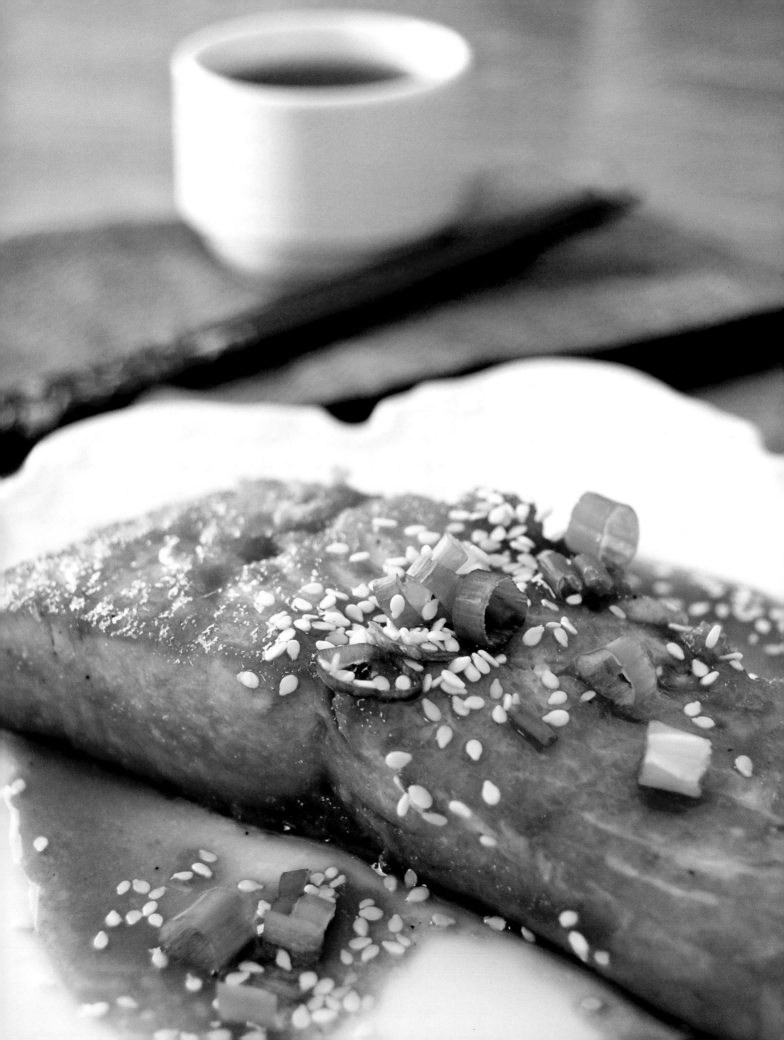

Filet O' GF Fish Sandwiches

Fish is a great, healthy protein source and should be on the menu a few times a week. However, tell my kids this and I can guarantee a revolt. They aren't big fish fans, unless of course I cut it into small pieces, drown it in ketchup, and call them "fish sticks." My solution is to get creative when cooking fish to get the whole family on board. One of our favorite recipes is this fun and incredibly tasty sandwich. With just a minimal crust on the fish you can feel good about serving this to your family knowing they are getting the good stuff, without the deep-fried, processed mess that comes with traditional boxed fish sticks. Crispy, cool slaw. Creamy, tangy tartar sauce. Crispy, flavorful fish. You won't "flounder" with this recipe. You should try it, just for the "halibut." OK, I'm done now.

Breading:

½	C (60 g) brown rice flour
2	Tbsp potato starch
1	tsp granulated garlic
1 ½	tsp granulated onion
1	tsp sea salt
~	Freshly ground pepper

Tartar Sauce:

½	C (120 mL) GF DF Mayo (Spectrum vegan mayo works well)
1	Tbsp sweet pickle relish
2	tsp grated yellow onion
~	Squeeze of lemon juice
~	Sea salt and freshly ground pepper to taste

Fish:

1	Tbsp oil (for cooking fish)
4	pieces halibut (or other firm white fish)

Slaw:

~	Recipe p. 204

Bun:

~	Your choice, but the English Muffins on p. 88 work great!

1. Mix breading ingredients together in a shallow dish.
2. Mix tartar sauce ingredients together in a small bowl. Set aside.
3. Heat oil in a large nonstick skillet over medium-high heat.
4. Wash fish and without patting dry, press into breading mixture, covering both sides of fish. Repeat for all pieces.
5. Place fish in hot pan and cook until browned on both sides and cooked through.
6. To serve, toast English muffins (or rolls) lightly. Spread a spoonful of tartar sauce on bottom bun, place cooked fish on top, then spoon a generous helping of slaw on top of the fish.

Serves 4

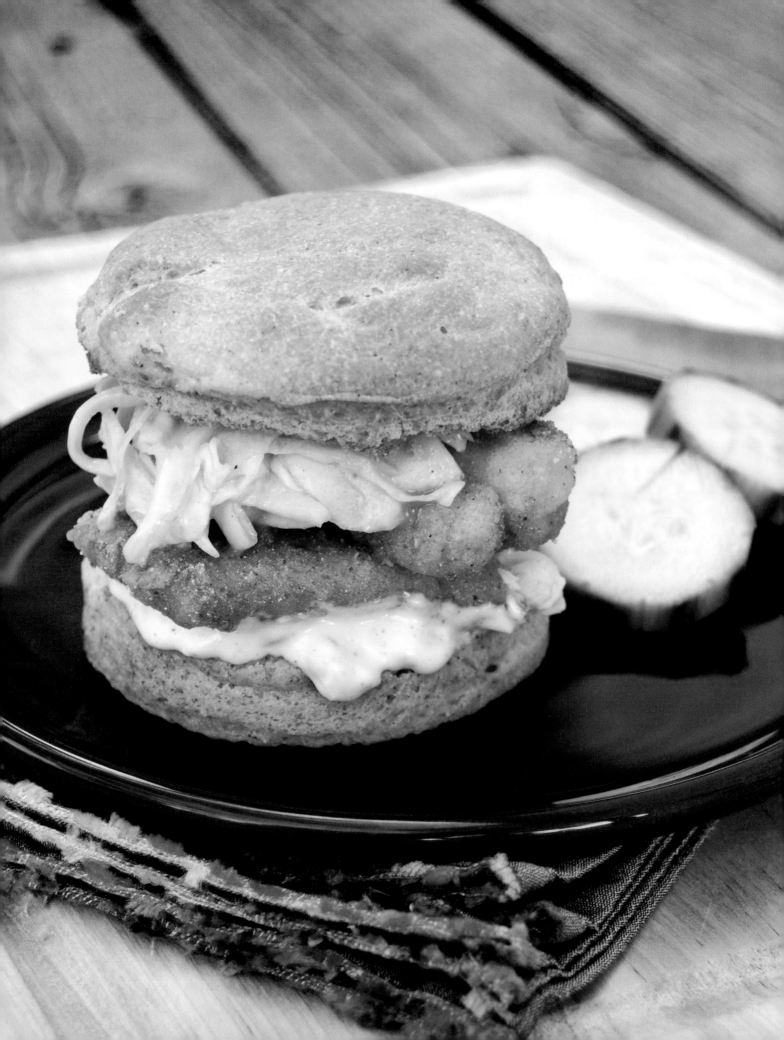

Bay Shrimp Veggie Salad

Here's another versatile dish that packs a nutritional punch! Loaded with healthy veggies and wild shrimp, this easy and light salad is great on picnics or at your next potluck. It's great as a light summer meal, or leave out the shrimp and add GF pasta for a filling side dish. Let your creative side shine with this recipe and see how many ways you can serve it up!

For the Salad:

2	C (300 g) wild bay shrimp, rinsed and drained
1	C (150 g) diced organic cucumber
1	C (150 g) diced organic celery
½	C (75 g) finely chopped organic red onion
1	C (150 g) diced organic radishes
1	C (150 g) diced organic Roma tomatoes
1	C (150 g) sliced black olives
¼	tsp granulated garlic
~	Freshly ground pepper to taste

For the Dressing:

4	Tbsp olive oil
4	Tbsp raw apple cider vinegar
1	small shallot, finely chopped
1	tsp Dijon mustard
1	tsp Italian seasoning
1	tsp granulated onion
½	tsp sea salt
~	Freshly ground pepper

1. In a large bowl, gently combine all salad ingredients. Set Aside.
2. In a jar with a tight-fitting lid, combine all dressing ingredients. Shake well. Drizzle over salad, toss to combine. Serve immediately or refrigerate until ready to serve.

Options:

~Eliminate shrimp and add cooked GF spiral brown rice pasta for a great summer side dish.

~Use diced chicken instead of shrimp.

~Try adding other veggies you love such as chopped broccoli or carrots!

Serves 4–6

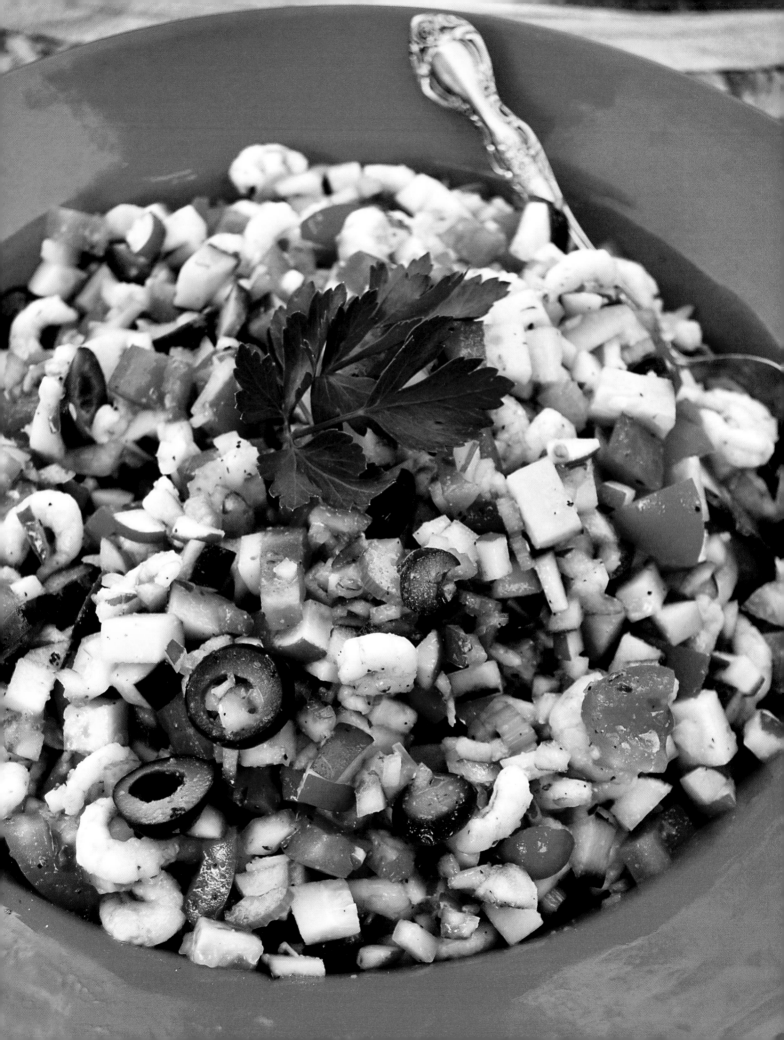

Baked Lemon Caper Salmon

I really like salmon fairly simply prepared, which is probably why I like this version so much. The lemon gives it a wonderful lift while the capers provide that tiny bite that really works well with the salmon.

4	wild salmon fillets
~	Sea salt
~	Freshly ground pepper
1	garlic clove, minced
2	tsp chopped fresh rosemary leaves
2	Tbsp lemon juice
1	Tbsp capers
2	organic lemons, sliced

1. Season salmon with salt and pepper. Place fillets in a greased 9" by 13" baking dish.
2. Sprinkle salmon with minced garlic, chopped rosemary, lemon juice, and capers. Place sliced lemons across each fillet.
3. Bake in a 375° oven for 10–15 minutes.

Serves 4

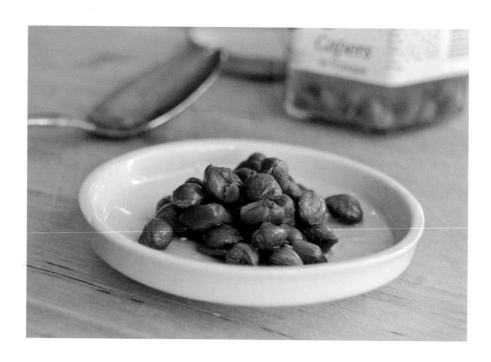

Entrées

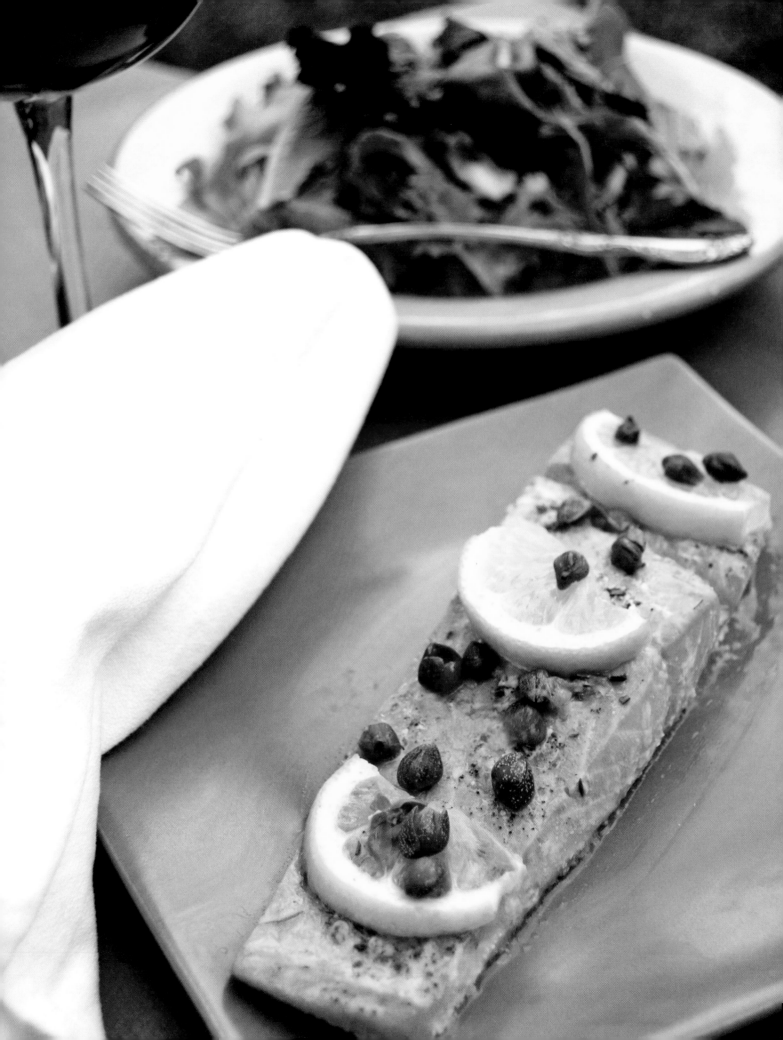

Batter Mix

This is one of those recipes that I feel a little bad about creating. Let's face it, fried foods, gluten-free or not, are not healthy options. But then I realized that there is the rare occasion that my kids and The Maniac want a crispy onion ring, or fish and chips, and we would never be able to have something out at a restaurant that was tasty and safe. That's when I realized that part of our overall health included reduced stress and peace of mind from not always relying on food establishments for a special occasion treat and by indulging in a past favorite food every once in awhile. So I created this recipe so we could have a "night out" in our own home, where we knew all of the ingredients were organic, high quality, fresh, and most of all, safe for all of us to consume. I've had many customers love this batter so much that they deep fry everything for weeks, which isn't the intent of this mix. I highly advise only eating fried foods occasionally, but enjoy every bite when you do, and enjoy the people you are with while you indulge. Then lose the guilt and move on. Life is meant for special occasions and food helps us celebrate those moments. It's OK, so enjoy! But not every day.

Chicken strips, fish fillets, onion rings, veggies, whatever you like! Makes enough batter to coat fish and onion rings for 5 or 6 people.

Dry Ingredients:

1	C (120 g) potato starch
¾	C (90 g) sorghum flour
1	tsp sea salt
1	tsp baking powder
½	tsp baking soda
¼	tsp xanthan gum
¼	tsp pepper
½	tsp paprika
1	tsp onion powder
⅛	tsp turmeric

Wet Ingredients:

1¼	C (300 mL) nondairy milk (see options below)

1. Add milk to dry mix. Whisk until smooth.
2. Let sit for 5 minutes to thicken.
3. Heat oil in nonstick skillet to 350°. Use enough oil so that it comes up the chicken/fish almost halfway.
4. Add chicken, fish, or onion rings to batter, coat completely, and add to hot oil.
5. Cook until golden brown on both sides and filling is cooked completely. Drain on a wire rack, sprinkle with salt to taste, and enjoy!

Options:

~Replace milk with gluten-free beer for delicious beer-battered onion rings or fish fillets!

~If you don't want to use that much milk, feel free to use ½ milk and ½ water.

~To make coconut shrimp, add unsweetened, finely-shredded coconut to the batter before dipping shrimp.

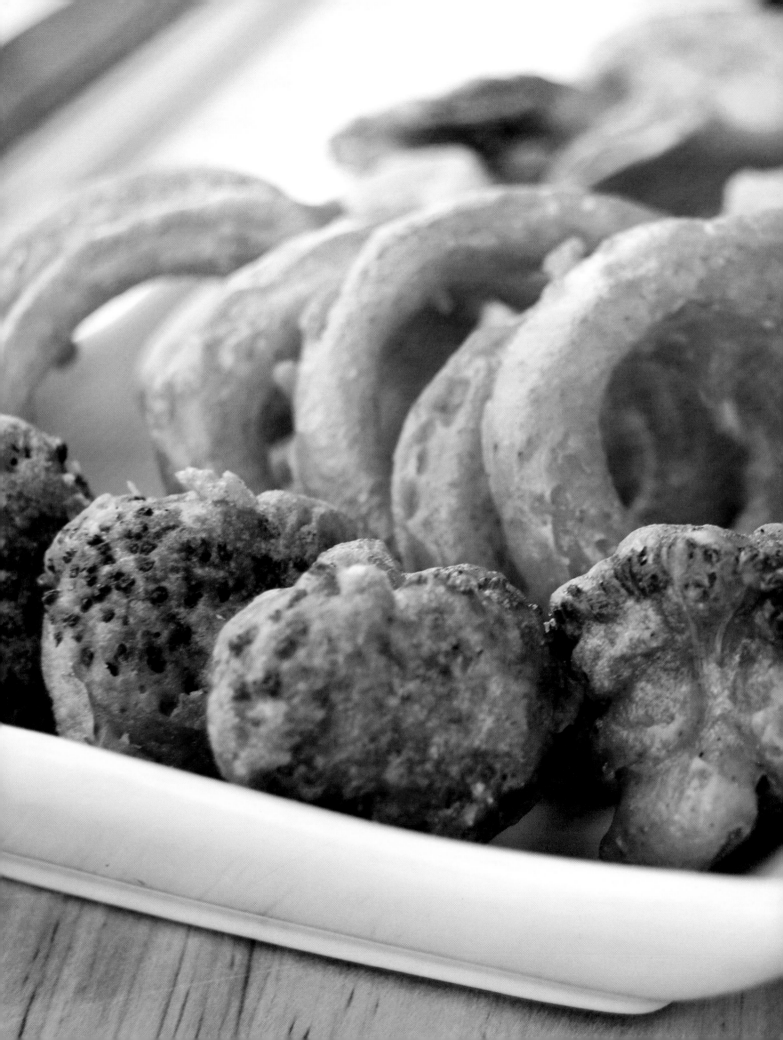

Corn Dogs

If you're looking for a more traditional corn dog, here you go! These dogs come out just like you remember, but without any nasty gluten or nitrites. And while they are fried, on occasion, it's OK to treat yourself to an old favorite. Again, sometimes maintaining health and happiness is not having to stress about eating a food that could be cross-contaminated at a restaurant. So enjoy these once in awhile in the safety of your home, and enjoy the memories!

1	C (120 g) Celiac Maniac Batter Mix (p. 188)
½	C (80 g) organic GF corn meal
½-1	C (120–240 mL) nondairy milk, or water
1	pkg grass-fed hot dogs, cut in half (Applegate Farms)
~	Coconut Oil for cooking

1. Mix batter mix, corn meal, and just enough milk together in a medium bowl until smooth and well blended, but very thick.
2. Pat hot dogs dry with a paper towel.
3. Heat a nonstick electric skillet to 345° and add enough oil to the pan so it comes halfway up the side of the hot dogs.
4. Place hot dogs in batter and turn to coat. Add batter-coated dogs to hot oil and cook until golden brown. Flip and cook until golden brown.
5. Remove from oil and let drain on paper towels placed over a wire cooling rack.

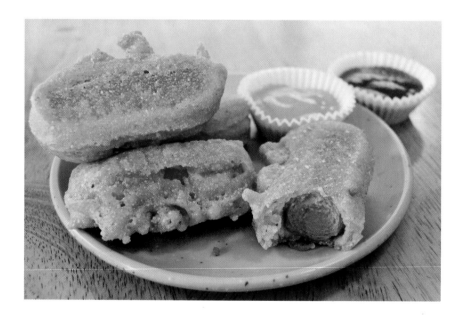

Serves 4

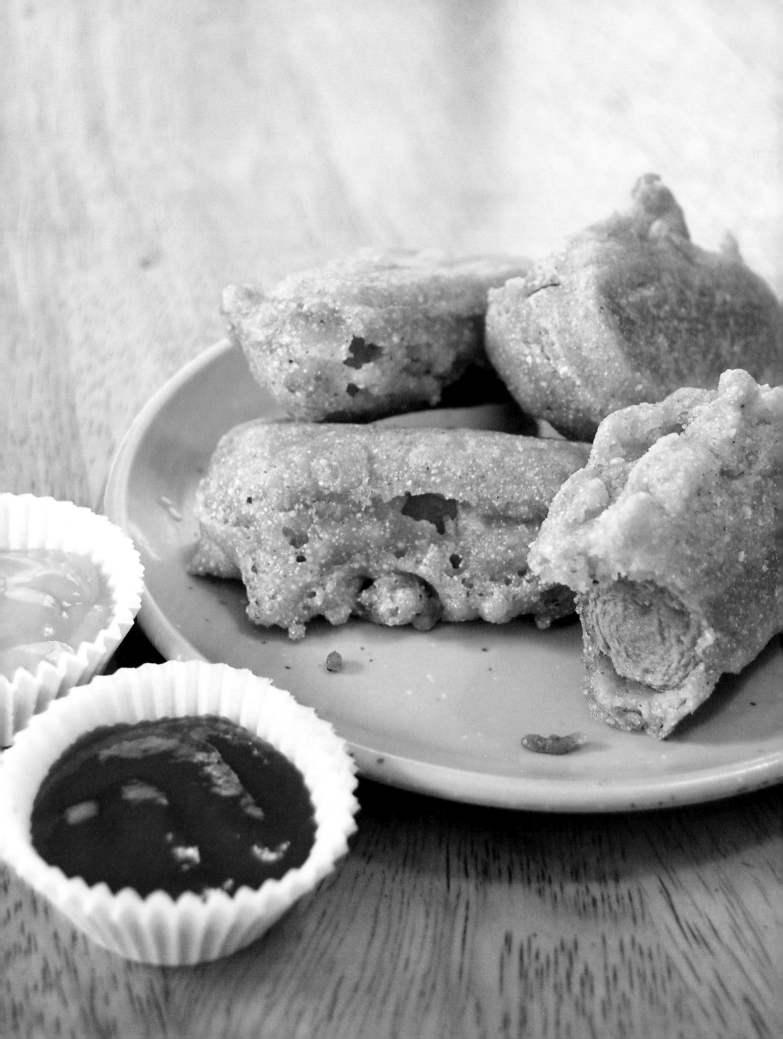

Pizza Crust

Once upon a time there was a guy who was diagnosed with a gluten issue and had a panic attack at the thought of never having pizza again. So he went to the store to find a GF pizza crust, only to start panicking again because each crust was worse than the next! Then one day his beautiful, loving and kind wife (aka: me) created The Celiac Maniac pizza crust (cue angels singing). And after just one blissful bite, they lived Happily Ever After! While the story is semi-accurate, the pizza crust lives up to the legend. This crust is crispy on the outside but tender and really bread-like chewy in the middle. This crust will leave you feeling like you've eaten the real thing. And one of my favorite things about this recipe is that I can make a whole bunch and freeze them for when I need them. They bake up just as perfectly from frozen as they do fresh! Need another reason to love this recipe? How about versatility! I've used it to make cinnamon rolls, bread sticks, and focaccia (see options below). But please, don't take my word for it. Try this crust for yourself and you too can live happily ever after!

For the Yeast:

1	Tbsp raw organic honey
1½	C (350 mL) warm water
1	Tbsp active dry yeast

Dry Ingredients:

½	C (60 g) amaranth flour
½	C (60 g) sorghum flour
1½	C (180 g) potato starch
1	C (120 g) tapioca starch
1½	tsp sea salt
1	rounded Tbsp xanthan gum

Wet Ingredients:

2	Tbsp olive oil
1	Tbsp raw apple cider vinegar
~	Organic palm shortening for greasing the pizza pan
~	Brown rice flour for dusting the pan and dough

1. In a small bowl, stir honey into warm water. Add yeast and stir gently. Set aside for 5 minutes to start foaming (this way you know it's working!).
2. In a stand mixer bowl combine dry ingredients. Add olive oil, vinegar, and yeast mixture.
3. Blend on low until a soft ball forms. Dough will be very soft.
4. Grease two 12-inch pizza pans with shortening. Place half of the dough on each pan.
5. Liberally dust dough with rice flour. With quick pats, press the dough into the pan, flattening into a circle. Continue to dust dough as needed to prevent sticking. But don't go too crazy—you don't want the dough to become grainy.
6. Preheat oven to 425°. Bake crusts for 12–15 minutes, until it begins to brown on the bottom, rotating trays halfway through.
7. Remove from oven and top with your favorite sauce and toppings. Place back in the oven, turn heat up to 450°, and bake for about 15 minutes (rotate again part way through), until sauce is bubbly and edges are browned. If desired, brush olive oil on edges of crust for flavor and to soften a bit.
8. Cool slightly, cut into slices, and enjoy!

Options:

~After baking crust initially, place on cooling rack to cool completely. Wrap each in plastic wrap and place in a freezer zip-top bag. Freeze until needed. To use, simply thaw crust on the counter and proceed with step 7 above.

~For focaccia bread: When pressing dough in step 5 above, leave dough a little bit thicker. Bake in step 6. Remove from oven, brush generously with olive oil. Top with favorite seasonings such as Italian herbs, garlic, and sun dried tomatoes. Bake in a 425° oven for about 10 minutes until hot and browned slightly on the edges.

Makes 2 crusts

Entrées

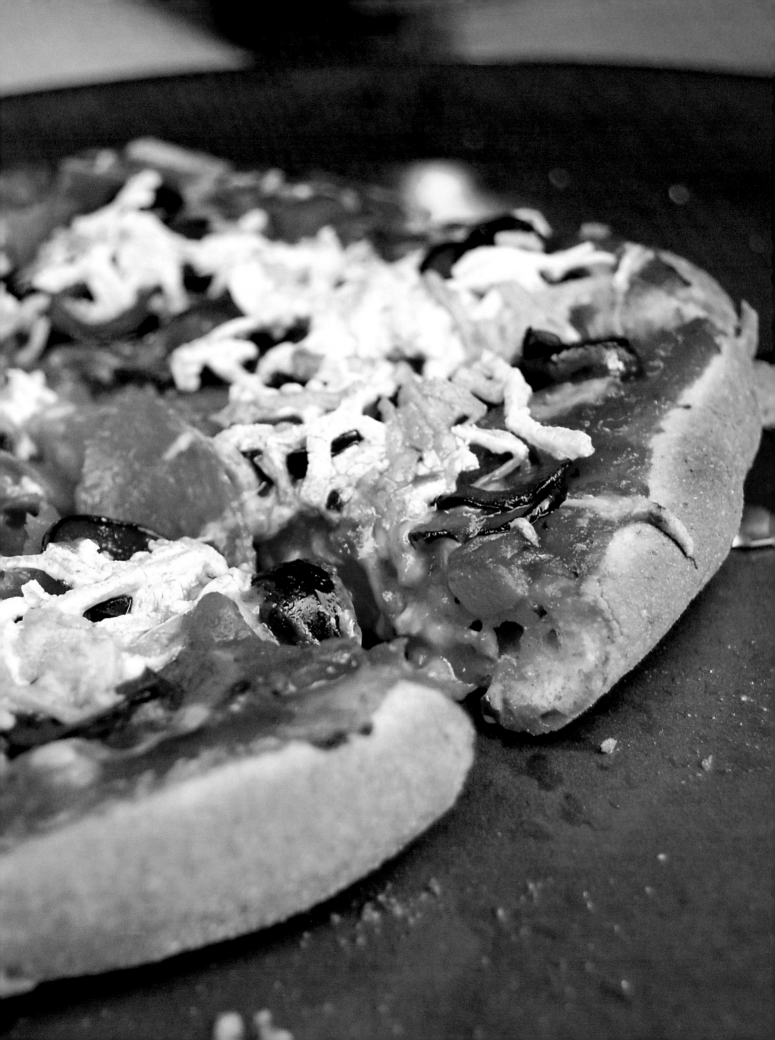

Corn Dog Cupcakes

This is such a fun one for the kiddos! A few ingredients and you've got yourself a great party snack, school lunch, or Family Fun Night Dinner. Homemade baked corndogs on a stick tend to be labor intensive and messy and never come out looking too good. But throw them in a cupcake liner and not only is it adorable, they are incredibly easy to make and eat. And the kids can help with this one! Let them use kid scissors to cut the hot dog into bite-size pieces and then push them into the filled liners.

~ **Cornbread batter (recipe p. 218)**
1 **pkg uncured hot dogs, such as Applegate Farms, sliced into bite-size pieces**

1. Make Cornbread batter according to directions.
2. Line a 12-cup muffin pan with paper liners. Spray liners lightly with nonstick spray.
3. Scoop cornbread batter into each cup, filling about ²/₃ full.
4. Place hot dog slices into each muffin cup, pushing into the batter, until each is evenly spaced with hot dog pieces.
5. Bake in a 350° oven for about 30 minutes, or until tops are browned and a toothpick inserted in the center comes out clean.

Makes 12

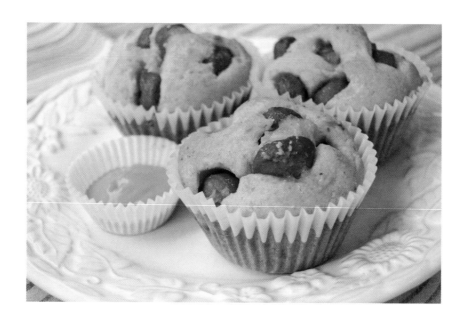

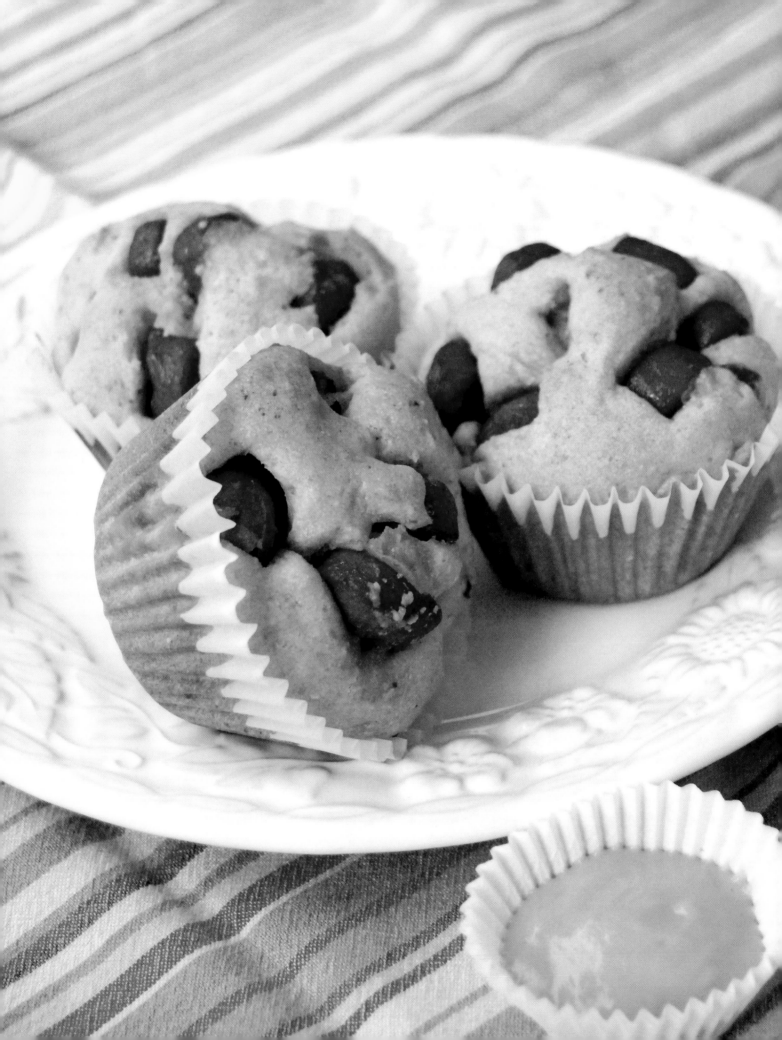

Black Bean Tostadas

The best thing about this tostada, other than the great flavors, is that it doesn't weigh us down like many Mexican dishes do with their heavy sauces and cheeses. It's light and flavorful, without any one overpowering spice. And while this meal is great as is, I find that we usually add shredded chicken or taco meat to this tostada to up the protein. As a matter of fact, this is a great meal to help use up just about any leftover meat you have on hand!

Shells:

4	organic GF corn tortillas
2	Tbsp coconut oil, divided

Filling:

1	small jalapeño, seeds and ribs removed, finely chopped
3	garlic cloves, minced
2	(15 oz) cans (about 900 g) organic black beans, rinsed and drained
½	C (120 mL) organic chicken broth
~	Sea salt
~	Freshly ground pepper

Topping:

3	C (125 g) shredded lettuce
2	organic Roma tomatoes, diced
1	tsp lime juice
~	Sea salt
~	Pepper

Add ons:

1	large Haas avocado, sliced
~	Nondairy cheese (Daiya)
~	Chopped fresh cilantro

1. Preheat oven to 400°. Brush corn tortillas with 1 Tbsp coconut oil on both sides. Place on a baking sheet (or 2) in single layers. Bake about 7 minutes, or until lightly browned and crisp. Set aside.
2. Heat 1 Tbsp coconut oil in a large skillet over medium heat. Add jalapeño and garlic. Sauté 1 minute.
3. Add beans to the pan and cook, stirring occasionally, until heated through, about 3 minutes.
4. Add broth, sea salt, and pepper to the beans. Stir. With a potato masher, smash up the beans until most are crushed but mixture is still chunky. Cover and set aside.
5. Meanwhile, in a large bowl toss lettuce with tomatoes, lime juice, sea salt, and pepper.
6. To serve, smear beans on each tortilla top with salad mixture and then garnish each with sliced avocado, cheese, and cilantro.

Option:

~Heat up leftover shredded chicken and add on top of the beans before topping with lettuce.

Entrées

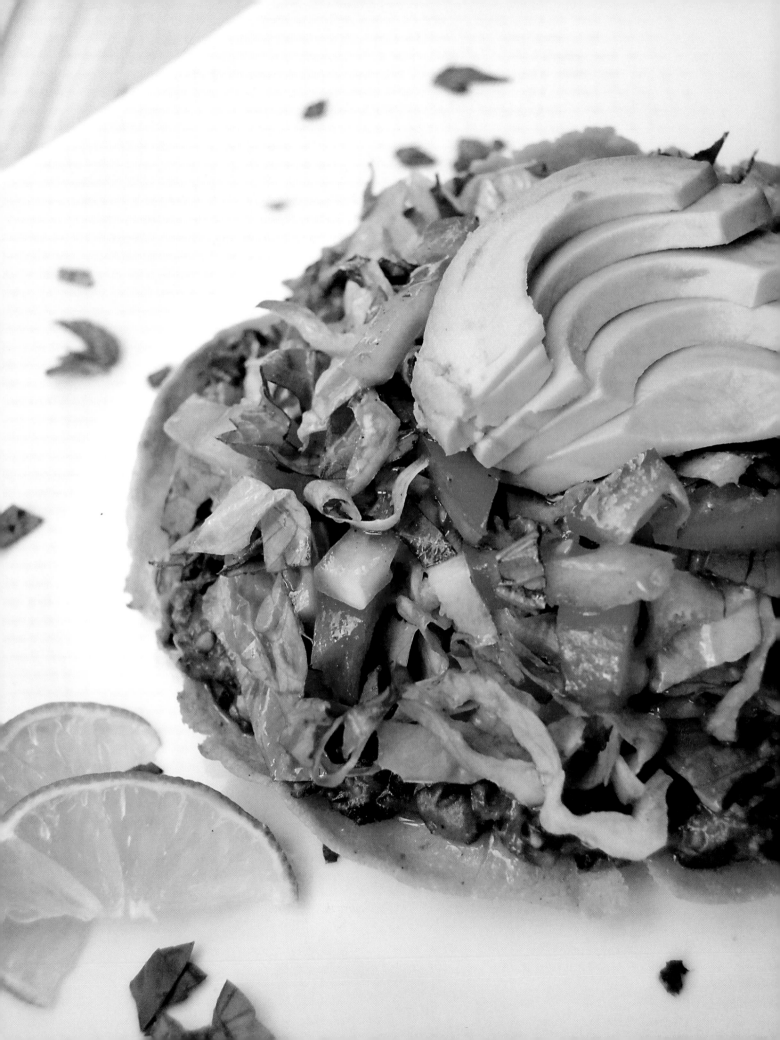

Butternut Squash Soup

As soon as the evenings turn cool and the first hint of color hits the leaves, I visit the farmers market for some butternut squash. It is such a mild but decadent squash that we make it a multitude of ways all winter long. But this soup is by far my favorite use of this gorgeous veggie. It's creamy without dairy, it's filling, and is incredibly healthy. Full of vitamin A and antioxidants, this soup will warm your tummy on a cool, crisp evening and help ward off those early season colds!

2	Tbsp olive oil (or coconut oil)
5	C (750 g) cubed peeled organic butternut squash
2	C (½ inch) cubed peeled organic russet potato (about 12 oz or 340 g)
1	tsp sea salt
½	tsp freshly ground black pepper
2	cups (300 g) sliced organic leek (about 2 medium)
4–6	cups (950–1,425 mL) homemade chicken or vegetable broth
½	C (120 mL) lite canned coconut milk

Garnish:

~ Chopped green onions

~ Toasted Pumpkin Seeds (see recipe p. 376)

1. Heat oil over medium-high heat. Add squash, potato, salt, pepper, and leek to pot. Sauté 5 minutes, stirring occasionally.
2. Stir in broth (enough to cover the potatoes and squash) and bring to a boil. Reduce heat and simmer about 20 minutes or until potato is tender, stirring occasionally.
3. With a hand immersion blender (or in your blender), blend until smooth.
4. Stir in coconut milk.
5. Spoon into bowls and garnish with chopped green onions and toasted pumpkin seeds. Sit back and enjoy this wonderful taste of fall!

Serves 6

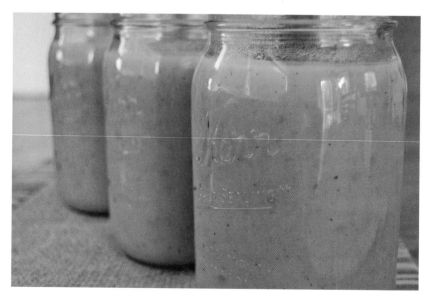

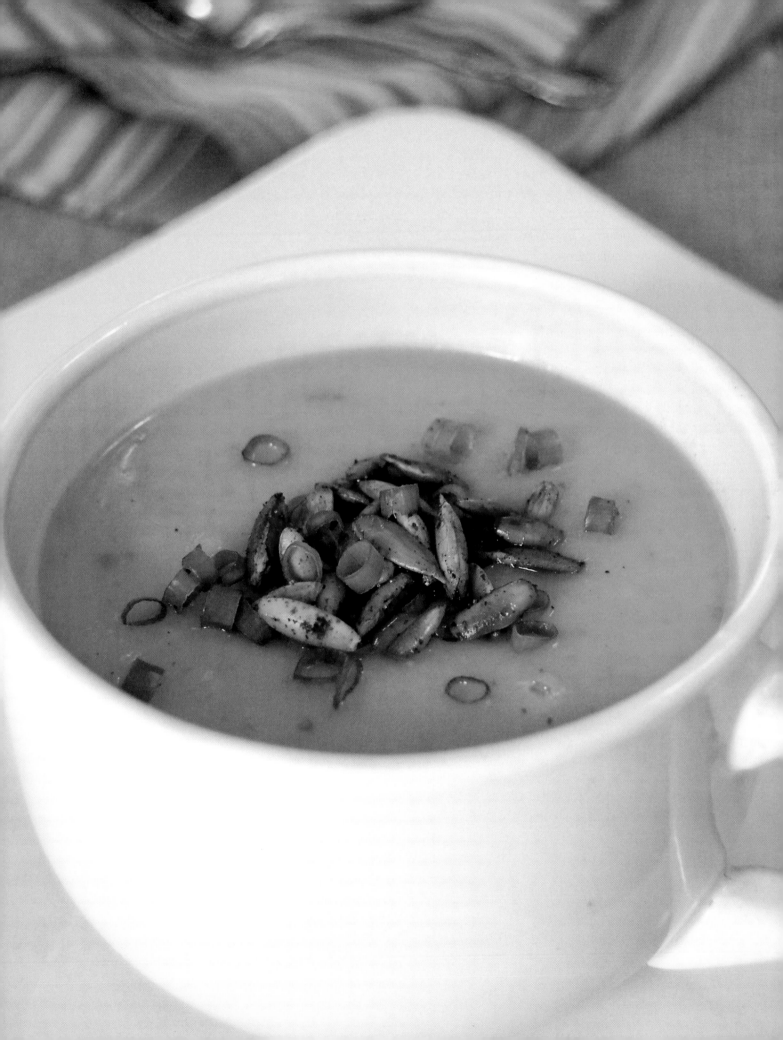

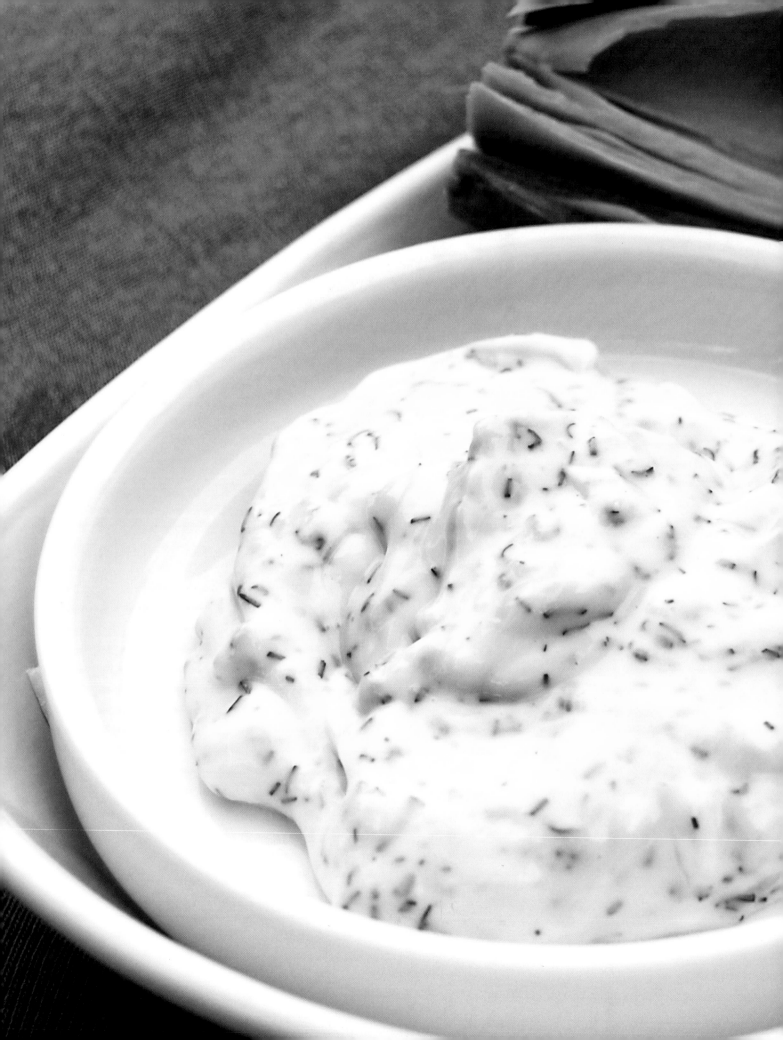

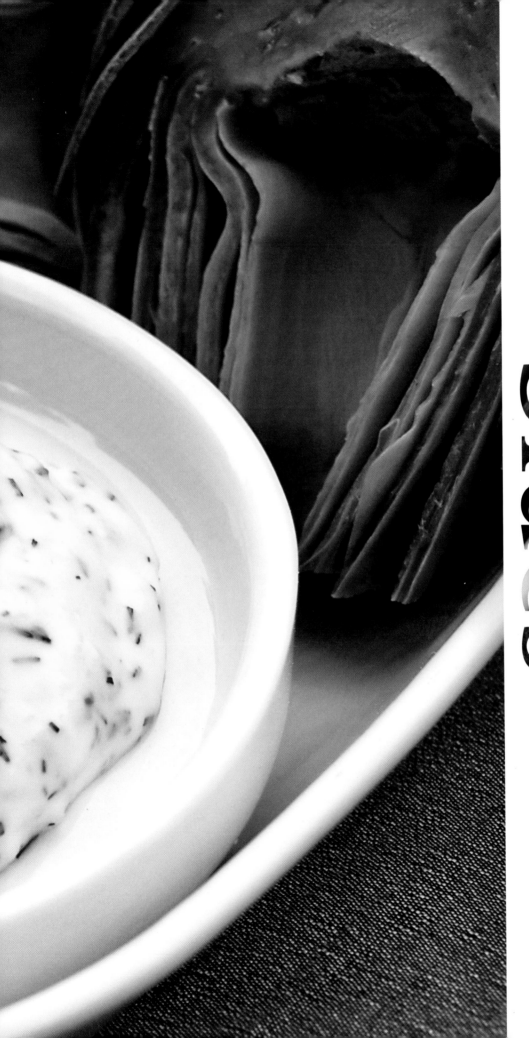

Sides

Cherry Tomato Salad

I love, love, love this refreshing and light tomato salad! A small ingredient list and three simple steps make this summer side even more appealing. Perfect with a grilled steak or chicken, this delicious and nutritious salad really tops off a summer meal nicely. Bring it to your next picnic or potluck, and feel free to tell everyone how you slaved over it in the kitchen!

Dressing:

2	Tbsp red wine vinegar
1	Tbsp olive oil
½	tsp coarse sea salt
~	Freshly ground pepper to taste

Salad:

2	pints (900 g) organic cherry tomatoes, halved
¼	C (40 g) organic red onion, finely chopped
2	Tbsp parsley, finely chopped

1. Whisk dressing ingredients in a bowl. Set aside.
2. Add salad ingredients to a medium bowl.
3. Pour dressing over tomato mixture and toss to combine. Even better after it sits in the fridge a few hours because the flavors develop!

Serves 4

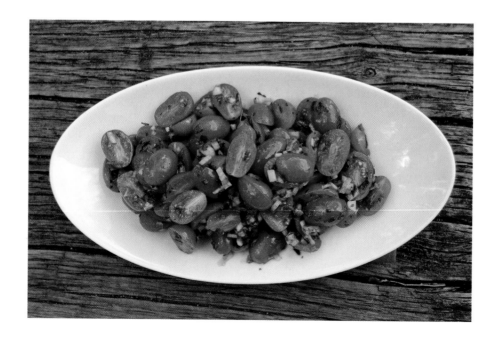

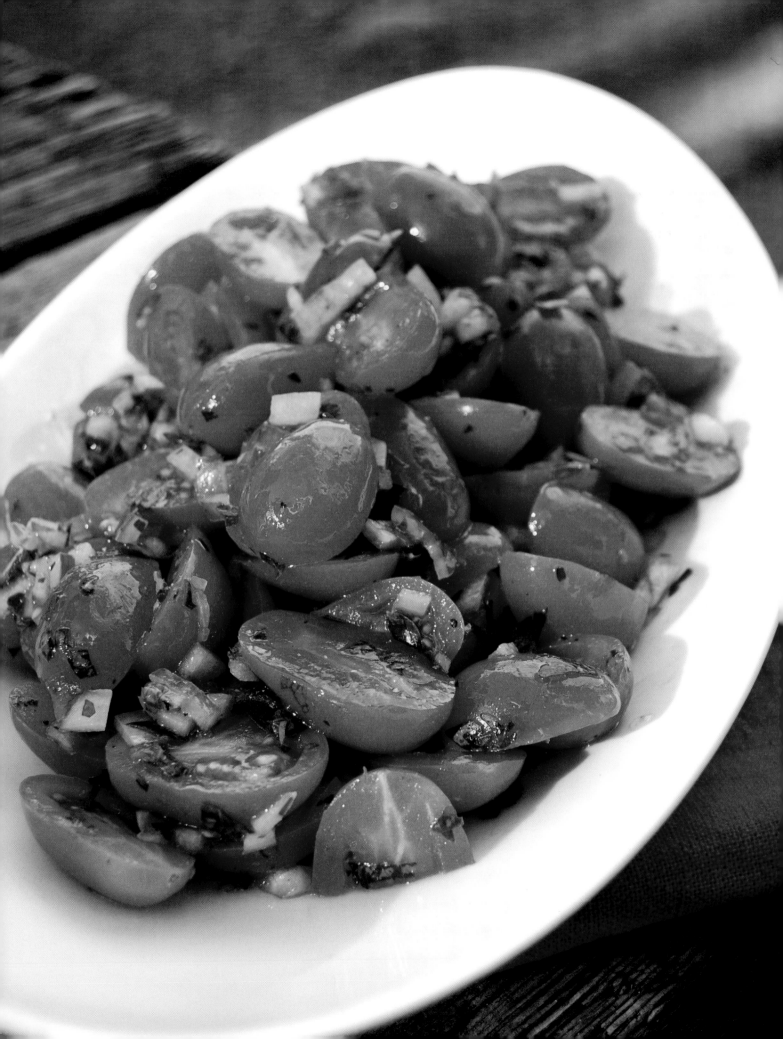

Simple Slaw

I was never a fan of coleslaw when I was a kid, mostly because no matter who made it, it was always drowning in a heavy mayonnaise dressing. No thanks. So when I really wanted a simple coleslaw recipe I could throw together at a moment's notice, that didn't call for an entire jar of mayo, I went to work. And finally, success! This very simple recipe came together nicely, delivering a tasty, light, slightly tangy and a little bit creamy slaw that every member of the family will like. I serve this as a summer side, or even on Pork Tacos (p. 174) with an extra squeeze of lime. Feel free to improvise with this one too. Add shredded carrots, shredded purple cabbage, some diced shallot, chopped broccoli, whatever you'd like!

~	Juice of 1 organic lime
2	tsp raw apple cider vinegar
2-3	Tbsp olive oil
3	Tbsp GF vegan mayo (Spectrum brand works well)
1	Tbsp raw organic honey
~	Sea salt and freshly ground pepper to taste
1	large package shredded organic cabbage

1. In a jar with a tight-fitting lid, combine lime juice, vinegar, oil, mayo, honey, salt, and pepper. Shake well to combine.
2. Place cabbage in a large bowl. Pour sauce over cabbage and toss to combine.
3. Refrigerate until ready to serve.

Serves 4

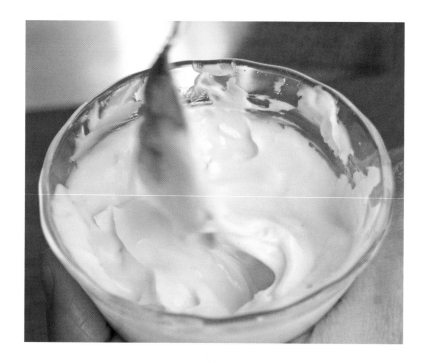

Sides

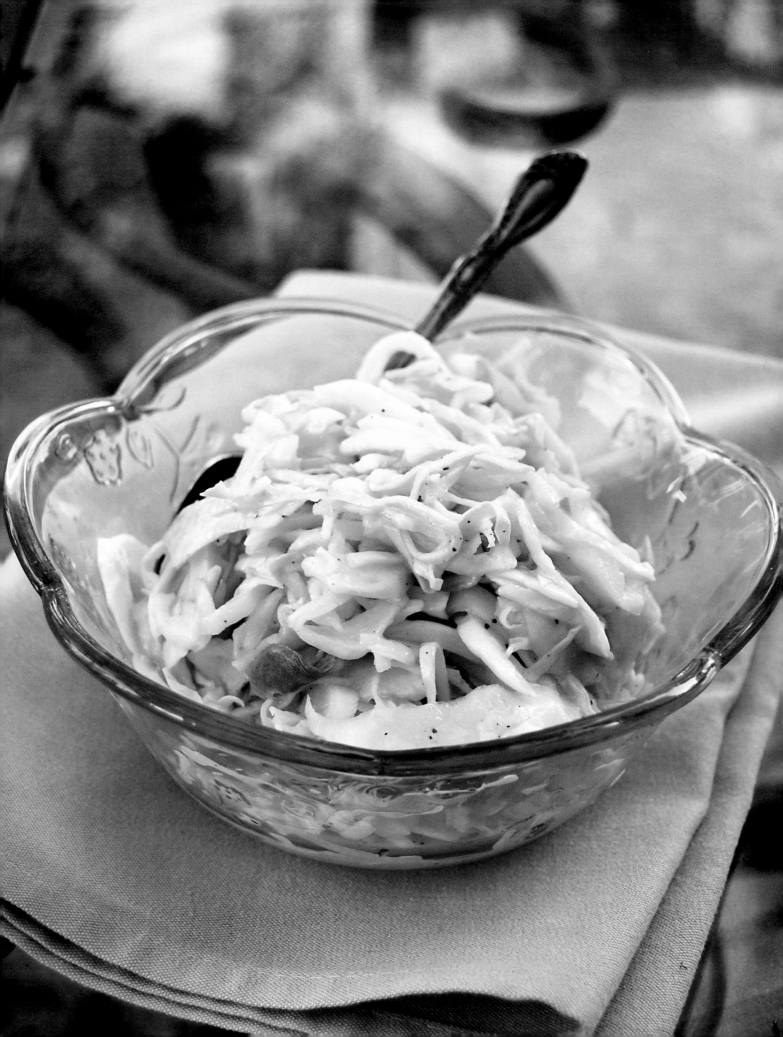

Fried Rice

Delicious, uses leftovers, fast, easy, and makes a great school lunch in the ol' thermos. Do I need to say more?

2	Tbsp coconut oil
1	C cooked brown rice (or white rice)—best if cooked the day before and stored in the fridge. Freshly cooked rice is very sticky and doesn't turn out as well.
½–¾	C (110 g) chopped cooked ham, bacon, chicken, pork or shrimp
2	green onions, chopped
¾	C (110 g) frozen organic peas (or peas and carrot blend), thawed
1–2	Tbsp GF tamari soy sauce or Bragg liquid aminos (or coconut aminos)
~	Toasted sesame seeds for topping

1. Heat oil in a large skillet over medium heat. Add rice and stir to coat with oil. Cook for 1–2 minutes to heat through.
2. Add your meat and most of the green onions, reserving some as a garnish. Stir.
3. Add peas. Stir and cook until peas are heated through, about 2 minutes.
4. Add tamari, a little at a time, until rice turns darker brown and is to your taste. Add more if desired, being careful not to add too much as it can get too salty very quickly.
5. To serve, place in a bowl and top with sesame seeds and remaining green onions.

Serves 4

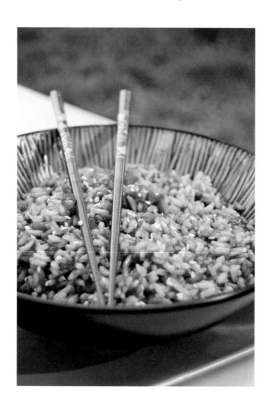

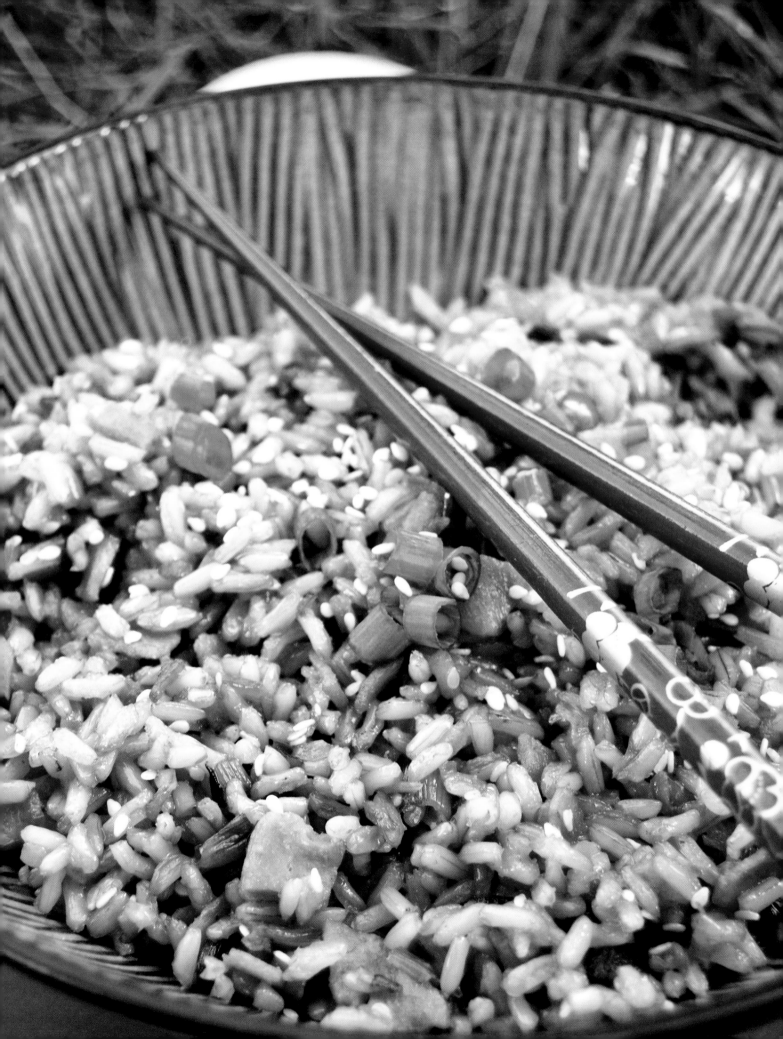

Zucchini Boats

All credit for this quick side dish goes to my hubby! Bored with the same old same old one night, he got a little creative and made one delish zucchini that the kids devoured in seconds. Tip: if you make anything slightly different and a little funky, the kids will eat it up—literally.

4	**medium organic zucchini, washed, ends removed, sliced in half lengthwise**
4	**tsp nondairy butter**
~	**Sea salt**
~	**Freshly ground pepper**
~	**Granulated garlic**
~	**Italian seasoning**

1. With a teaspoon, scoop out the seeds from each zucchini halve, making sure to not take out too much flesh, and not breaking through the ends.
2. Place zucchini on a baking sheet. Place 1 tsp butter in each scooped-out zucchini. Sprinkle salt, pepper, garlic, and Italian seasoning on tops.
3. Bake in a 400° oven for 15 minutes, or until butter is melted and zucchini is tender.

Serves 4

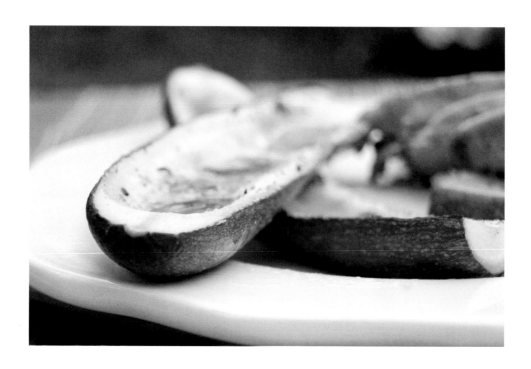

Sides

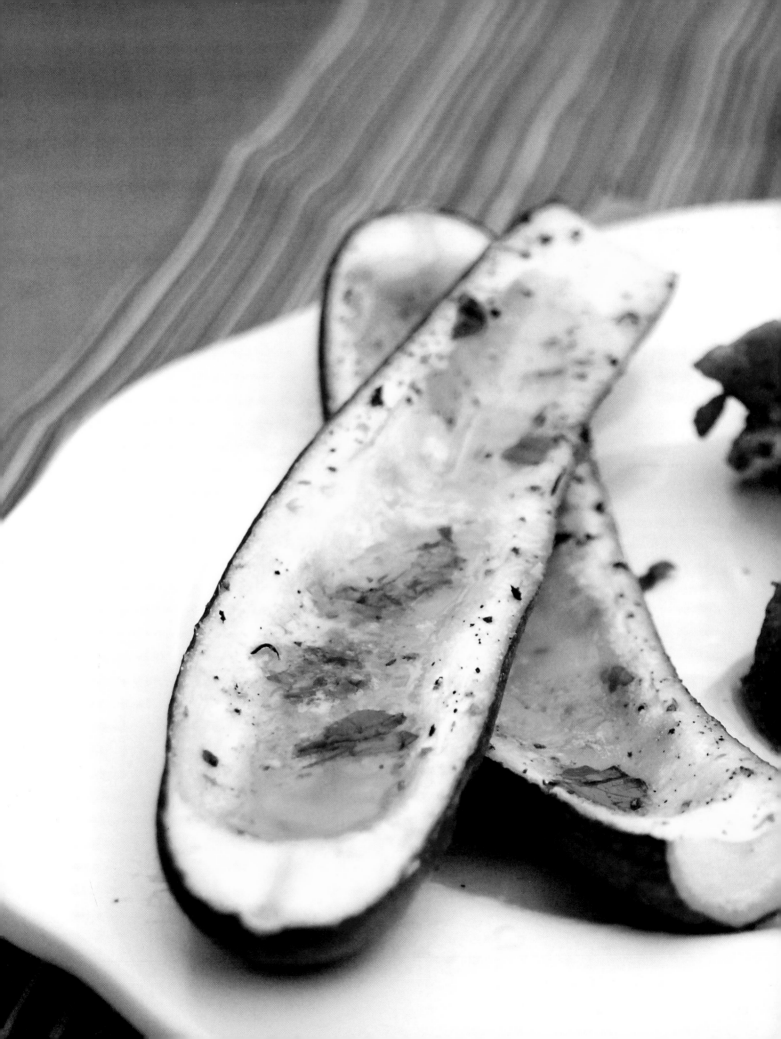

Sweet Potato Biscuits

Not a Thanksgiving goes by that we don't share these tender sweet potato biscuits at the table. Another old recipe with a successful conversion to gluten-free, and boy am I thankful it worked! The sweet potato keeps the biscuit moist while the shortening still gives it a flaky texture. Pure turkey day perfection paired with Honey Butter (p. 270).

Dry Ingredients:

1	C (120 g) sorghum flour
½	C (60 g) teff flour
¾	C (90 g) potato starch
¾	C (90 g) tapioca starch
2	tsp xanthan gum
1½	tsp baking powder
½	tsp baking soda
1½	tsp sea salt

Wet Ingredients:

1	C (190 g) organic shortening (Spectrum), chilled
¼	C (60 mL) nondairy milk, chilled
2	Tbsp raw organic honey
2	C (300 g) cooked, mashed organic sweet potato (I actually use yams—I like the orange color)
¼	tsp pumpkin pie spice

Tops:

2	Tbsp melted coconut oil
~	Sea salt

1. In a medium bowl, whisk together dry ingredients.
2. With a pastry blender, cut in shortening until pea size crumbs form.
3. In a separate bowl stir together milk, honey, sweet potato, and pumpkin pie spice.
4. Add sweet potato mixture to the dry ingredients and mix until a dough ball forms. Don't over mix! You want those pieces of shortening to stay pieces and not become smashed into the dough.
5. Drop by spoonfuls onto a parchment-lined baking sheet, or scoop with an ice cream scoop and shape by hand into "biscuit" shapes.
6. Brush tops with melted coconut oil and sprinkle tops with sea salt.
7. Bake in a 375° oven for 17–20 minutes, or until tops and bottoms are browned and biscuits are cooked through.

Makes about 15

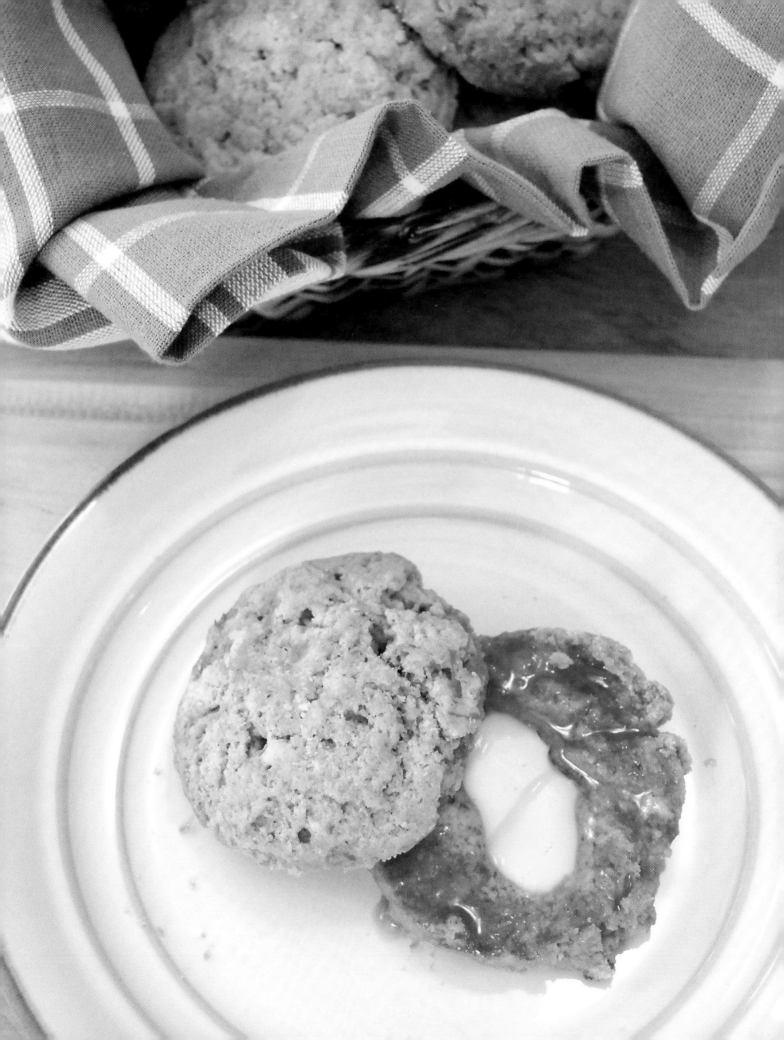

Garlicky Green Beans

The best part about these garlicky green beans is the dark, caramelized pieces that get a little more heat from the pan than the rest. Try to keep the pan fairly hot, without burning, to get as many of those beans as you can! They are delicious.

2	Tbsp coconut oil
3	big handfuls of frozen organic green beans (about 3 C or 450 g)
3	cloves garlic, minced
2	Tbsp coconut aminos (or Bragg liquid aminos or GF tamari soy sauce)
~	Freshly ground pepper

1. Heat oil in a large skillet over medium heat. Add green beans, stirring to coat in oil.
2. Let beans cook for about 10 minutes, stirring occasionally.
3. Add minced garlic, aminos, and pepper. Stir.
4. Cook an additional 5 minutes or until beans have browned slightly and are tender.

Serves 4

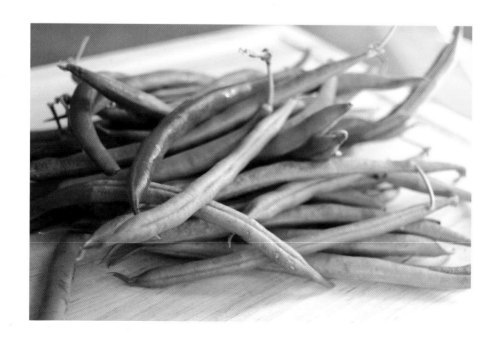

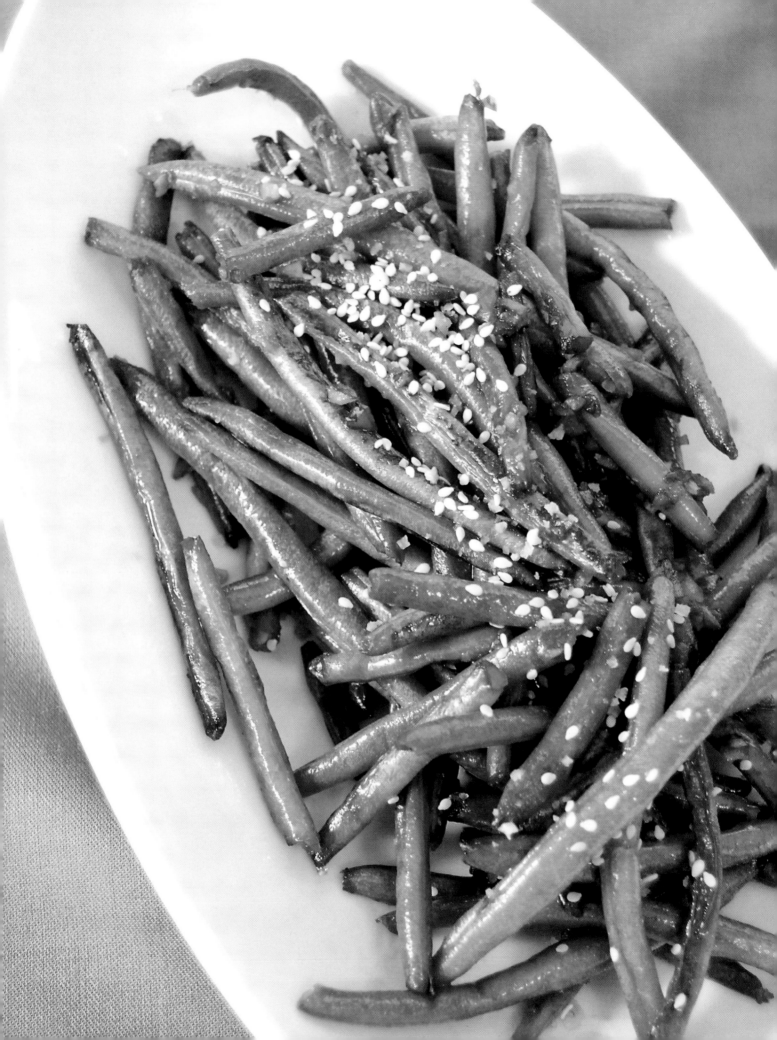

Roasted Cauliflower

A really hot oven is the key for nicely caramelized cauliflower bottoms. And who doesn't love a good caramelized bottom? I love oven-roasting most vegetables because it really concentrates the flavors without turning them into mush. And if you ever get the chance to try any of the various colored cauliflowers out there, please do so, especially the orange-hued cheddar cauliflower. The flavor will knock your caramelized bottoms off!

1	head of organic cauliflower
¼	C (60 mL) coconut oil, melted
~	Sea salt
~	Freshly ground pepper

1. Rinse and break apart cauliflower. Cut larger crowns into smaller, bite-size pieces. Put cauliflower in a large bowl.
2. Pour oil over cauliflower. Add salt and pepper to taste. Mix well to coat all of the pieces with the oil.
3. Spread cauliflower evenly on a parchment-lined baking sheet.
4. Bake in a 450° oven for 20 minutes, or until cauliflower is tender and browned on the edges.

Option:

Try sprinkling granulated onion or garlic on cauliflower before baking for additional flavor. For a smoky kick, sprinkle on a touch a cumin and chili powder before baking. Cauliflower is neutral in flavor so you can use it as a blank canvas for flavor!

Serves 4

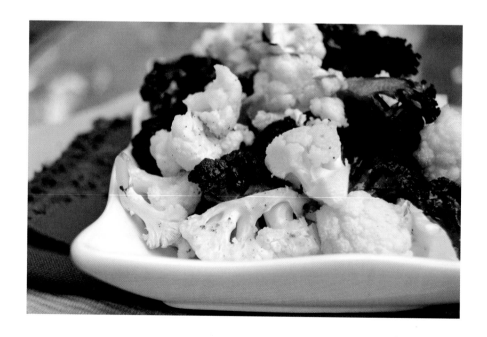

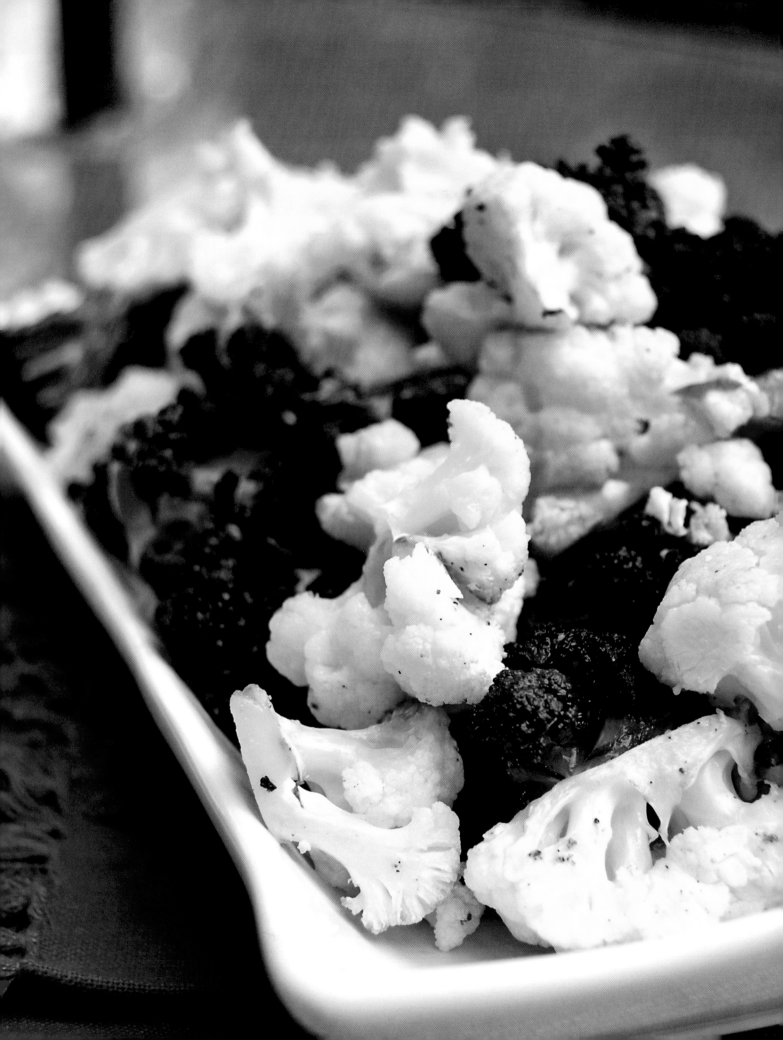

Artichokes with Garlic Dill Mayo

This garlic dill mayo gives you that something extra to turn simple steamed artichokes into an elegant side. Be sure to mince garlic finely with a knife and not through a garlic press, as it can be too strong that way.

4	large artichokes
~	Juice of 1 lemon
½	C (120 mL) vegan mayo (Spectrum)
1	garlic clove, minced
¾	tsp dried dill

1. Heat a large stock pot with water to boiling.
2. Wash and trim artichoke leaves. Cut off the top 1 inch or so of the artichokes.
3. Cut chokes in half, from top to bottom. Spoon out the "choke," or the fuzzy part.
4. Reserving 1 tsp lemon juice, drizzle remaining juice over cut artichokes to help prevent browning.
5. Place artichokes in boiling water and cook until fork tender at the base, about 20 minutes.
6. Meanwhile, in a small bowl, combine mayo, garlic, dill, and 1 tsp lemon juice. Refrigerate until ready to use.
7. To enjoy, dip leaves and artichoke heart in garlic dill mayo.

Serves 4

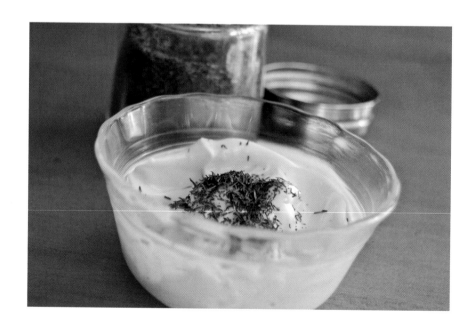

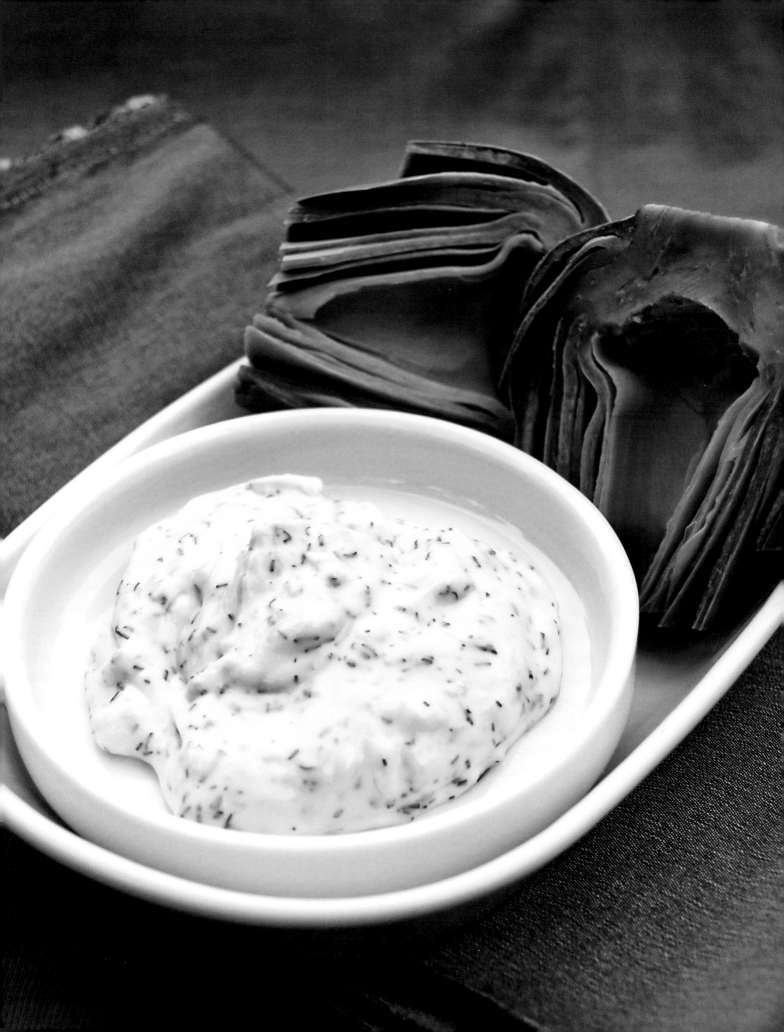

Cornbread

Perfectly golden with a hint of sweet, this cornbread goes well with easy beans (p. 238), or bake in large muffin tins, slice in half, and use as a bun for sloppy joes (p. 156).

Dry Ingredients:

1¼	C (200 g) organic cornmeal
½	C (60 g) brown rice flour
½	C (60 g) potato starch
¼	C (30 g) tapioca starch
1	tsp xanthan gum
3	tsp baking powder
1	tsp sea salt

Wet Ingredients:

⅓	C (80 mL) raw organic honey
1	C (240 mL) coconut milk (or nondairy milk of choice)
¼	C (60 mL) coconut oil, melted
½	C (120 mL) organic unsweetened applesauce
1	Tbsp flax meal mixed with 3 Tbsp hot water

1. Whisk together dry ingredients. Set aside.
2. In a stand mixer combine the wet ingredients until blended.
3. Slowly add in dry ingredients, until fully incorporated. Batter should be thick but thin enough to pour into the pan.
4. Bake in a large (10-inch) Lodge cast-iron skillet, or nonstick 10" by 10" baking pan.
5. Bake in a 350° oven for 15 minutes. Remove pan and brush top of cornbread with melted dairy-free butter or coconut oil. Return to oven and continue baking another 15–20 minutes or until top springs back to the touch and is golden brown.
6. If you are using a wedge pan or muffin pans, baking time will need to be reduced to about 20 minutes.

Serves 4-6

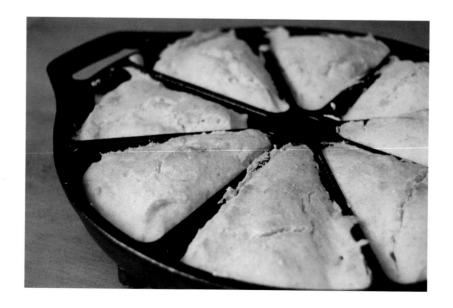

Sides

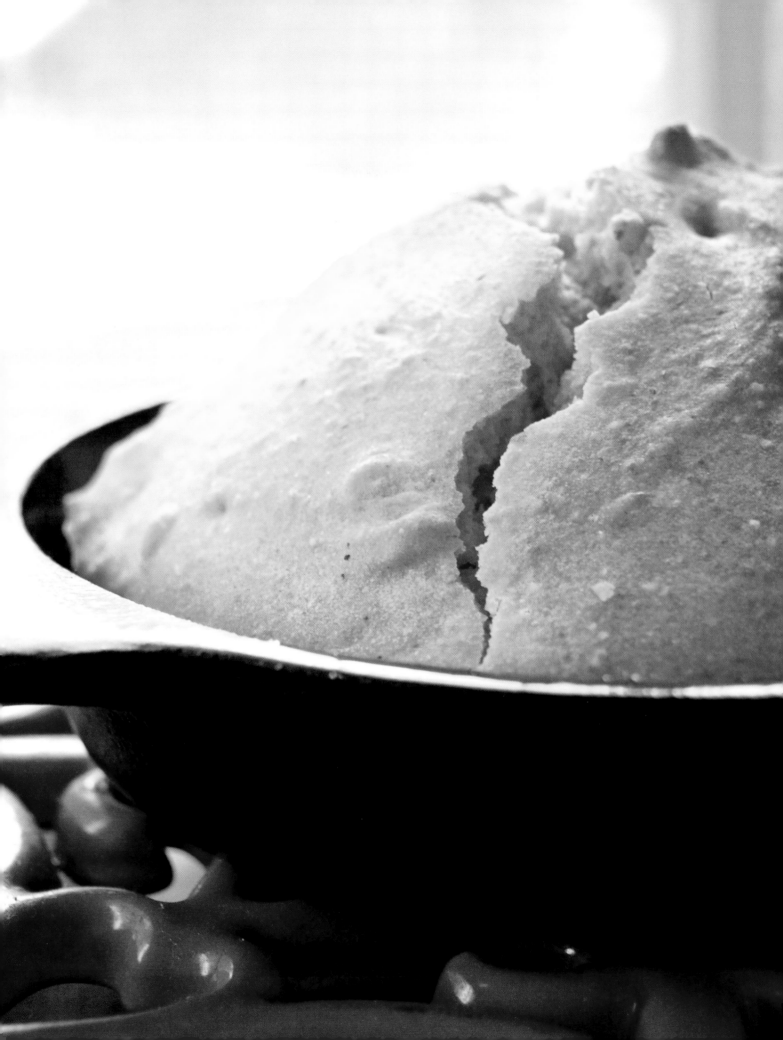

Pan-Roasted Brussels Sprouts

I can't believe how much I despised the Brussels sprout when I was a kid. Couldn't stand the smell of them cooking, let alone the taste. Now? I can't get enough! When the season rolls around and they hit stores, I eat Brussels sprouts every day it seems. This version is from a fantastic restaurant in my town that makes amazing food with a staff that knows how to keep food-allergic customers safe and happy. Of course, their Brussels sprouts are a notch above perfection, but this is a pretty close rendition that I think you'll enjoy.

2	Tbsp Coconut oil
1	lb (450 g) organic Brussels sprouts, washed, tough outer leaves and stems removed, cut in half
~	Sea salt and freshly ground pepper to taste
2	garlic cloves, minced
2	Tbsp roasted, salted, shelled pistachios
2	Tbsp pomegranate seeds

1. Heat oil in a large skillet over medium heat.
2. Add sprouts and brown, stirring occasionally to prevent burning, about 15 minutes. Season with salt and pepper. Add garlic in the last 2 minutes of cooking.
3. Garnish with pomegranate seeds and pistachios.

Serves 4-6

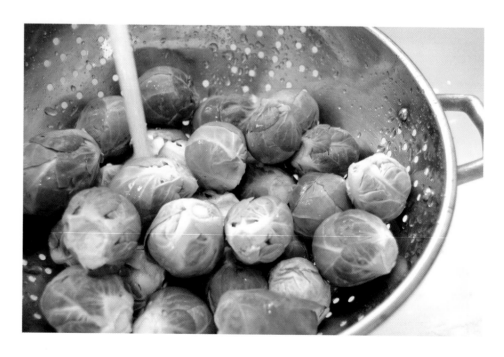

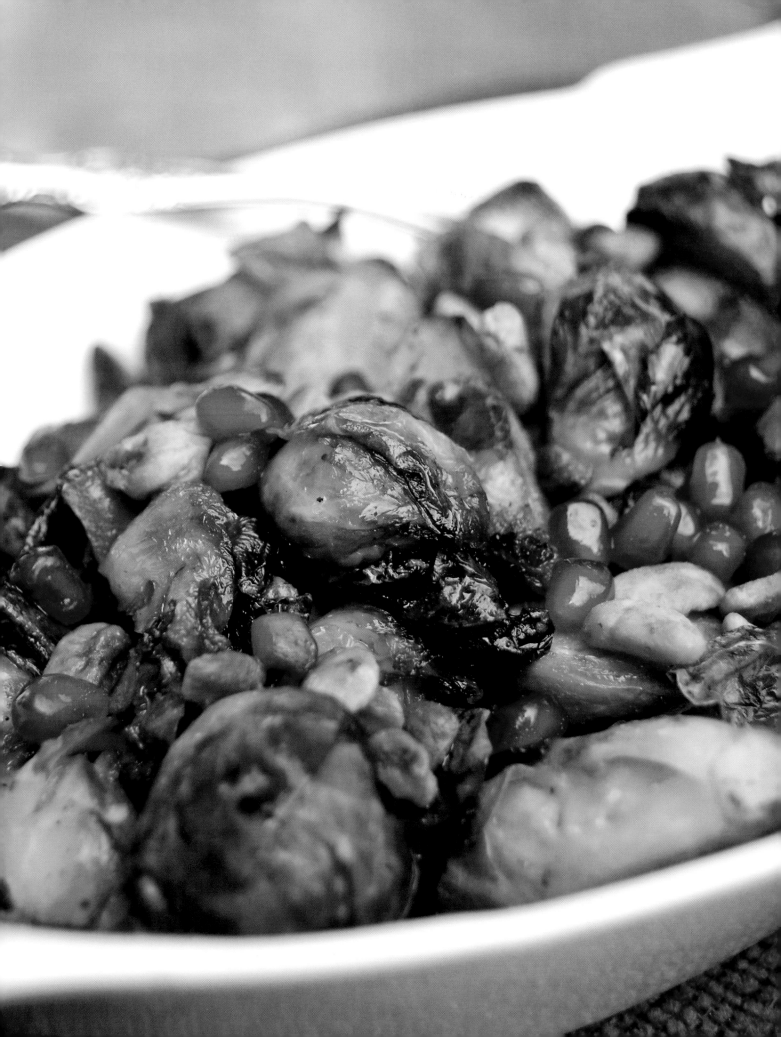

Spanish Rice

My big sis gets credit for this recipe. I can always count on her to recreate dishes like this as a tasty and economical way to enjoy it at home. We use it as a side dish for taco night, and we add chicken to any leftovers for a school lunch the kids really love.

1	Tbsp coconut oil
1	small organic yellow onion, diced
~	Sea salt
~	Freshly ground pepper
1	tsp cumin
1	tsp granulated garlic
1	C (190 g) organic brown rice
1	(14.5) oz (about 475 ml) can organic stewed tomatoes
1 ½	cans (from tomatoes) water

1. Heat oil in a large pan over medium heat.
2. Sauté diced onion with sea salt, pepper, cumin, and garlic for 1 minute.
3. Add rice and sauté for about 4 minutes.
4. Add canned tomatoes and 1½ cans of water. Bring to a boil.
5. Cover, reduce heat to low, and simmer for about 30–45 minutes or until rice is tender and most of liquid is absorbed.

Option:

Make it a meal! Add diced cooked chicken, steak, or pork, reheat for a thermos, and use for school lunches or a great workday lunch!

Serves 4-6

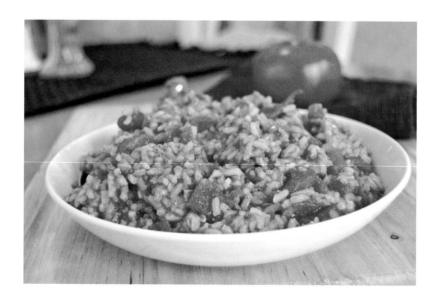

Sides

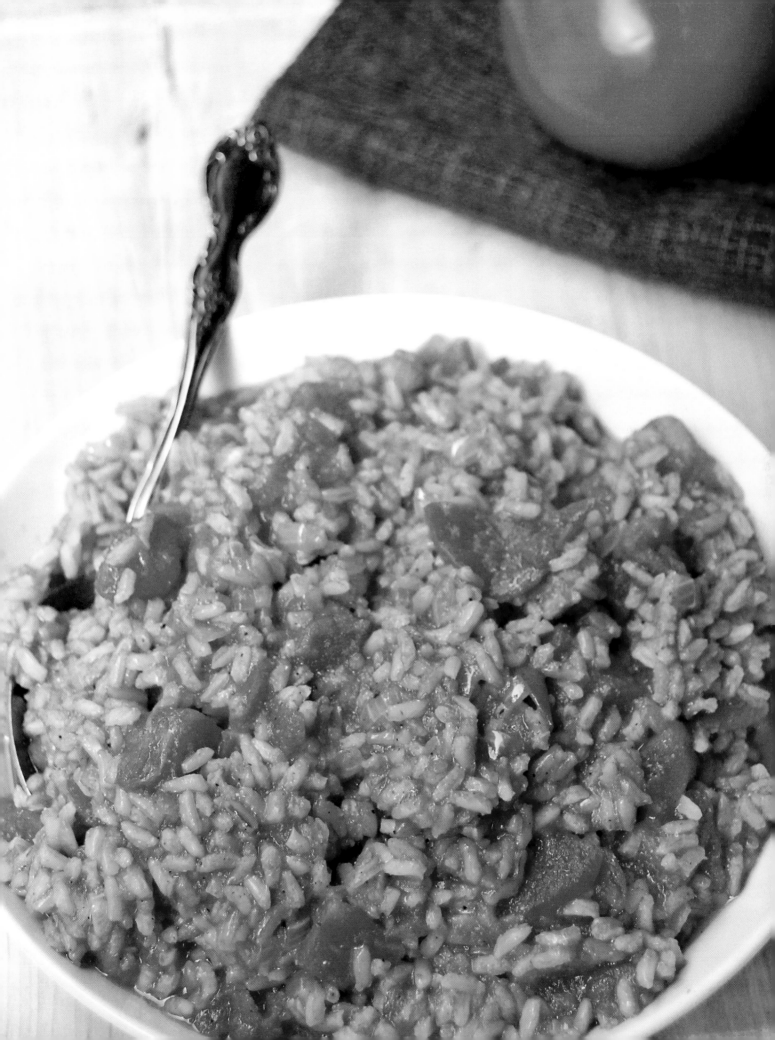

Flour Tortillas

I'm not sure how these came about, because I never would have attempted to make tortillas prior to being gluten-free. I believe it all stems from cravings and/or necessity at this point! Either way, I'm so glad my adventurous spirit kicked in post-GF because there is something so satisfying about a doughy warm tortilla smothered in (nondairy) butter. We've used these as wraps for lunch, as the beautiful vessel for a "cheese" quesadilla, and for burritos. I've even broiled them with "butter" and cinnamon and sugar for dessert. This is also a good recipe to help gain confidence cooking/baking in the gluten-free kitchen... it's very difficult to mess this one up, so go for it!

Dry Ingredients:

⅓   C (40 g) sorghum flour

½   C (60 g) teff flour

⅓   C (40 g) brown rice flour

½   C (60 g) potato starch

½   C (60 g) tapioca starch

2   tsp xanthan gum

1   tsp baking powder

½   tsp organic evaporated cane juice

1   tsp sea salt

Wet Ingredients:

2   heaping Tbsp Spectrum organic shortening, chilled

1   tsp apple cider vinegar

¾   C (180 mL) warm water

1. Whisk together dry ingredients.
2. Cut chilled shortening into dry ingredients with a pastry blender until pea-size crumbs form.
3. In a measuring cup, combine the apple cider vinegar and the warm water. Add a little at a time to the dry mix, stirring until a soft dough is formed. If dry, add a little more water until it comes together.
4. Heat a large electric skillet to 400°.
5. Form small balls of dough with your hands and place one dough ball between 2 sheets of wax paper. Roll with a rolling pin until about 1/8-inch thick.
6. Cook tortillas in skillet, a few minutes per side, until it just starts to bubble and brown. Be careful not to overcook or they can become crispy.
7. Keep warm on a plate covered with foil. Serve warm or use in your favorite recipe!

Makes about 9

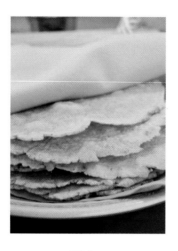

Sides

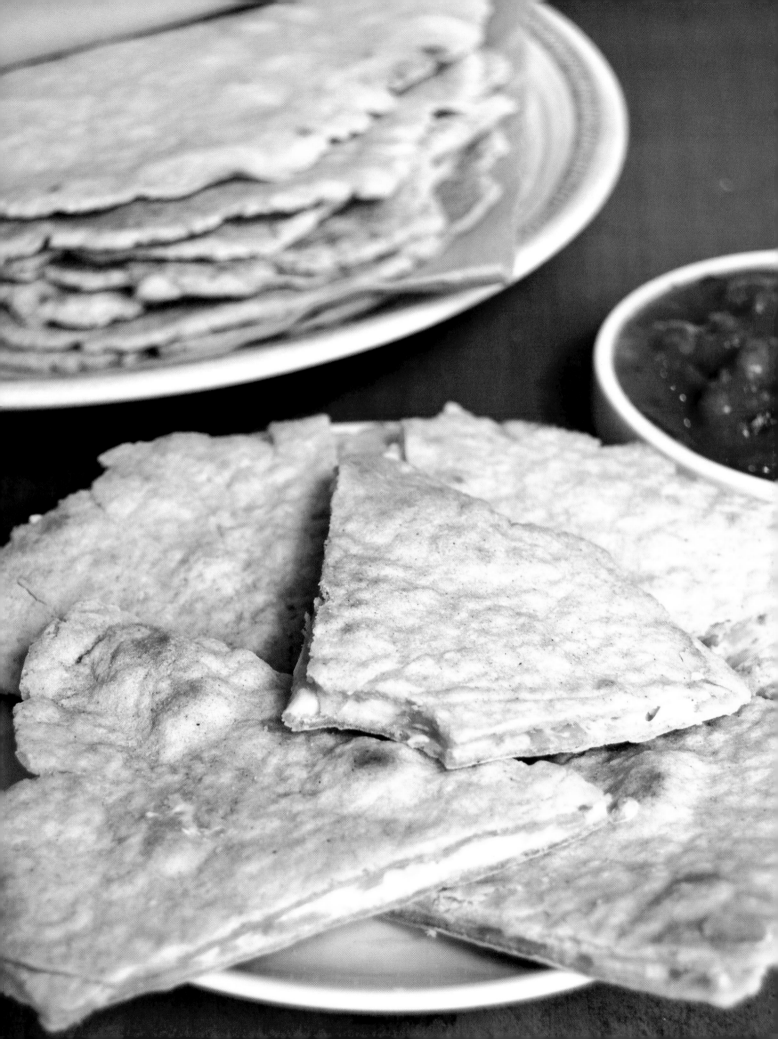

Cucumber Salad

This quick salad makes a wonderful, cool summer side dish. Perfect for a picnic, potluck, Tuesday... anytime really. My kids say it tastes like fresh dill pickles. I say it takes 5 minutes to prepare so I can make it as often as I want!

Salad:

2   large organic English cucumbers, sliced (you can peel cucumbers fully or partially if desired)

Dressing:

2   Tbsp GF rice vinegar

1   Tbsp olive oil

1   tsp organic raw honey (warmed slightly if needed to help it dissolve)

Finishing Touch:

~   Pinch of sea salt

~   Freshly ground pepper to taste

1   tsp dried dill (or about 1 Tbsp chopped fresh dill)

1. Place sliced cucumbers in a large shallow dish.
2. Whisk together dressing ingredients. Pour evenly over cucumbers.
3. Sprinkle tops of cucumbers with sea salt, pepper, and dill.

Serves 4

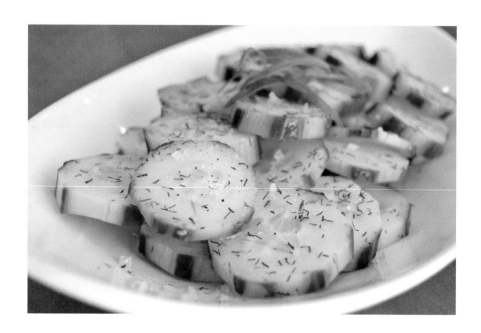

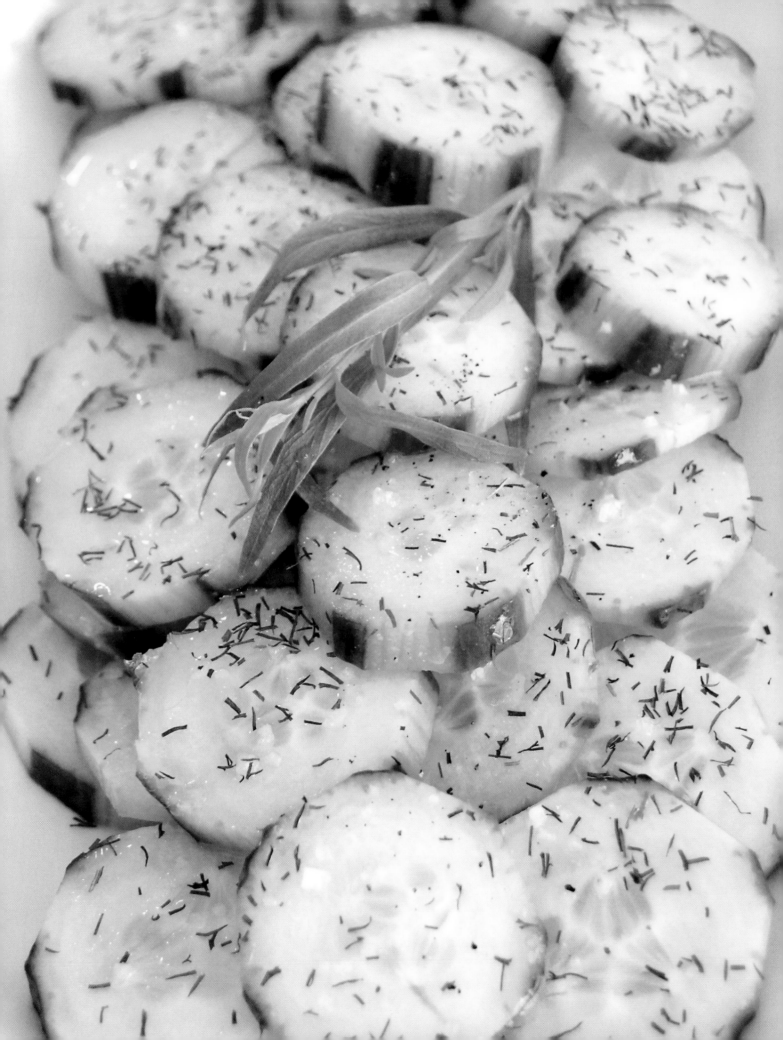

Sweet and Sour Cabbage

Cabbage has been proven to have cancer-preventative properties, which is just one more reason to enjoy this sweet and tangy dish. The fact that it is ready in minutes only makes it that much better.

For the Sauce:

1	Tbsp oil of choice
2	Tbsp coconut aminos (or Bragg liquid aminos)
¼	C (60 mL) rice vinegar
2	Tbsp raw honey

For the Cabbage:

1	Tbsp coconut oil
1	large head organic Napa cabbage, sliced
1	C (150 g) shredded organic purple cabbage
~	Sea salt
~	Freshly ground black pepper

1. In a small bowl, stir together sauce ingredients. Set aside.
2. Heat oil in a large skillet over medium heat. Add cabbages and toss occasionally, cooking until slightly browned and just wilted.
3. Sprinkle cabbage with sea salt and pepper. Add sauce to pan, remove from heat, and stir to combine.
4. Serve!

Serves 4

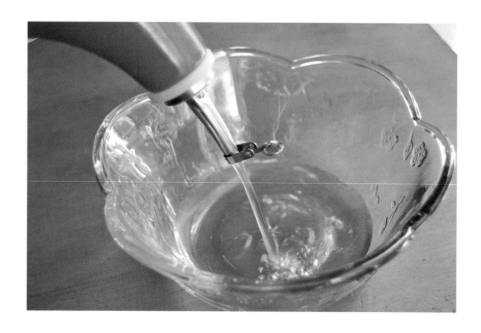

Sides

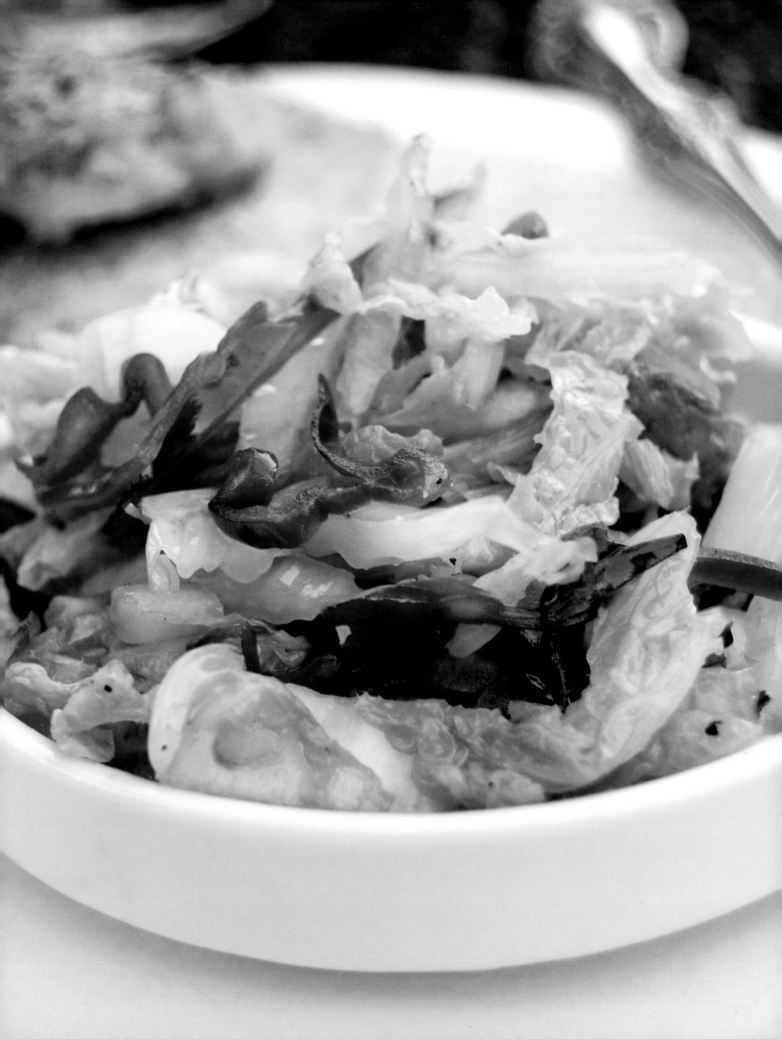

Easy Peasy Carrot Salad

Just the vibrant colors of this quick and easy salad make me happy! The kiddos love this one too, "because it's so much more fun eating shredded carrots than big carrot sticks." At least, I've been so informed by my six-year-old. Whatever gets them eating the veg is what I say! Freshly shredded carrots pack the most flavor and nutrition, but if you're in a rush, feel free to use pre-bagged shredded carrots found in your local supermarket's produce section.

1	small shallot, finely chopped
3	Tbsp red wine vinegar
2	C (300 g) shredded organic carrots (about 6 large carrots, shredded in your food processor)
1	C frozen organic peas (150 g), thawed by running under cold water in a colander
¼	tsp granulated onion
1	tsp sea salt
~	Freshly ground black pepper
¼	C (60 mL) olive oil

1. In a small bowl, combine chopped shallots and vinegar. Let sit for 15 minutes.
2. Meanwhile, place shredded carrots in a serving bowl.
3. Sprinkle peas over top of carrots.
4. For dressing, add granulated onion, salt, and pepper to the bowl of shallot and vinegar. Slowly whisk in olive oil until fully incorporated.
5. Drizzle dressing over the carrot salad and serve!

Serves 6

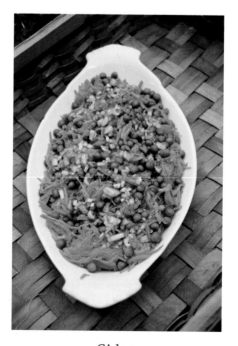

Sides

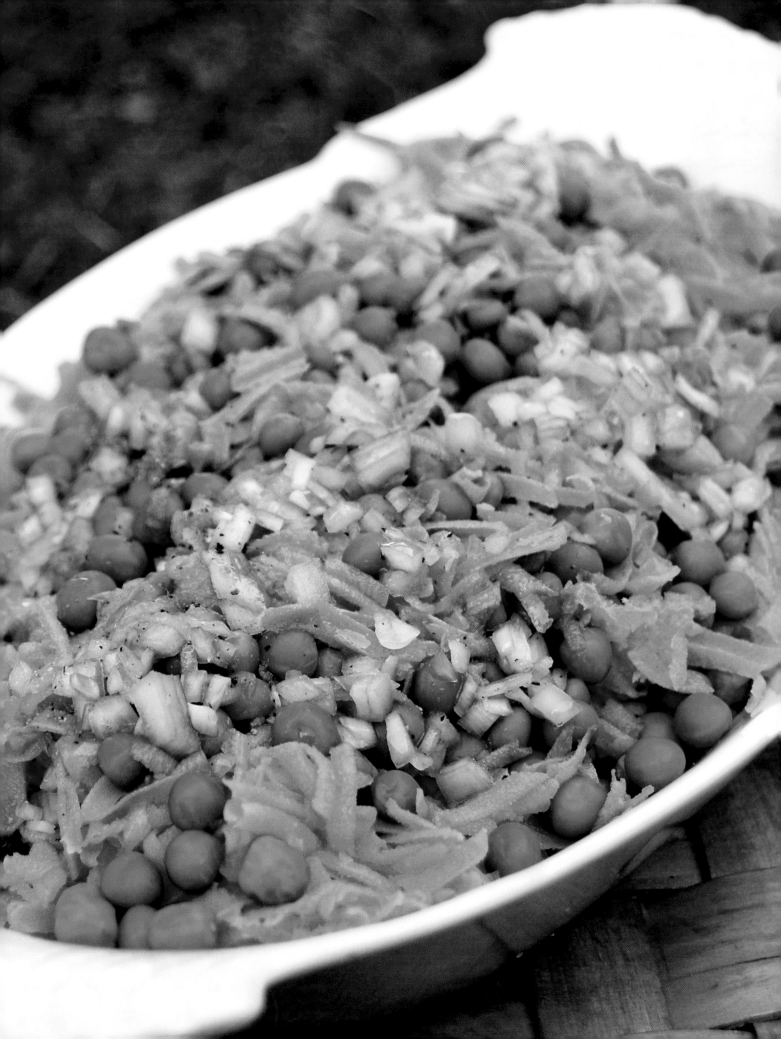

Corn Tortillas

Corn tortillas are so easy to make and the ingredients couldn't be simpler. As a matter of fact, just about any corn tortilla recipe calls for the same two ingredients: masa harina and water. Masa harina, in simple terms, is dried and ground corn with hydrated mineral of lime, which gives it its distinct flavor. The only trick here is to make the dough pliable and not too wet. Yes, organic corn tortillas are easy to purchase, but as a special treat now and again, nothing beats the flavor and texture of homemade corn tortillas.

2   C (240 g) GF masa harina (I like Bob's Red Mill)

1½–2   C (350–475 mL) warm water

1. In a medium bowl, mix together masa harina and warm water until combined.
2. If dough is too sticky, add more masa harina; if it begins to dry out, sprinkle with water. Cover dough tightly with plastic wrap and allow to stand for 15 minutes.
3. Preheat a medium Lodge cast-iron skillet or nonstick electric skillet to medium-high.
4. Divide dough into small balls. Using your hands, press each ball of dough flat between two sheets of parchment paper.
5. Place tortilla in preheated pan and allow to cook for approximately 30 seconds, or until browned and slightly puffy. Turn tortilla over to brown on second side for approximately 30 seconds more, then transfer to a plate. Repeat process with each ball of dough. Keep tortillas covered with a towel to stay warm and moist until ready to serve.

Makes 12–15

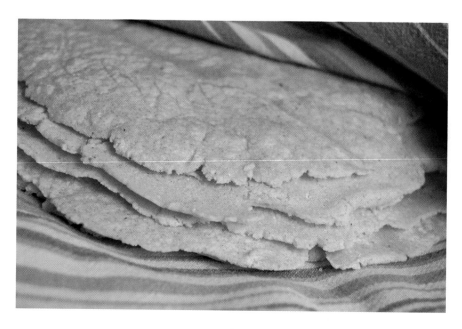

Sides

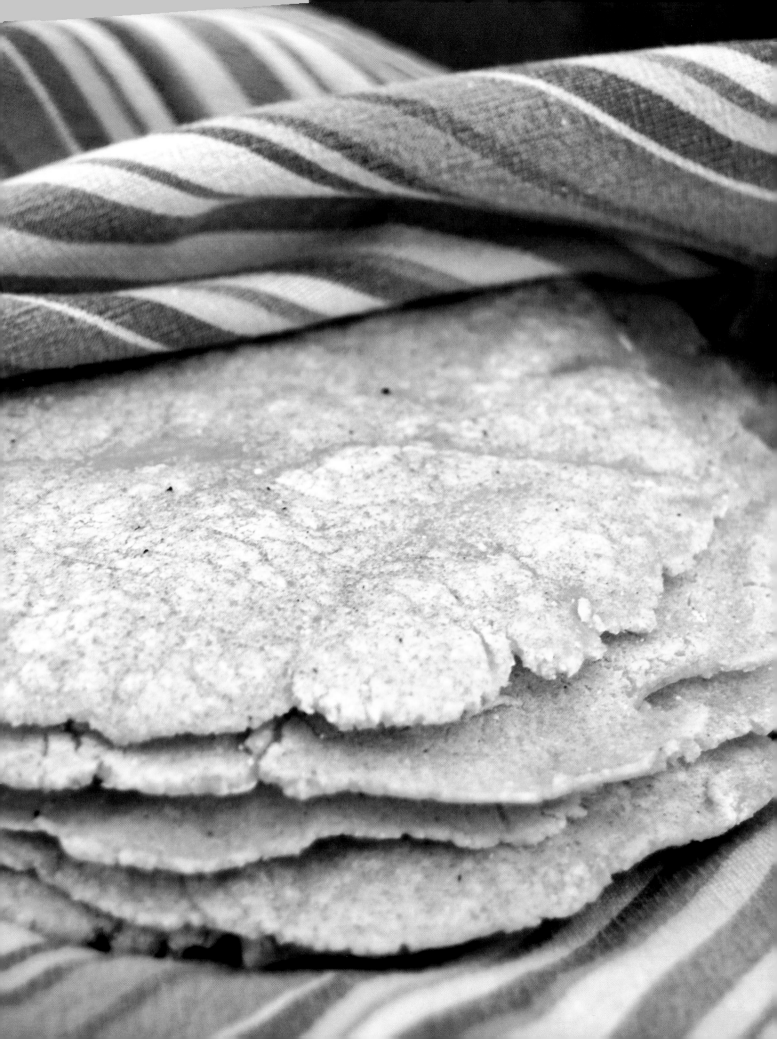

Sausage Veggie Stuffing

Enjoy this savory and traditional stuffing at your next holiday meal, either in a casserole dish or make it "Wow!" by serving in individual stuffed acorn squash. Your guests will be impressed and no one will know it's gluten-free!

1	lb (450 g) GF Italian sausage, casings removed
3	Tbsp coconut oil
1	large leek, chopped (white and pale green parts only)
1	large organic apple (Granny Smith, Pink Lady) peeled, cored and chopped
1	C (150 g) chopped organic celery
2	medium organic carrots, peeled and chopped (can use parsnips)
½	medium organic yellow onion, chopped
8	oz (230 g) white button mushrooms
1½	tsp poultry seasoning
2	Tbsp coconut flour
1	tsp chopped dried rosemary
⅓	C (50 g) chopped organic Italian parsley
~	Sea salt
~	Freshly ground pepper
5	C (about 700 g) Quick Bread Cubes (p. 390) toasted lightly (or any toasted bread cubes of your choice)
½	C (120 mL) organic chicken broth
1	C (150 g) pecans, coarsely chopped and lightly toasted

1. Brown sausage in 1 Tbsp oil in a skillet. Transfer to a large bowl.
2. In same skillet, heat 2 Tbsp oil over medium heat. Add leeks, apples, celery, carrots, onions, mushrooms, and poultry seasoning. Sauté until leeks and carrots soften, about 6 minutes.
3. Add veggies to the bowl of sausage. Stir to combine.
4. Add coconut flour, rosemary, parsley, salt, pepper, and bread cubes. Stir to combine.
5. Pour broth over sausage mixture and stir gently.
6. Spoon stuffing into a greased baking dish, sprinkle top with pecans, and cover with foil.
7. Bake in a 350° oven for 30 minutes.
8. Uncover and bake an additional 10 minutes to brown the top.

Option:

Or spoon stuffing into acorn squash halves (seeds removed), place all in a 9" by 13" baking dish. Add 1 C of water to the pan, cover with foil and proceed with step 7, or until squash is tender.

Serves 4-6

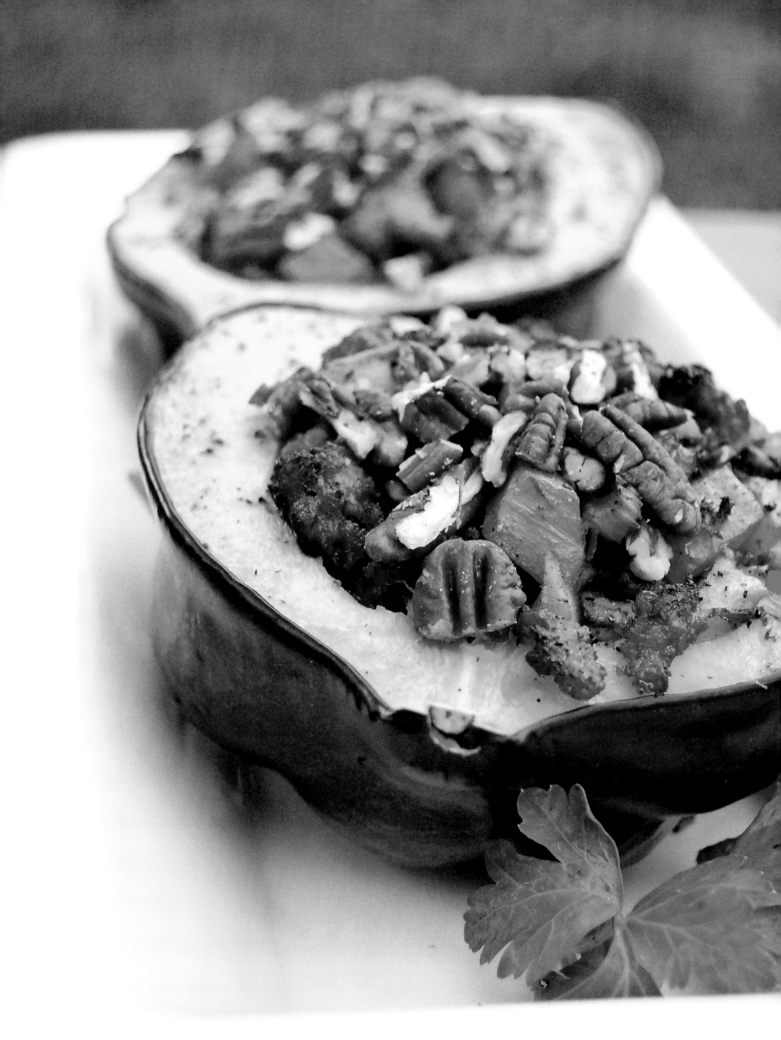

Broccoli Salad

I have three words... simple... summer... salad... wait, make that four words.... Picnic! And Potlucks! And—oh, forget it. It's great, take my five or so words for it.

Dressing:

3	Tbsp rice vinegar
¼	C (60 mL) olive oil
3	Tbsp vegan mayo (Spectrum)
2	Tbsp raw organic honey
~	Sea salt
~	Freshly ground pepper

Salad:

3	large organic broccoli crowns, washed and chopped
½	C (75 g) diced organic red onion
6	slices uncured bacon, chopped and cooked crisp (US Wellness Meats)
¾	C (110 g) roasted, salted sunflower seed kernels
1	8 oz can sliced water chestnuts
¾	C (110 g) organic raisins

1. To make the dressing, combine all ingredients in a jar with a tight-fitting lid and shake well until fully combined. You can also blend in a blender or Bullet food blender. Set aside.
2. Combine salad ingredients in a large bowl, top with dressing and stir to coat.

Serves 4-6

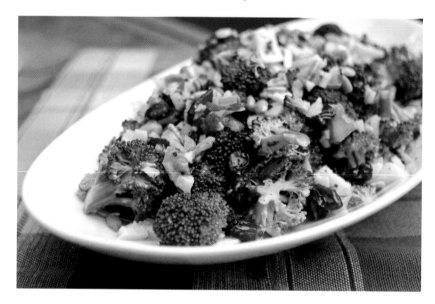

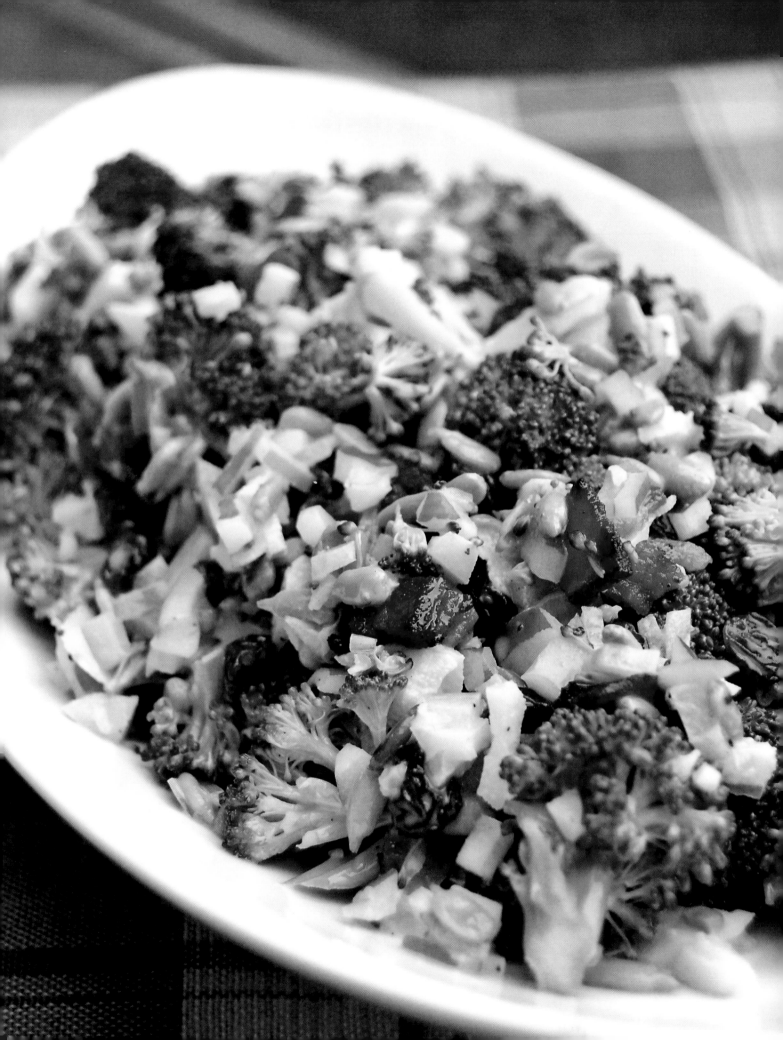

Easy Beans

Who says beans have to take days to prepare? For those occasions you need a fast side dish without much fuss, this is the recipe for you! Just a few ingredients, a quick stir, and you're all set. This recipe is so quick and versatile you can serve it with the Cornbread (p.218) for a filling winter dinner or dish it up alongside Grilled Steak (p.262) to complete a tasty summer BBQ. Either way you'll love it!

½	medium organic yellow onion, diced
1	Tbsp coconut oil
2	cans organic pinto beans, 1 rinsed and drained, the other use the beans and the water (you can substitute another favorite bean, such as kidney, great northern, or black beans for 1 can)
⅓	C (80 mL) GF ketchup
2	Tbsp raw organic honey
2	Tbsp GF tamari soy sauce (or Bragg liquid aminos or coconut aminos)
2	tsp granulated onion
1	tsp granulated garlic
1	tsp chili powder
~	Sea salt and freshly ground pepper to taste

1. In a medium sauce pan, sauté diced onion in oil until translucent.
2. Add remaining ingredients to pan, stir until combined.
3. Heat over medium heat until it starts to boil. Turn down heat to low and simmer for about 10 minutes until flavors are combined and beans are heated through.

Serves 4

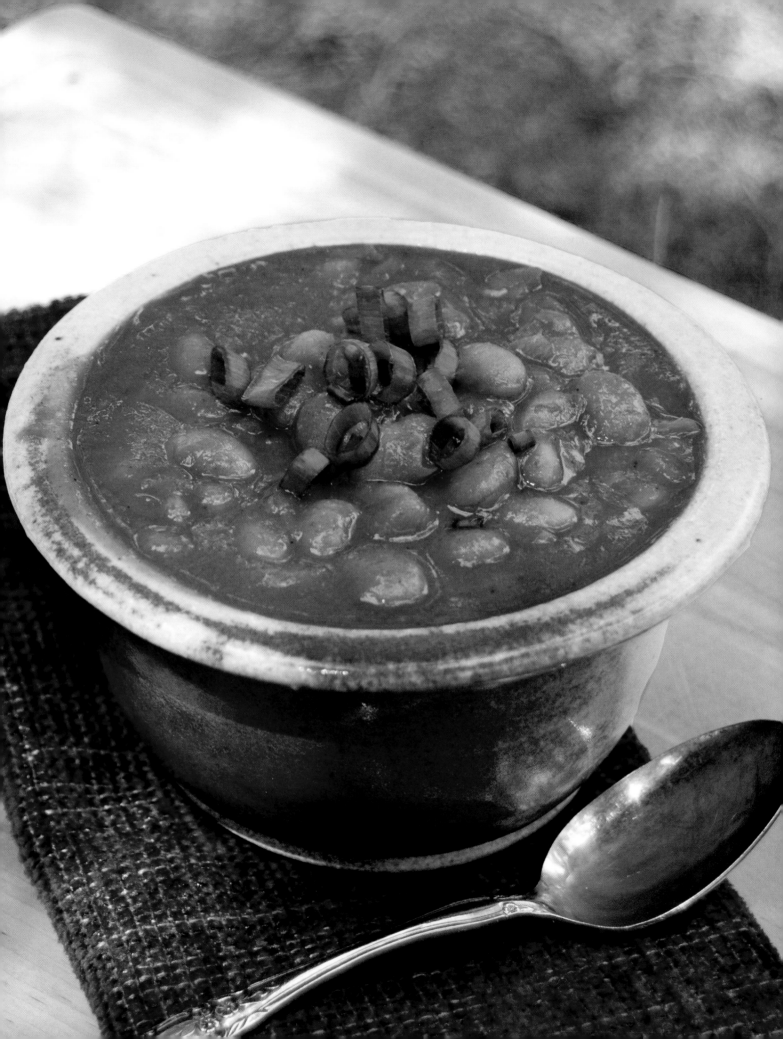

Honey Glazed Carrots

Who loves fast and easy side dishes? Who loves fast, easy side dishes that your family will actually eat? Me! Me! Me! I absolutely will not make a side dish that takes longer to prepare than the main part of the meal. Call me crazy. Which is why I love these yummy glazed carrots so much. They look like a million bucks and taste like it too. I also like to use real maple syrup in place of the honey, especially in the fall.

1	Tbsp coconut oil
10	large organic carrots, cut into coins
2	Tbsp organic raw honey
~	Sea salt
~	Freshly ground pepper

1. Heat oil in a large skillet over medium-high heat. Add as many carrots as will fit and do not stir. Let them sit and get caramelized and browned before stirring. Then set them aside and do the same for the remaining carrots until all are browned and softened, about 10 minutes.
2. Add all the carrots back to the pan, and turn heat to medium-low. Add honey, salt, and pepper to carrots. Remove from heat and serve.

Serves 4

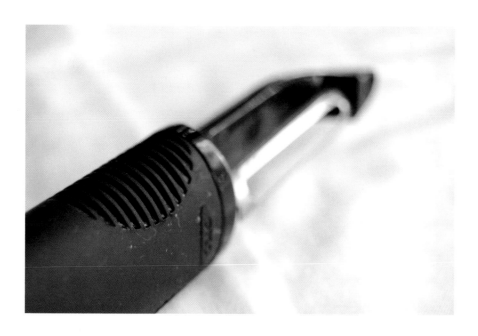

240 Sides

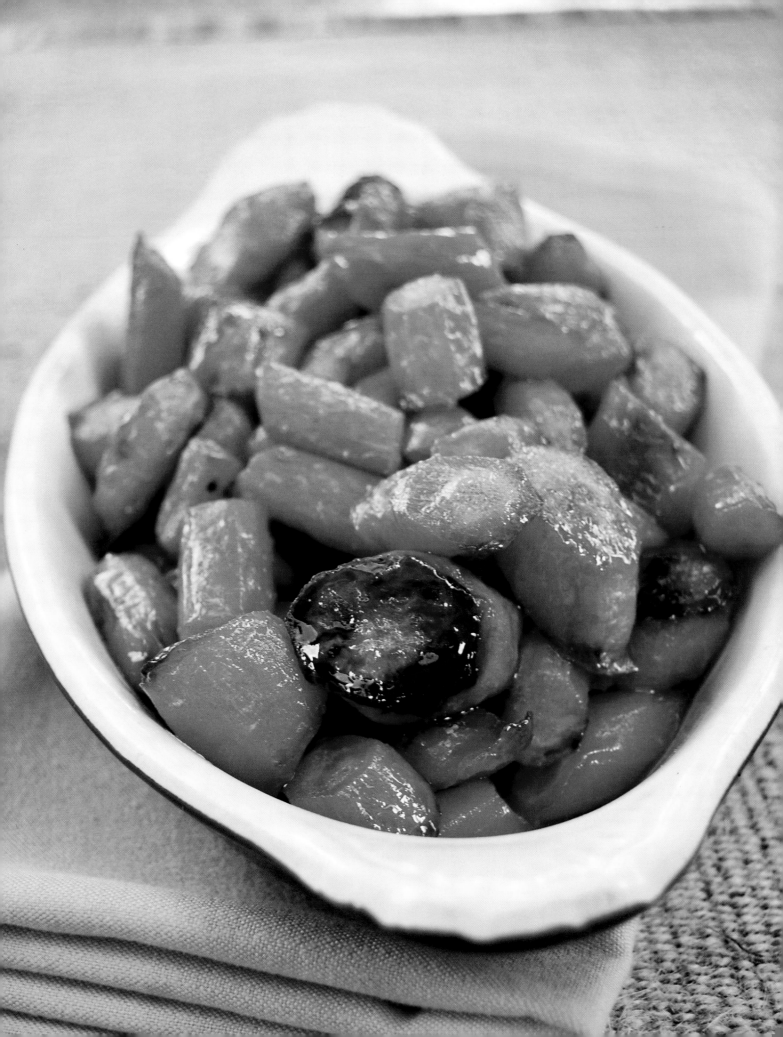

Zucchini with Mushrooms

I don't know about you, but side dishes in my house seem to be an afterthought most nights. I'd love for them to be elaborate, but I just never seem to have the energy or brain power by 5 PM to give it my all. So sides must be speedy and easy or they don't make the cut. This one fits the bill, with lots of flavor and nutrients to boot!

~	**5 medium organic zucchini**
1	**Tbsp olive oil**
½	**small organic yellow onion, chopped fine**
½	**C (75 g) chopped mushrooms**
~	**Sea salt**
~	**Pepper**

1. Wash and slice zucchini lengthwise, then slice into large pieces.
2. Heat large skillet over medium-high heat. Add olive oil and onions. Cook for about 3 minutes, until translucent.
3. Add mushrooms to pan and cook until soft, about 2 minutes.
4. Add zucchini to pan and cook, stirring occasionally until zucchini is soft, about 5 minutes.
5. Season with sea salt and freshly ground pepper to taste.

Serves 4

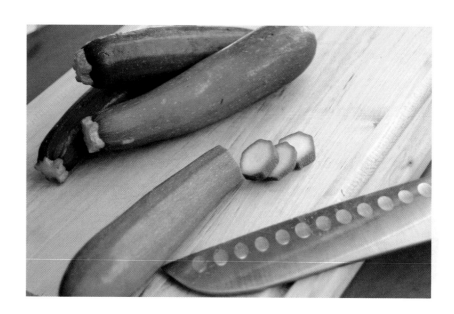

Sides

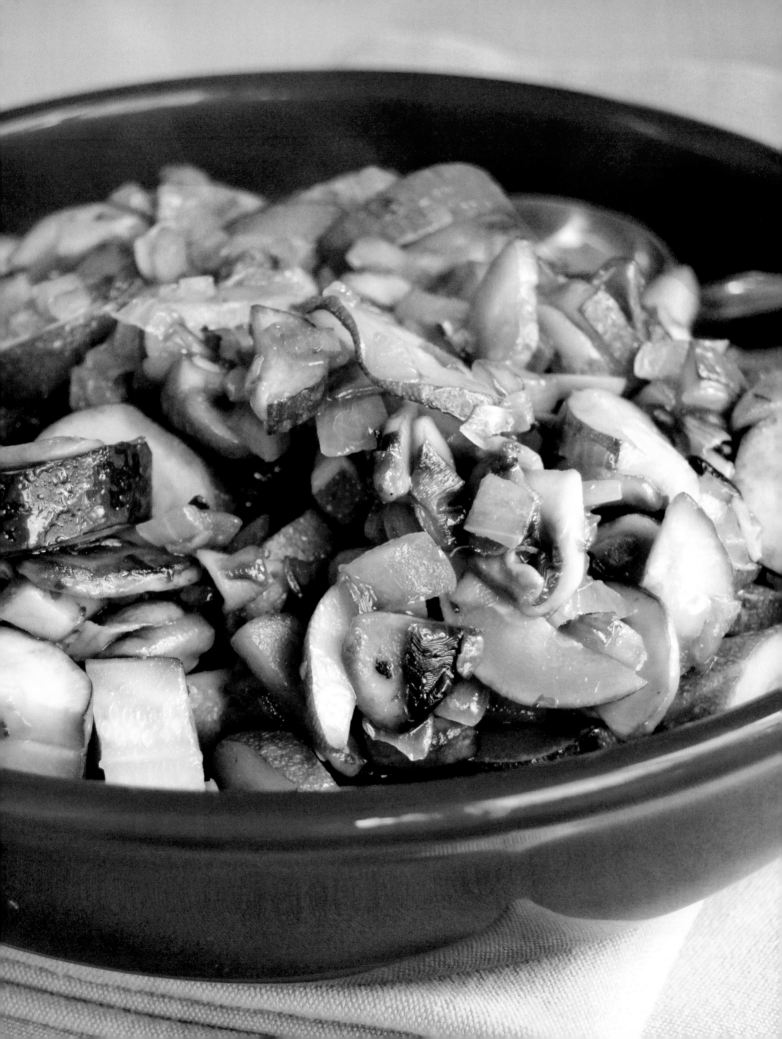

Famous Mashed Potatoes

Someone made this combo of mashed potatoes famous.... I'm not sure who it was, but it wasn't me. Seems like it has been around awhile but I thought I'd revive it with a nice dairy-free version. My family loves this side dish because it tastes like potato skins from the restaurant without all the yucky stuff.

6	medium organic russet potatoes, washed and cubed
½	C (120 mL) coconut milk, or nondairy milk of choice
4	garlic cloves, crushed
¼	C (60 g) nondairy butter
~	Sea salt to taste
~	Pepper to taste
6	slices uncured bacon, diced and cooked crisp (US Wellness Meats)
½	C (75 g) nondairy cheese (I like Daiya Cheddar for this)
~	Sliced green onions for garnish

1. Place potatoes in a saucepan and cover with water. Cover and bring to a boil.
2. Cook for about 25 minutes, or until potatoes are very tender.
3. Meanwhile, in a small saucepan, heat coconut milk and garlic to warm.
4. Drain potatoes and place back in pan.
5. Add in milk mixture, butter, and salt and pepper to taste.
6. Blend with a hand blender until smooth and creamy. If needed, add more coconut milk until desired consistency is reached.
7. Fold in bacon pieces and cheese.
8. Garnish with green onions and serve immediately.

Serves 4

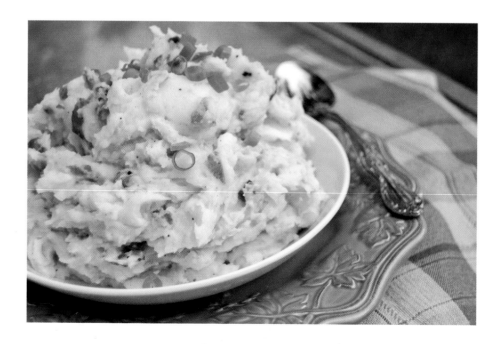

Sides

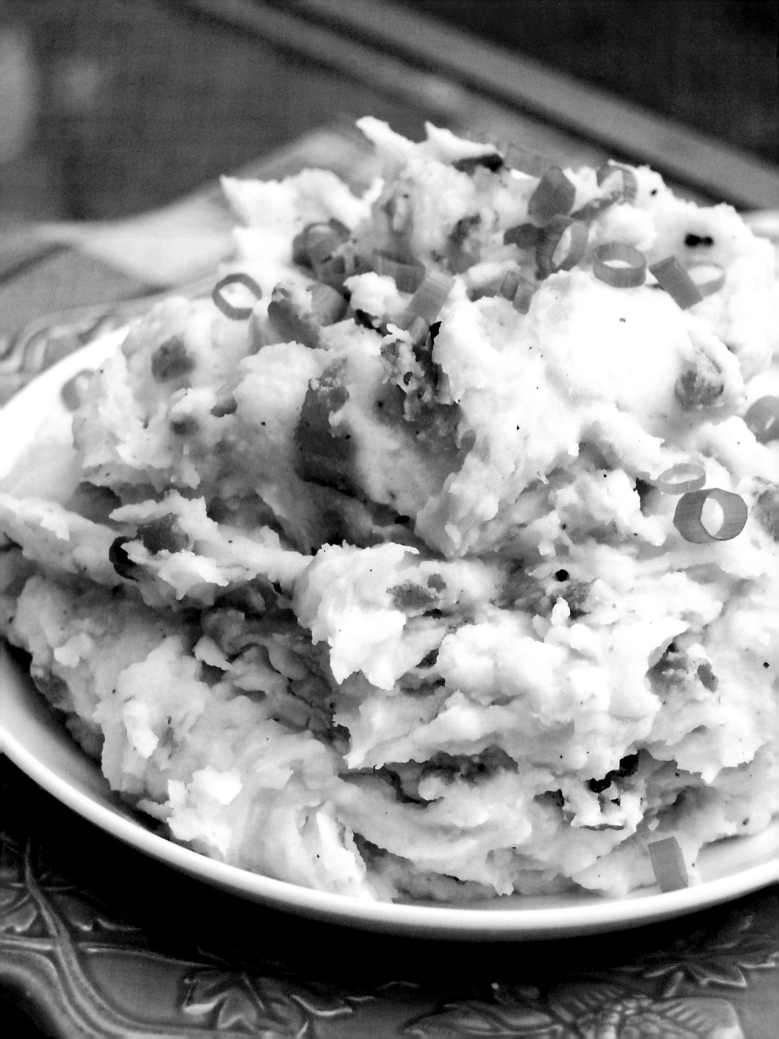

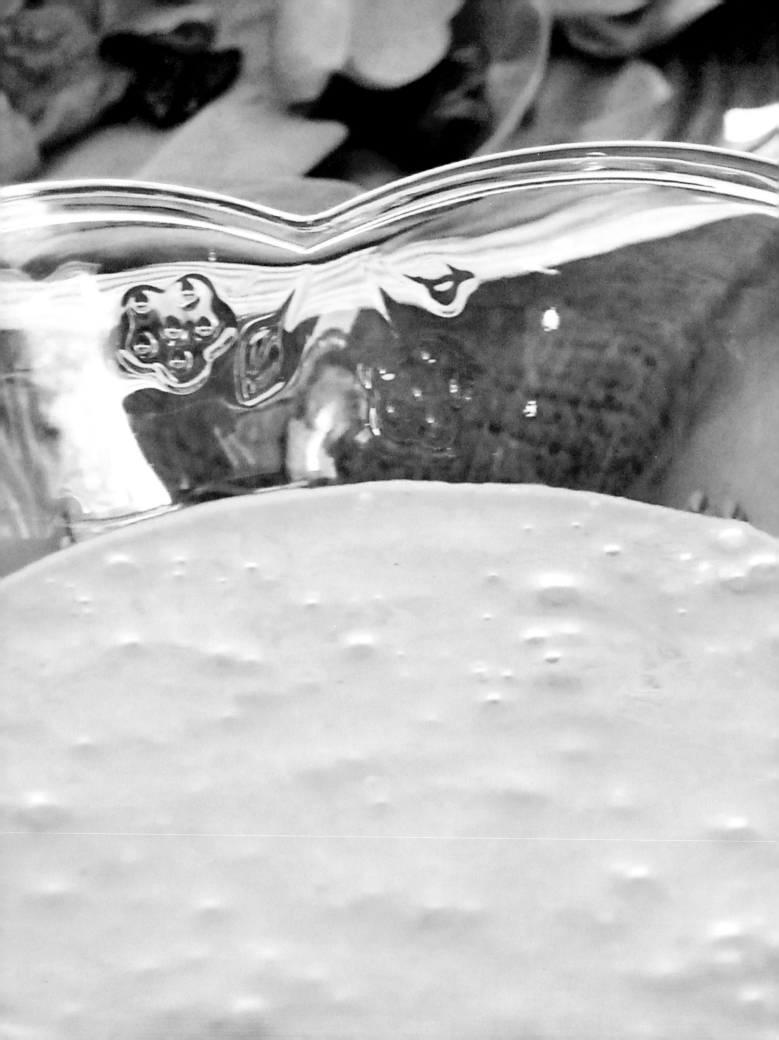

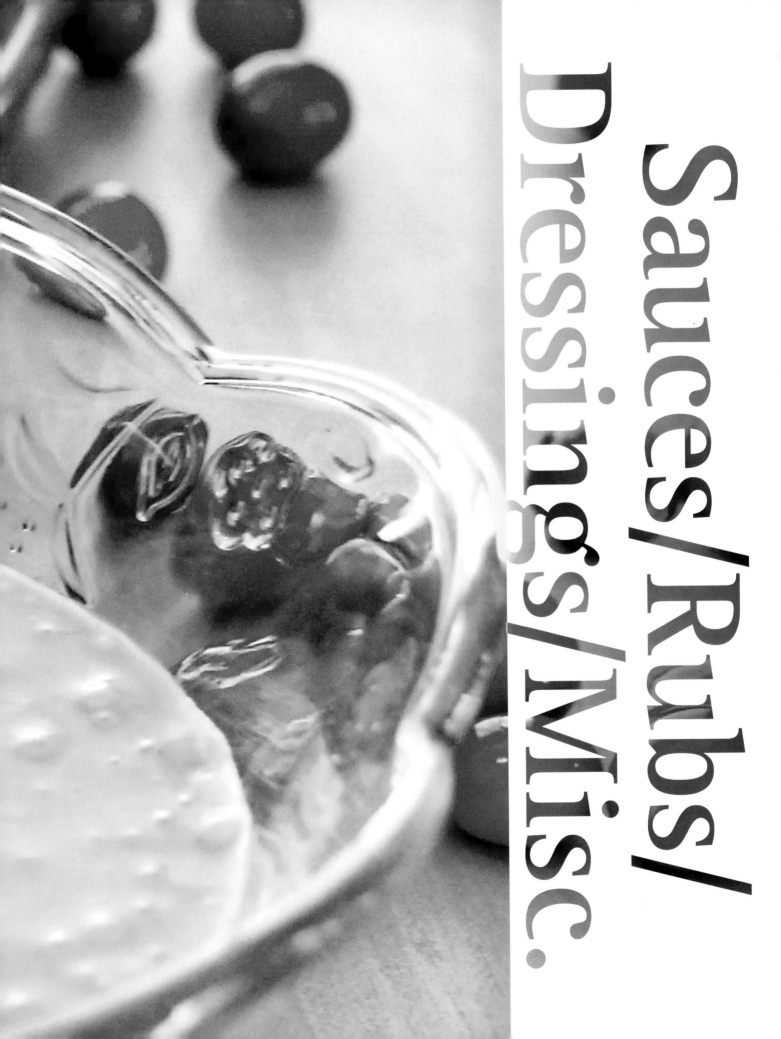

Sauces/Rubs/
Dressings/Misc.

Spaghetti (and Pizza) Sauce

I've included both a "Make Ahead and Freeze"—size recipe, and a more manageable "Just Enough" recipe. When I can, I like to make a large pot of this sauce and store leftovers in the freezer. And really, isn't it just as easy to chop three onions as it is to chop one? So if you're going to do the work, might as well do it efficiently and make enough for a few months. Because, trust me, you will never want a store-bought sauce again after trying this one.

Make Ahead and Freeze

1	C (240 mL) olive oil
3	small organic yellow onions, chopped
1	small bunch of organic Italian parsley, chopped
3	large cloves of garlic, minced
3	(4 oz) cans (about 400 g) organic tomato paste
115	oz can (3l, 414 ml) organic tomato sauce (warehouse store size)
115	oz can (3l, 414 ml) organic diced tomatoes (warehouse store size)
1½	tsp oregano
1½	tsp basil
½	tsp rosemary
1½	tsp freshly ground black pepper
1	Tbsp sea salt

1. Heat oil in a very large stock pot over medium heat. When it's hot, add in chopped onion. Let onion cook, stirring occasionally, until it turns translucent and softens, about 5 minutes.
2. Add chopped parsley and garlic. Stir and cook for 1 minute.
3. Add in tomato paste, stirring well to blend it into the onion, parsley, and garlic.
4. Add tomato sauce, diced tomatoes, and remaining spices, stir well.
5. Bring sauce to a simmer and cook on low, covered, for about an hour.
6. Serve or let cool in mason jars, refrigerate, and then freeze for later use.

To make pizza sauce: reserve about 4 Cups of the sauce in the pan. Add another can of tomato paste. With a hand immersion blender, blend sauce until smooth. Store in smaller mason jars in the freezer until needed for your favorite homemade pizza!

Just Enough Sauce

¼	C (60 mL) olive oil
1	small organic yellow onion, chopped
¼	C organic Italian parsley, chopped
1	large clove of garlic, minced
1	(4 oz) can (113 g) organic tomato paste
1	large (28 oz) can (831 ml) organic tomato sauce
1	large (28 oz) can (831 ml) organic diced tomatoes
½	tsp oregano
½	tsp basil
~	Pinch of rosemary
½	tsp freshly ground black pepper
1	rounded tsp sea salt

1. Follow instructions above.

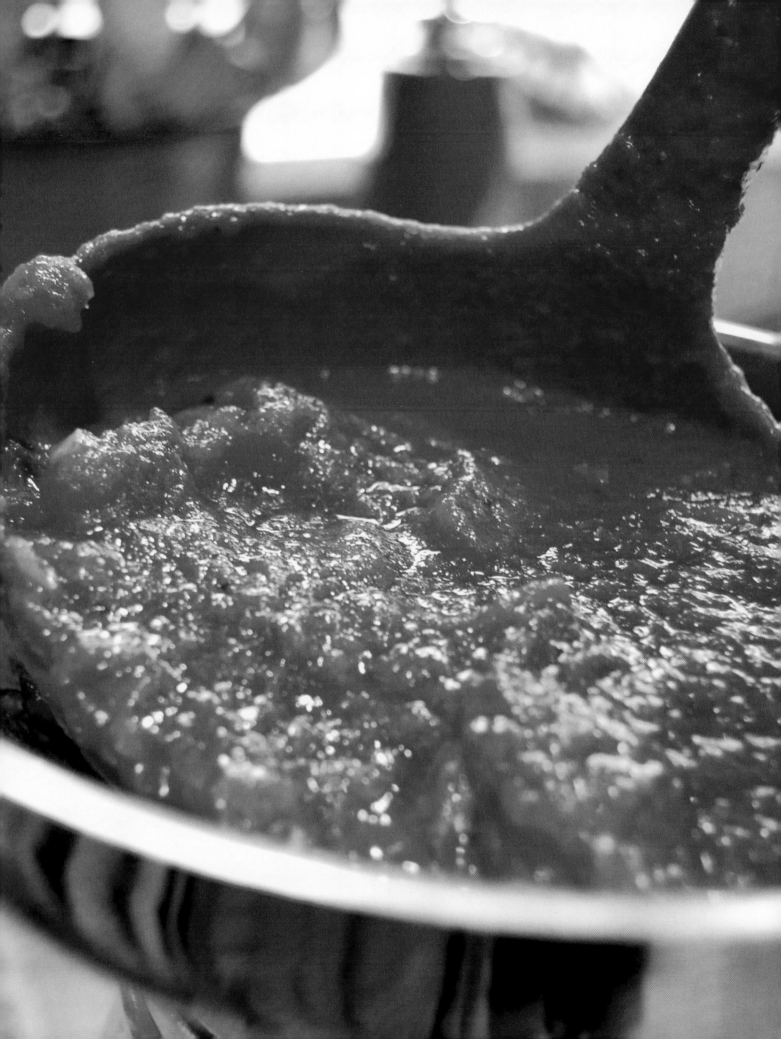

Honey Mustard Dipping Sauce

Not particularly fancy or involved, this dipping sauce is quick and simple, and it uses ingredients you always have on hand. Sometimes the difference between a "chicken again?" lunch and "this lunch was great!" is a little sauce for dipping. Feel free to adjust the amount of honey depending on how sweet you like it.

2	Tbsp yellow mustard
1	Tbsp raw organic honey
¼	tsp granulated onion
~	Pinch of sea salt
~	Freshly ground black pepper

1. Mix all ingredients in a small bowl until combined. Use as a dipping sauce for Coconut Chicken Strips (p. 106) or Steak Bites (p. 160).

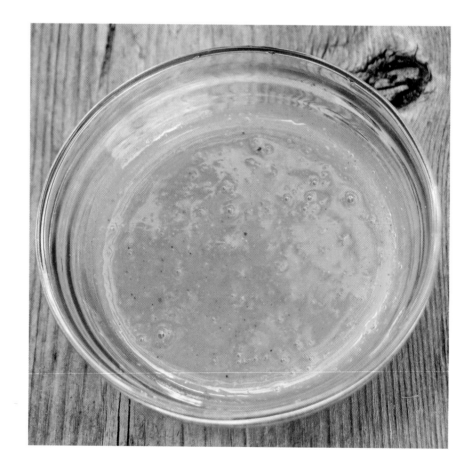

Sauces / Rubs / Dressings / Misc.

BBQ Sauce

One of the hardest things with food allergies is never knowing who to trust. Does that bottle say gluten-free? What does "no gluten ingredients used" mean? It's hard to know and keep on top of what company is trustworthy and has a safe product. That's why for many simple items, I just make it myself. I can make much more for much less, store the leftovers, and know exactly what's in it at all times. I like control.

1	shallot, finely chopped
1	garlic clove, finely chopped
1	(15 oz) can (about 475 mL) organic tomato sauce
1	(4 oz) can (120 mL) organic tomato paste
½	tsp granulated garlic
1	tsp granulated onion
1	Tbsp raw apple cider vinegar
½	tsp Wright's liquid smoke flavoring (this is a great gluten-free addition to your pantry!)
3	Tbsp raw organic honey
1	tsp sea salt
~	Freshly ground pepper

1. Mix all ingredients in a bowl until combined. Cover and refrigerate for about an hour before using to let flavors come together. Enjoy on meatballs, chicken, chicken wings, steaks, and burgers! Store leftovers in an airtight container in the fridge for 1 week, or freeze for up to 3 months.

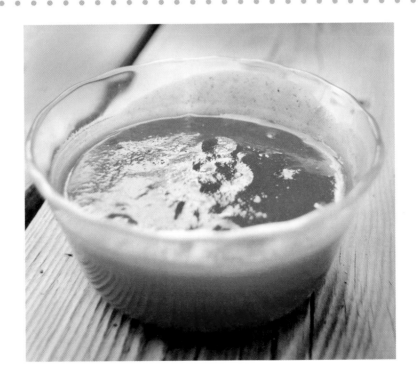

Sugar-Free Cranberry Sauce

I love cranberry sauce for its tangy goodness, high antioxidants, and its versatility. We use this sugar-free sauce for the holidays and then use leftovers to make Cranberry Chicken Fingers (p. 136), or we spoon it over vanilla ice cream (p346), and I even use it to make zesty cranberry vinaigrette (p. 257). With so many ways to enjoy this healthy little berry, you might want to double this recipe!

4	C (600 g) fresh or frozen organic cranberries (about two 12 oz bags)
2	C (475 mL) 100% organic apple juice
1	C (240 mL) pure maple syrup (or coconut nectar or ½ C of each)
~	Zest of 1 orange
~	Juice of 1 orange

1. Combine all ingredients in a large saucepan over medium heat. Bring liquid to a boil.
2. Turn heat to medium-low and simmer about 18 minutes, stirring occasionally, until cranberries have "popped" and sauce starts to thicken.
3. Remove from heat and let cool to allow sauce to thicken more.

Tips:

~Make sure to zest your orange before juicing it!

~If you like your sauce even thicker, make a slurry of 1 Tbsp arrowroot starch and a little cold water. Add to sauce the last 1 minute of cooking. Do not add too soon or the sauce will thicken and then thin out again.

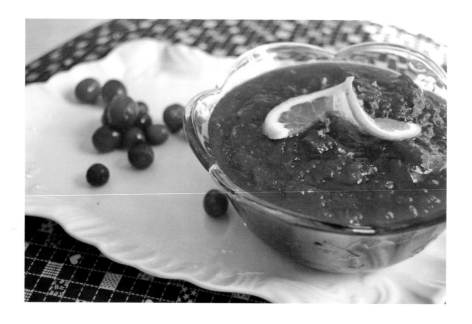

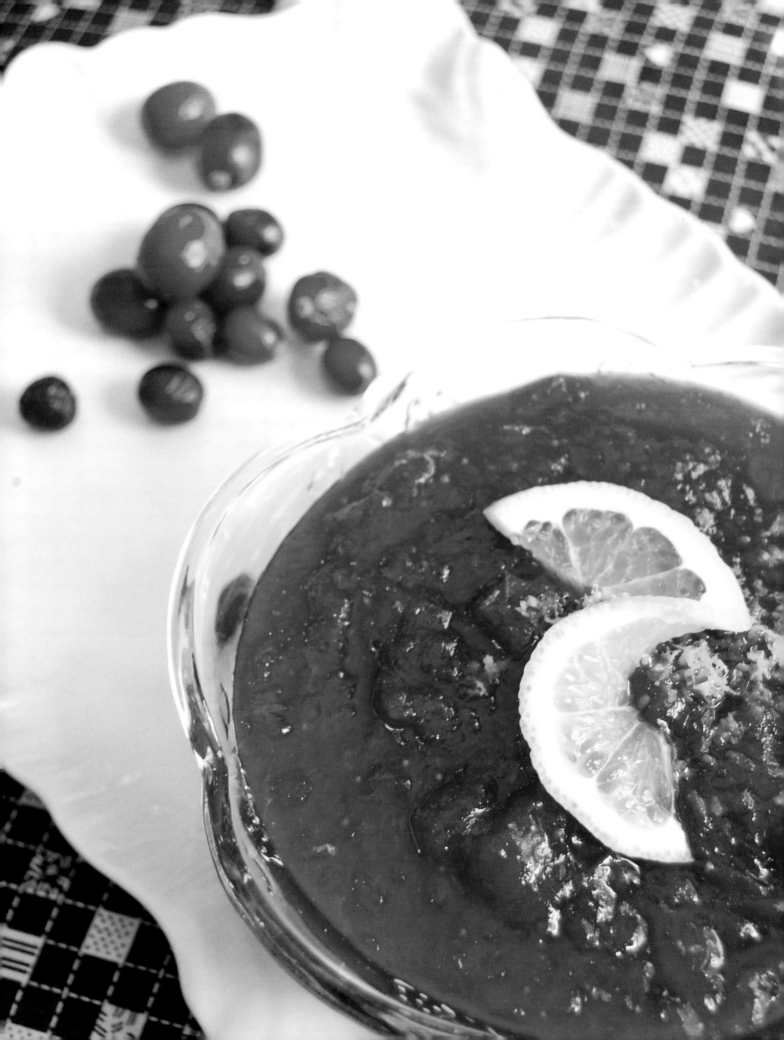

Balsamic Vinaigrette

There are a few basic salad dressings everyone should know how to make. Partly because they're so easy, partly because they taste so much better than anything in a bottle. And it doesn't hurt that it's much more economical to do so as well. Here's one of those basic vinaigrettes that you'll come back to time and again.

½	C (120 mL) olive oil
¼	C (60 mL) balsamic vinegar
1	clove garlic, minced
1	tsp organic Dijon mustard
½	tsp sea salt
~	Freshly ground pepper
⅛	tsp oregano
⅛	tsp basil

1. In a food processor or Bullet blender, mix ingredients until emulsified. Serve immediately.
2. Store leftovers in a jar with a tight-fitting lid for up to a week. If the oil solidifies in the fridge, simply let it sit on the counter for 15 minutes or so to warm up before shaking and using.

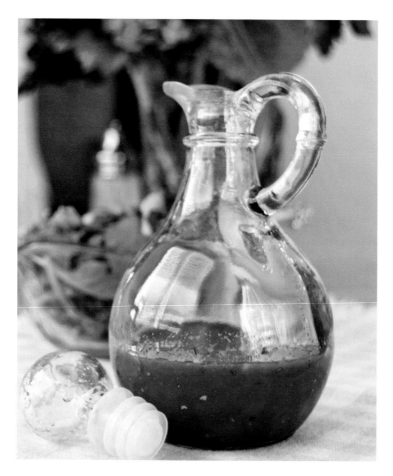

Sauces / Rubs / Dressings / Misc.

Poppy Seed Dressing

My mom loves poppy seed dressing and had a recipe she loved, but it was primarily mayo and sugar. I revamped it a bit to make it healthier and allergy friendly, but it still tastes as good as the original.

⅓   **C (80 mL) white wine vinegar**
3   **Tbsp raw organic honey**
¾   **C (180 mL) olive oil**
¼   **C (40 g) finely chopped onion**
1   **Tbsp organic Dijon mustard**
½   **tsp sea salt**
2   **tsp poppy seeds**

1. Process all ingredients in a blender or Bullet food blender until fully incorporated. Serve immediately and store leftovers in an airtight container in the fridge for up to a week.

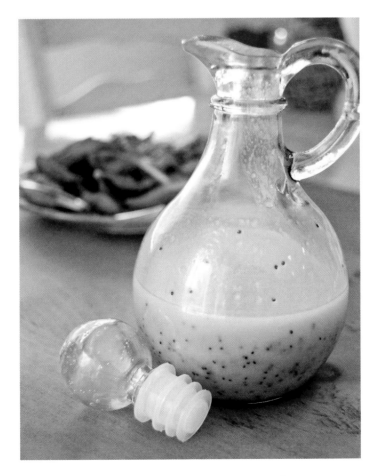

The Healthy Gluten-Free Life

Garlic Vinaigrette

There is an amazing restaurant in my town that serves one incredible steak salad. It is enhanced by a flavorful garlic salad dressing that I'm pretty sure I could suck straight from the bottle if they'd let me. But they won't. So I had to come up with my own, and here it is! But be warned, you may actually want to eat a few extra salads with this dressing in your repertoire!

½	C (120 mL) olive oil
¼	C (60 mL) white wine vinegar
2	cloves garlic, crushed
2	tsp Dijon mustard
⅛	tsp tarragon
⅛	tsp dill
⅛	tsp marjoram
⅛	tsp basil
⅛	tsp thyme
1	tsp raw organic honey
⅛	tsp sea salt
~	Freshly ground pepper

1. In a jar with a tight-fitting lid combine all ingredients. Shake vigorously until fully mixed. Serve over your favorite salad!

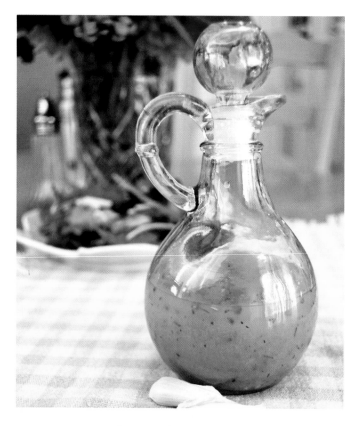

Cranberry Vinaigrette

Made with leftover cranberry sauce (p. 252) from the holidays, this dressing couldn't be easier. It really livens up salads and gives them a festive touch.

⅓ C (80 mL) balsamic vinegar

¾ C (180 mL) olive oil

¼ C (60 mL) Cranberry Sauce (see recipe p. 252)

1 tsp organic Dijon mustard

1 clove garlic, minced

¼ tsp sea salt

¼ tsp pepper

1 Tbsp raw organic honey

1. Blend all ingredients in a blender or Bullet blender until fully combined. Use immediately. Store leftovers in an airtight container in the fridge for up to a week.

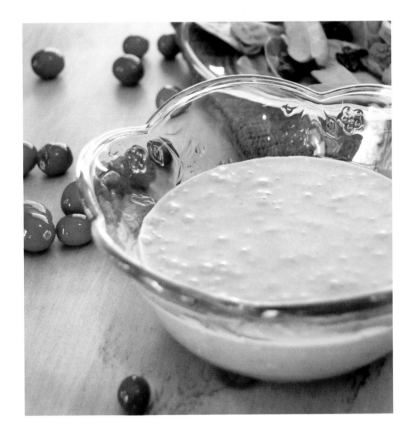

Italian Vinaigrette

A great Italian dressing is so easy to make at home, and so much tastier than its bottled counterparts. A few simple ingredients whisked together and you're ready for a great salad, or even marinade for chicken!

½ C (120 mL) olive oil
¼ C (60 mL) white wine vinegar
1 shallot, finely chopped
1 tsp organic Dijon mustard
1 tsp Italian seasoning
1 tsp granulated onion
½ tsp sea salt
~ Freshly ground pepper

1. In a food processor or Bullet blender, mix ingredients until emulsified. Serve immediately.
2. Store leftovers in a jar with a tight-fitting lid for up to a week. If the oil solidifies in the fridge, simply let it sit on the counter for 15 minutes or so to warm up before shaking and using.

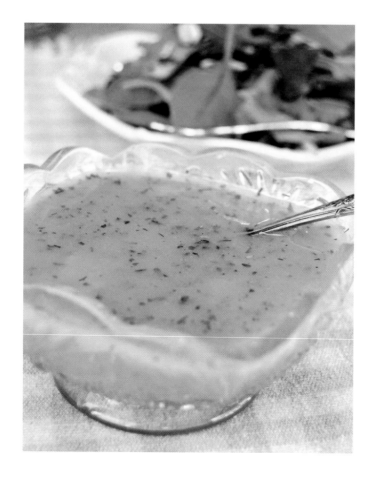

Salad Seasoning

I created this seasoning as an impromptu way of flavoring my salads without the fuss of always making a full-on dressing. For a busy weekday lunch, I like to just drizzle oil and vinegar on my salads to get back out the door quickly, but that can be bland and tasteless. I like to make a batch of this seasoning and store it in an airtight container. Then I just sprinkle on a little bit over my oil and vinegar and there you have it! A great seasoned salad without the fuss!

1	tsp sea salt
¼	tsp granulated onion
⅛	tsp granulated garlic
⅛	tsp Italian seasoning
~	Freshly ground pepper

1. Mix all ingredients in a small bowl. Store in an airtight container.
2. To use, sprinkle vinegar and olive oil on your salad, then a pinch of this seasoning on top.

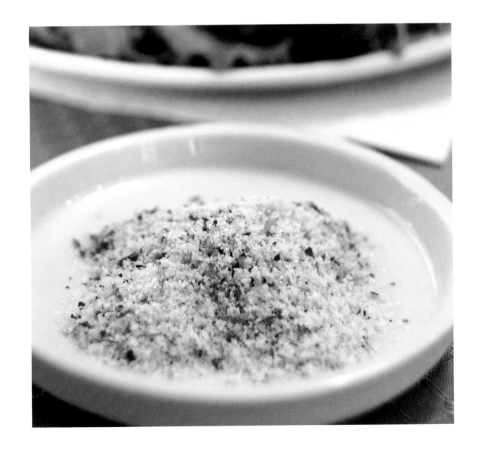

Taco Seasoning

Thanks to my ingenious sister, again, for coming up with this blend! Now we know exactly what's in our spice mix without the worry of hidden gluten or chemicals. Plus, I can control the flavor profile. Like it spicy? Add more cayenne. Like it garlicky? Sprinkle in more granulated garlic. The options are endless!

2	Tbsp chili powder
1½	Tbsp paprika
1	Tbsp cumin
1	Tbsp granulated onion
2½	tsp granulated garlic
1	Tbsp sea salt
~	Pinch of cayenne

1. In a small bowl, mix ingredients until well blended. Store in an airtight container for up to 6 months.
2. To use, season 1 pound ground beef with 1½ Tbsp of seasoning mix. (1½ Tbsp mix = 1 packet store bought taco seasoning).

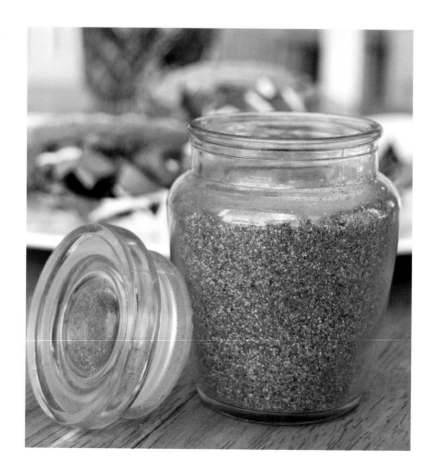

Sauces / Rubs / Dressings / Misc.

Italian Seasoning

Why spend money on this wonderfully versatile spice when you can make your own at home for a fraction of the cost? I use this blend on everything from salads to chicken to breads. Make a big batch, store some in an airtight container for you, and put the rest into a few fancy jars for your friends!

2	Tbsp basil
2	Tbsp marjoram
2	Tbsp oregano
1	Tbsp rosemary (preferably ground)
2	tsp thyme
2	tsp granulated onion
2	tsp granulated garlic

1. Mix together all ingredients and store in an airtight container for up to 6 months.

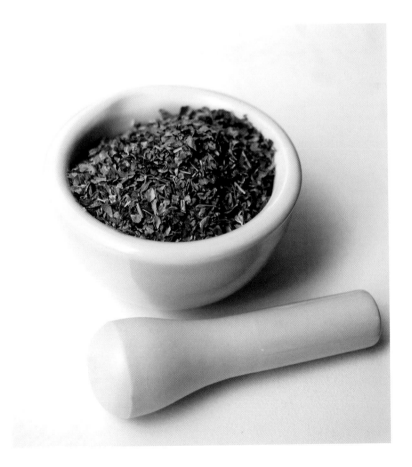

Steak Rub

This is our go-to seasoning blend anytime we grill steaks. It's easy but super-flavorful, and the honey gives it just the slightest touch of sweet that goes well with the spices. If you're feeling motivated, double or triple the recipe and keep the rub in an airtight container so it's ready when you need it.

Steaks:

4	grass-fed steaks (US Wellness Meats)
2–3	Tbsp raw organic honey

The Rub

1	Tbsp granulated onion
½	Tbsp granulated garlic
2	tsp sea salt
1	tsp pepper
1	tsp paprika
1	tsp basil
1	tsp parsley
1	tsp marjoram
¼	tsp rosemary
¼	tsp smoked paprika
¼	tsp celery seed
¼	tsp oregano
¼	tsp cumin
~	Pinch cayenne

1. In a small bowl, mix together rub ingredients until combined.
2. Drizzle honey over both sides of steaks and rub it in evenly with your hands to coat.
3. Sprinkle about 1 tsp of the rub on each side of the steaks, making sure to coat well and evenly.
4. Grill steaks, about 4 minutes per side (depending on cut of meat and thickness) or until done and still pink in the center.
5. Let steaks rest for 10 minutes. Serve and enjoy!

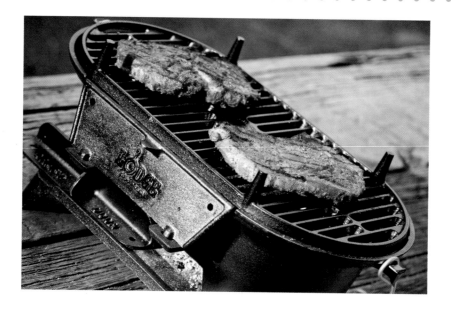

Sauces / Rubs / Dressings / Misc.

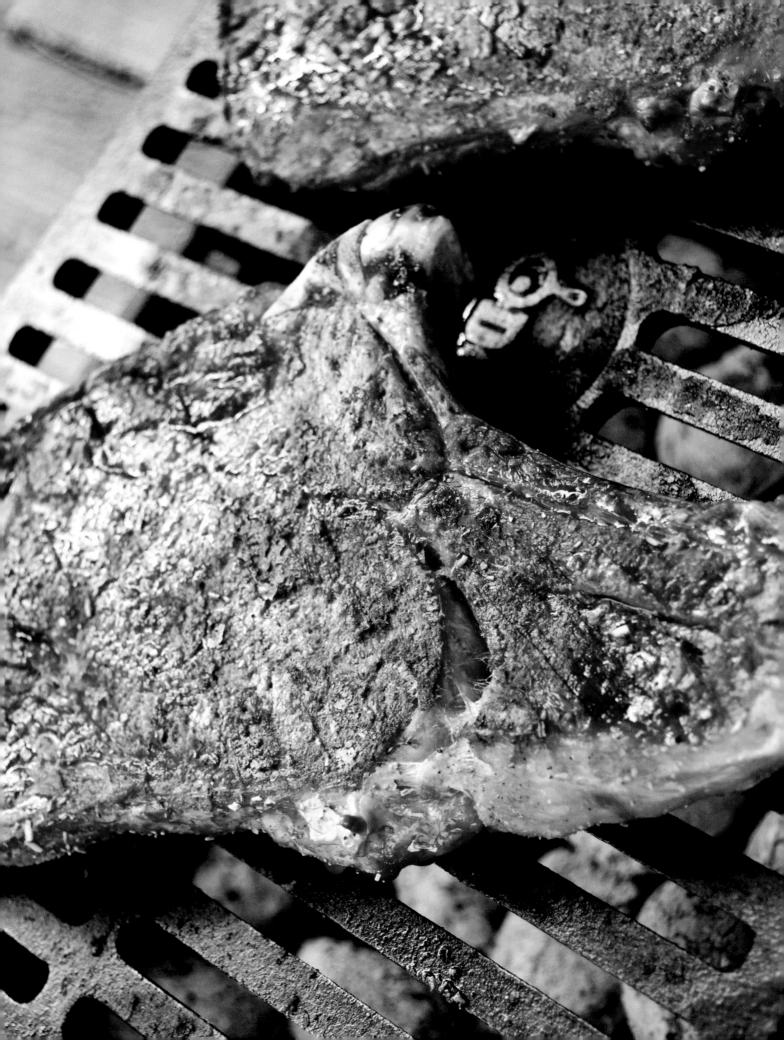

Pork Tenderloin Rub

My sister found the original version of this recipe somewhere... we really aren't sure where. But after tweaking it to fit her taste she blessed my kitchen with its yumminess. And I'm so glad she did! As a regular performer at our house, this rub is sure to become a favorite for you as well.

Pork:

2–3 lb (900–1350 g) organic pork tenderloin (US Wellness Meats)

Rub:

2	**Tbsp organic brown sugar**
1	**tsp yellow mustard**
1½	**tsp paprika**
1½	**tsp cumin**
1½	**tsp sea salt**
1	**tsp black pepper**
1	**tsp granulated garlic**
1	**tsp granulated onion**
1	**tsp rosemary**
½	**tsp sage**
½	**tsp thyme**

1. In a small bowl combine all rub ingredients.
2. Place tenderloin in a large zip-top bag. Add rub mixture. Seal top and squish loin around to cover it with the rub.
3. Refrigerate loin for at least 2 hours or overnight.
4. Bake loin in a 9" by 13" baking dish in a 375° oven for 30–45 minutes (depending on the size of the loin) or until the internal temperature reaches 160°. Let meat rest for 10 minutes and then slice and serve.

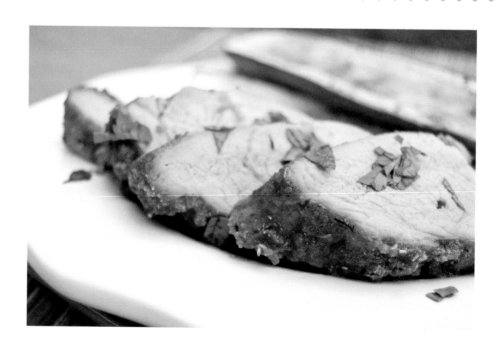

Sauces / Rubs / Dressings / Misc.

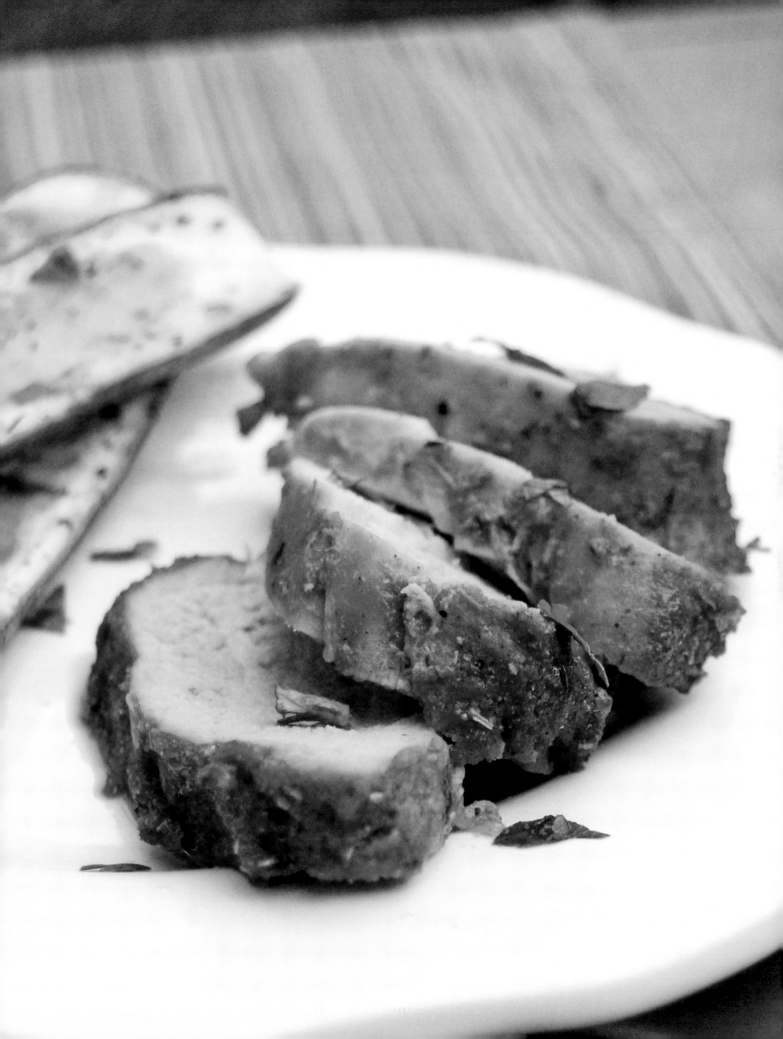

Speedy Guacamole

There are much more complicated and "proper" ways to make guacamole, but when I'm whipping this out for my kid's lunch, the last thing I want to do is spend 30 minutes dicing and chopping. This recipe, like most of mine, was born out of necessity. Healthy, quick, flavorful, and my kids love it. Good enough, I say! Try to keep salsa on hand at all times to add to various dishes for a kick of flavor, and to add that little somethin'-somethin' to this guacamole without any extra effort. Not that extra effort is a bad thing . . . except on a Monday morning at 7 AM prior to coffee. Then, not so much.

1	large ripe organic avocado
2	Tbsp of your favorite GF salsa
½	tsp granulated garlic
½	tsp granulated onion
½	tsp sea salt
⅛	tsp cumin
⅛	tsp chili powder
~	Freshly ground pepper to taste
~	Squeeze of lime juice

1. Scoop out avocado flesh into a medium bowl. Mash with a fork until fairly smooth, with some small chunks of avocado still in there.
2. Add remaining ingredients and stir to combine.
3. Enjoy as a veggie dip, with your favorite GF tortilla chips, or even as a dip for Steak Bites (p. 160) or Coconut Chicken Strips (p. 106)!

Serves 4–6

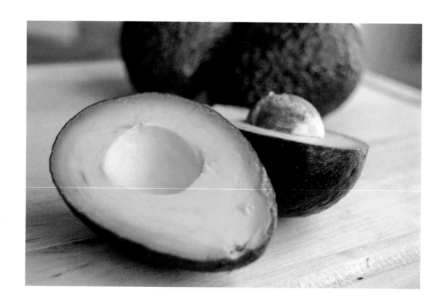

Sauces / Rubs / Dressings / Misc.

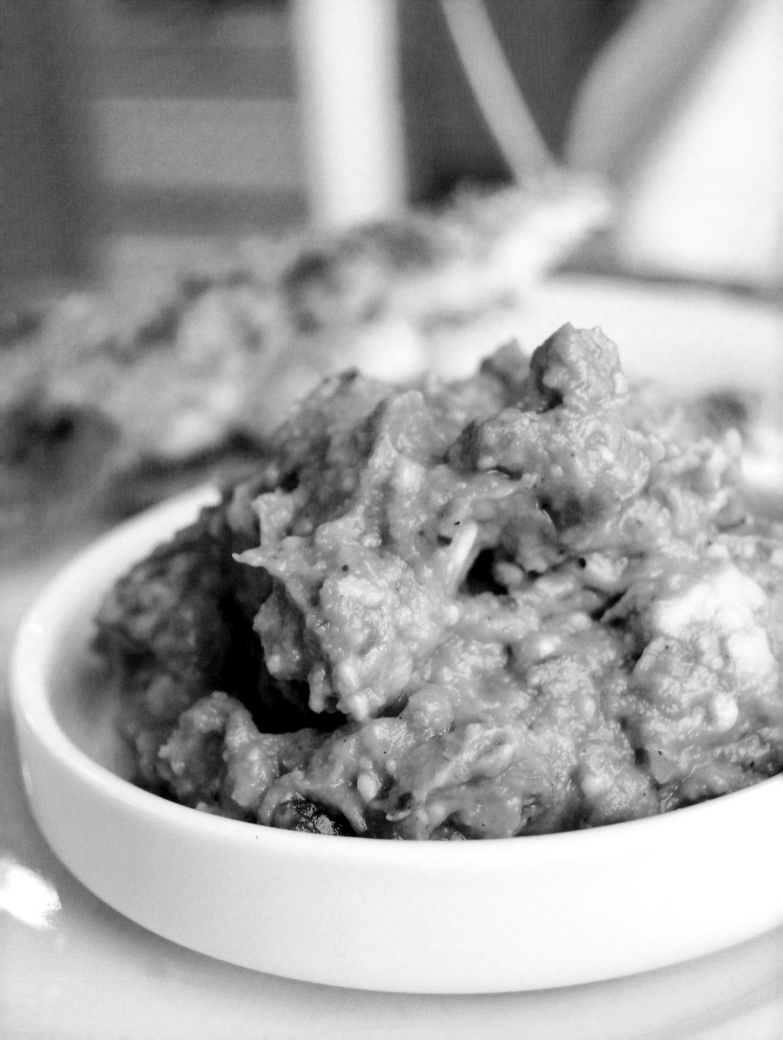

Shortcut Chicken Stock

While you can make chicken stock from a whole chicken, which is the preferred method, I'm often short on time, so I go for this quick and easy process. I still get quality chicken stock for a fraction of the cost, without wondering what strange things may have been added to it in the process.

1	**leftover organic chicken carcass (see tips)**
1	**large organic onion, quartered**
3	**large organic carrots, peeled and cut into chunks**
4	**ribs organic celery, washed and cut into chunks**
1	**handful fresh organic Italian parsley, roughly chopped**
1	**tsp thyme**
2	**bay leaves**
2	**whole garlic cloves, peeled and sliced**
~	**Sea salt**
~	**Pepper**
~	**Cold water**

1. Place all ingredients, except for water, in a large stock pot. Fill pot with cold water until it covers the chicken and vegetables, pretty much to the top.
2. Cook on high until it begins to boil. Turn heat to medium and simmer gently as long as you can, at least 3 hours.
3. Let stock cool a bit and strain it into glass canning jars. Let cool completely and freeze until needed. Make sure you only fill jars to the bottom of the curved neck to avoid cracking the glass as the liquid freezes and expands.

Tips:

~Whenever I make a whole chicken I keep the chicken carcass wrapped tightly in the freezer until I have time to make stock. Just throw it in frozen!

~Save leek tops, asparagus ends, etc. and freeze. When making stock, just throw in frozen pieces to add tons of flavor at no extra cost.

~My favorite, no-brainer way to make stock is with my extra-large slow cooker. I follow the same steps, but place it in my slow cooker on low and let it go for 24 hours. The stock is amazing!

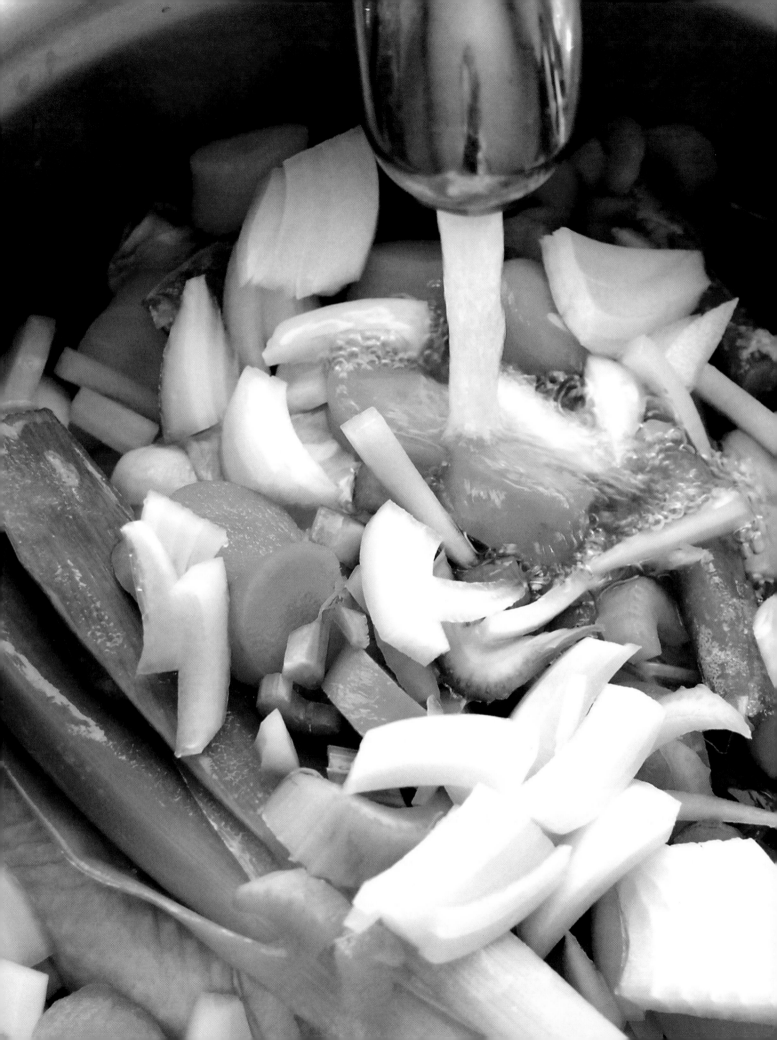

Honey Butter

No two words were ever better together. This honey butter was made specifically for my Sweet Potato Biscuits (p. 210), but it's also great on Quick Dinner Rolls (p. 386) or Blueberry English Muffins (p. 92).

½   **C (120 g) Earth Balance soy-free "butter"**

2   **big Tbsp of raw organic honey**

⅛   **tsp pure vanilla extract**

1. Whip all ingredients with a hand blender until light and fluffy and well blended. Don't mix too long or butter will start to separate. Serve immediately.

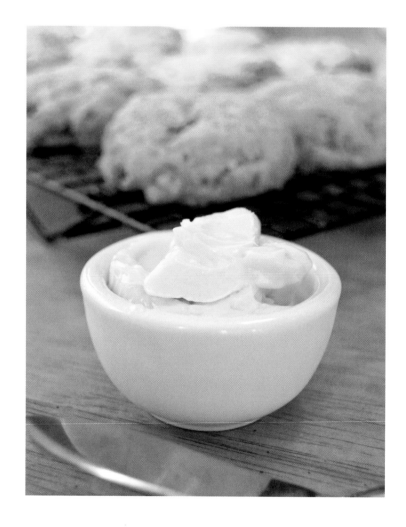

Strawberry Honey Butter
A Christmas morning treat!

A berry twist on my original honey butter. We like to have this butter on pancakes with maple syrup for Christmas morning. Makes it just a little bit more special with a dollop of this beautiful butter on top.

¾   C (180 g) nondairy butter, softened
     (Earth Balance Soy Free Spread)

⅓   C (50 g) minced organic strawberries

1   Tbsp softened raw organic honey

1   tsp fresh lemon juice

¼   tsp orange zest

1. With a hand mixer blend all ingredients in a medium bowl until smooth. Do not over mix!

2. Transfer butter to a pastry bag with tip, and then pipe into rounds on a parchment-lined baking sheet.

3. Freeze until firm and store in an airtight container in the fridge until needed, up to 2 days. Let the butter soften a bit before serving.

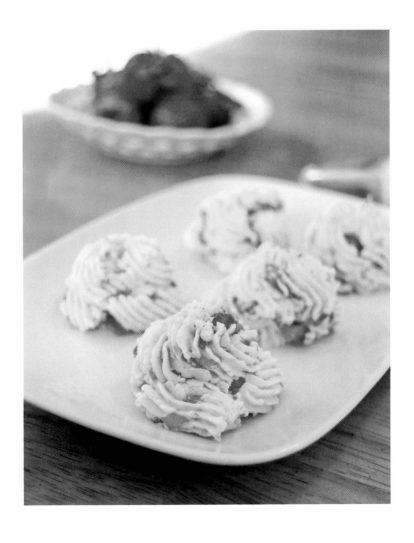

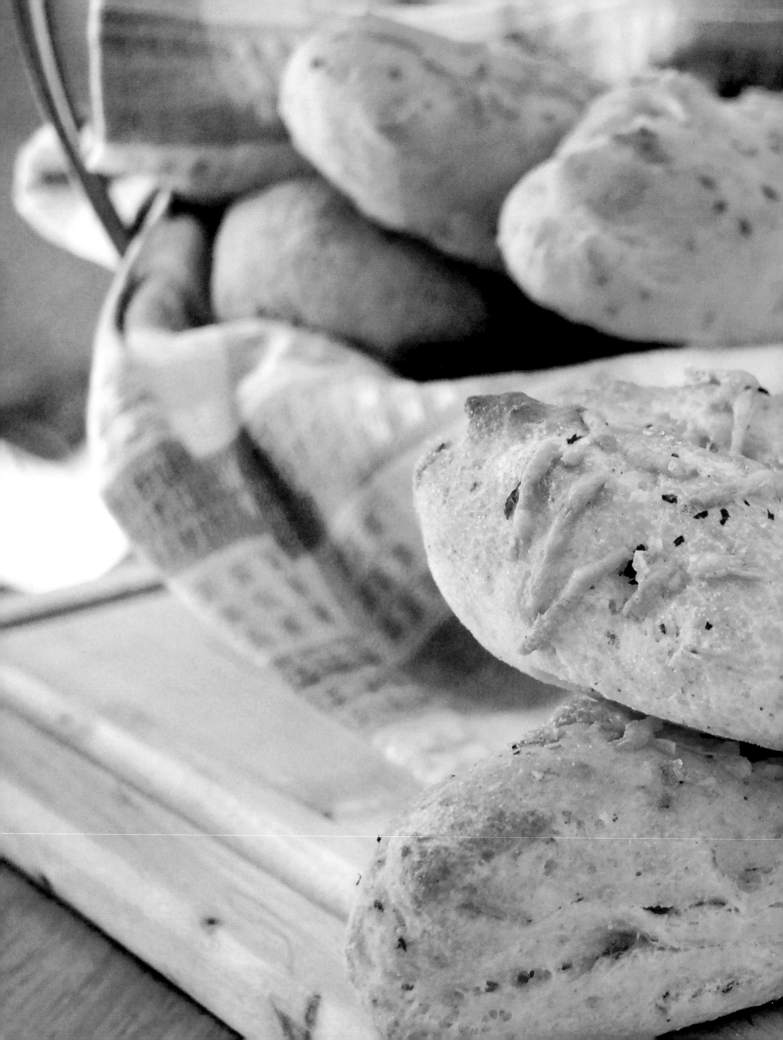

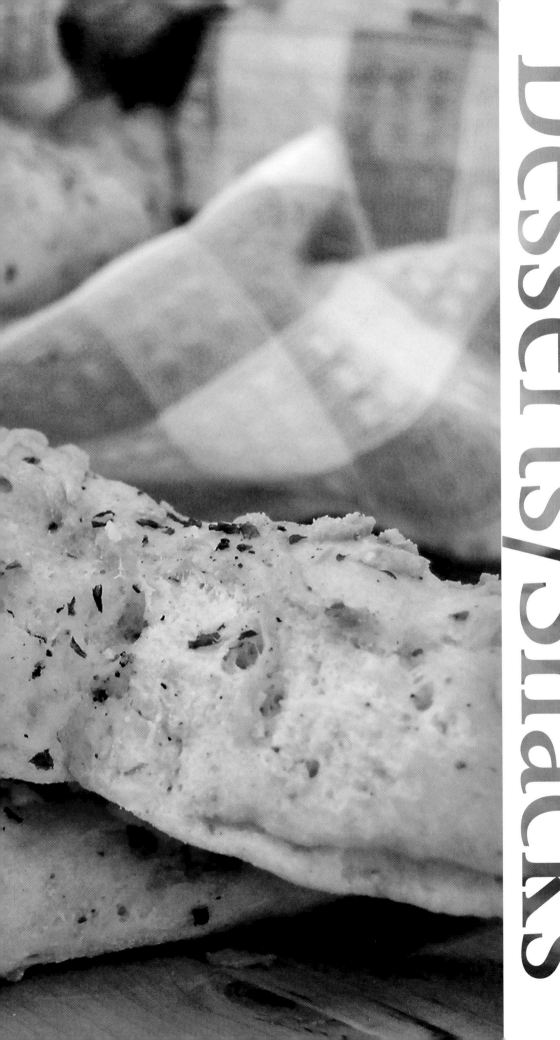

Baking/Desserts/Snacks

As Needed Chocolate Chip Cookies

This is where it all started for me. The love affair. The improper thoughts. The desire to assemble blah, boring dry ingredients from my pantry into something amazingly delicious. The love of baking and the almighty Chocolate Chip Cookie! I call these "as needed" because when it comes to a chocolate chip cookie, there is no want. It is a need, and when you need one, you need one, am I right? So mix up a batch or two. Or three. Freeze the dough until needed, then simply soften on the counter for an hour or so and scoop and bake as you normally would! Or, if you're like me and my children, you can thaw the dough and eat it straight from the container. Remember, no raw eggs, so you can eat as much as you like... or at least as much as your skinny jeans will allow.

Dry Ingredients:

1¼	C (150 g) sorghum flour
½	C (60 g) teff flour
¼	C (30 g) amaranth flour
¾	C (90 g) potato starch
¾	C (90 g) tapioca starch
2	tsp xanthan gum
1½	tsp baking soda
1	tsp baking powder
1½	tsp sea salt

Wet Ingredients:

2	Tbsp flax meal mixed with ⅓ C hot water
¾	C (180 g) nondairy butter
½	C (120 mL) organic shortening or coconut oil
1	C (180 g) packed organic brown sugar
½	C (100 g) organic evaporated cane juice (or ½ C [120 mL] organic raw honey or ½ C pure maple syrup)
1	Tbsp organic, unsweetened apple-sauce
1	Tbsp pure vanilla extract
10	oz bag (about 300 g) GF DF SF choco-late chips (Enjoy Life brand)

1. Whisk together dry ingredients.
2. In a small bowl, mix flax meal with hot water and set aside.
3. In a large mixing bowl, cream together butter, shortening, brown sugar, and sugar.
4. Add flax meal, applesauce, and vanilla. Mix until combined.
5. Slowly add the dry ingredients, about ½ cup at a time, to the wet ingredients, until fully incorporated. If for any reason the dough is too dry and doesn't stick together, slowly add in a little water until it comes together and looks like traditional cookie dough. Mix for 1 minute.
6. Stir in chocolate chips.
7. For best results, cover and refrigerate dough for 1 hour or overnight. Firm dough makes the best cookies. But if you can't wait (no judgment here) drop by teaspoonfuls onto parchment-lined baking sheets.
8. Bake at 350° for 11–12 minutes. The edges will be slightly browned, but they will not look done in the center. This is OK! Do not overbake. The trick here is to leave them doughy in the center. Once cool, the texture is moist, chewy, and perfect, plus they stay softer for a few days this way.

Tips:

See Kitchen Tips at the beginning of the book (p. 40) for directions on freezing cookie dough or making a dry mix ahead of time!

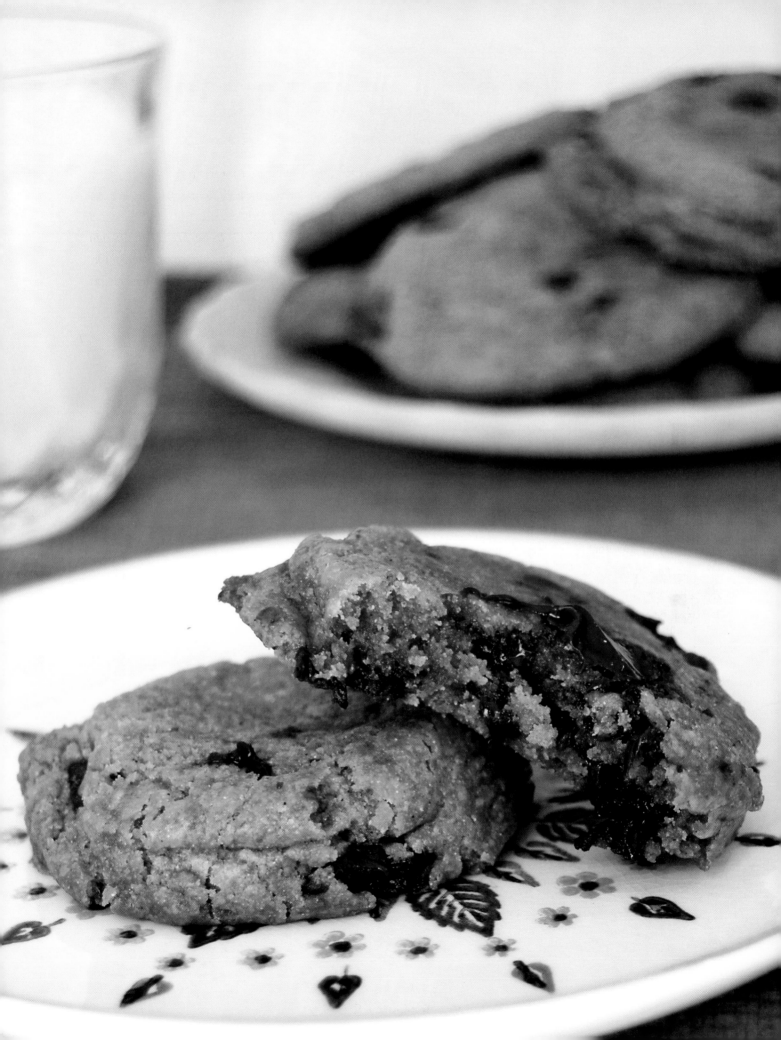

Grain-Free Lemon Cookies

Lemon is such a wonderful, light, tangy addition to many desserts and treats, including this cookie! Chewy, sweet, and a little bit of that lemon zing make this cookie wonderful on its own or with a cup of tea. They remind me of those lemon cooler cookies that were popular when I was a kid, except I can pronounce all of the ingredients for these.

1	**C (120 g) almond meal**
1	**Tbsp coconut flour**
¼	**C (30 g) organic unsweetened coconut flakes (coarsely chopped)**
¼	**C (60 mL) organic raw honey**
2	**Tbsp coconut oil (or nondairy butter)**
~	**Zest of 1 organic lemon**
2	**tsp fresh lemon juice**
~	**Powdered sugar for dusting**

1. In a medium bowl, combine all ingredients and mix well.
2. Place ½- Tbsp scoops of dough on a parchment-lined baking sheet.
3. Pat down each cookie with the palm of your hand.
4. Bake in a 350° oven for 10–11 minutes or until edges are lightly browned and center is set.
5. Let cool on baking sheet for 5 minutes, then transfer to a wire cooling rack to cool completely.
6. Dust cookies with a light sprinkle of powdered sugar. Enjoy!

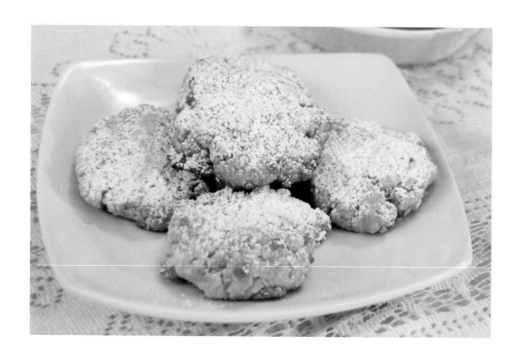

Baking / Desserts / Snacks

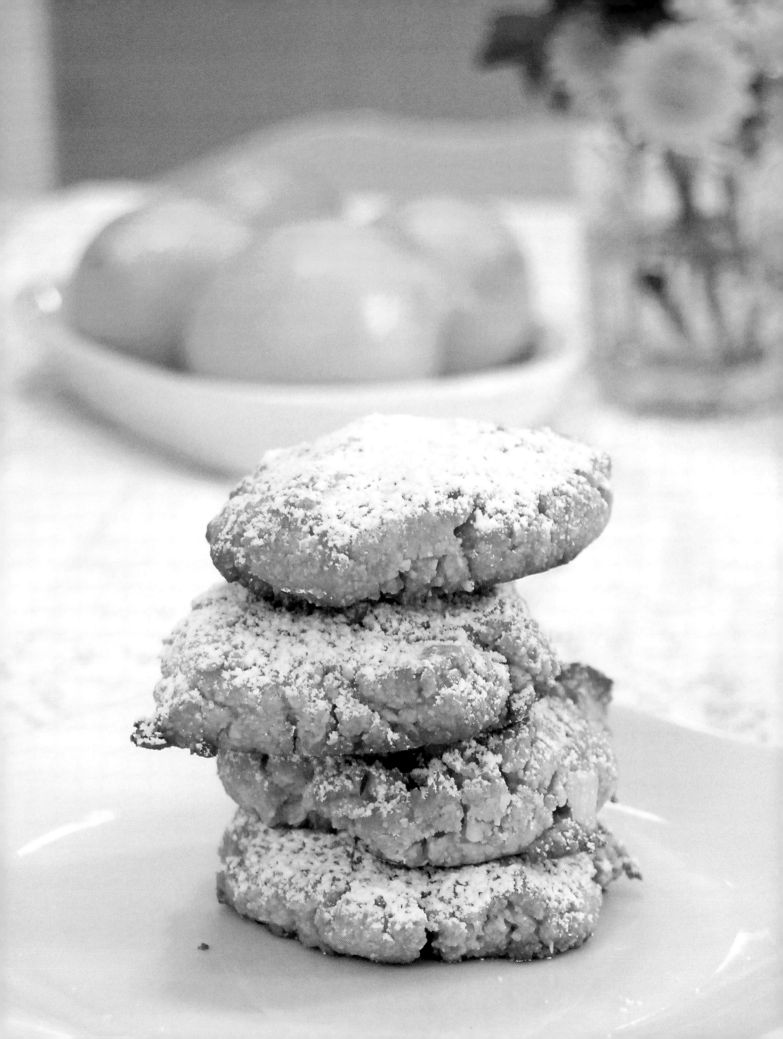

High Desert Cookies

This cookie was modeled after the cowboy cookie, which includes a lot more sugar and loads of oats. And because oats are such a gray area for most gluten-intolerant people, we didn't include any oats in this book, or in this cookie. And you know what? You won't miss them at all! The wonderful hint of orange, with the coconut and pecans, fill this big cookie up like nobody's business. By far our best selling cookie at any farmers market or event, one bite and you'll be a fan of the High Desert as well.

Dry Ingredients:

1¼	C (150 g)	sorghum flour
½	C (60 g)	teff flour
¼	C (30 g)	amaranth flour
¾	C (90 g)	potato starch
¾	C (90 g)	tapioca starch
2	tsp	xanthan gum
1½	tsp	baking soda
1	tsp	baking powder
1½	tsp	sea salt

Wet Ingredients:

¾	C (180 g)	nondairy butter
½	C (95 g)	organic shortening
1	C (180 g)	packed organic brown sugar
½	C (100 g)	organic evaporated cane juice (or ½ C [120 ml] organic raw honey or ½ C pure maple syrup)
2	Tbsp	flax meal mixed with ⅓ C hot water
1	Tbsp	organic unsweetened applesauce
1	Tbsp	pure vanilla extract

Add Ins:

2	C (300 g)	chopped toasted pecans
1	C (150 g)	nondairy chocolate chips
1	C (90 g)	organic unsweetened coconut flakes
¼	tsp	orange zest

1. Whisk together dry ingredients.
2. In a large mixing bowl, cream together butter, shortening, brown sugar, and sugar.
3. Add flax meal, applesauce, and vanilla. Mix until combined.
4. Slowly add the dry ingredients, about ½ cup at a time, to the wet ingredients, until fully incorporated. Mix for 1 minute.
5. Stir in pecans, chocolate chips, coconut, and orange zest. Mix to combine.
6. For best results, cover and refrigerate dough for 1 hour or overnight.
7. Drop by large teaspoonfuls onto parchment-lined baking sheets.
8. Bake at 350° for about 11–12 minutes, until edges are slightly brown. Do not overbake.

Options:

Be sure to check out our tips on freezing cookie dough or making a dry mix ahead of time, in the front section of the book.

Baking / Desserts / Snacks

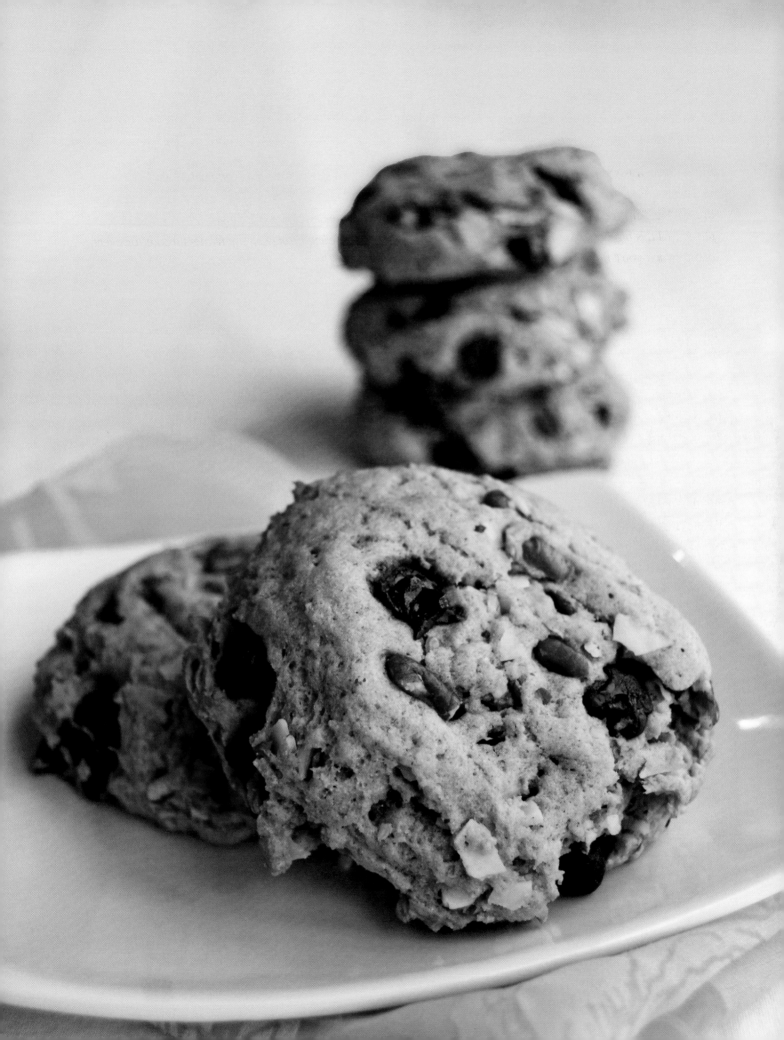

Chocolate Almond Cookies

If there were ever two words that belonged together when describing a cookie, its "chocolate" and "almonds." Fudgy in the middle, crispy on the edges, with bits of melted chocolate chips, and that hint of almond extract that leaves people saying, "What's in this cookie? It's delicious!" And this little beauty is just fancy enough to give as gifts or take to your next holiday cookie exchange. With a cookie this good, no one will be able to guess it is gluten-free, dairy-free, and egg-free!

Dry Ingredients:

¼	C (30 g) almond meal
¾	C (90 g) sorghum flour
½	C (60 g) brown rice flour
¾	C (90 g) potato starch
¾	C (90 g) tapioca starch
1	Tbsp xanthan gum
1	tsp baking soda
1	tsp baking powder
1	tsp sea salt
¾	C (90 g) organic cocoa powder

Wet Ingredients:

2	Tbsp flax meal mixed with ⅓ C hot water
1	C (240 g) nondairy butter
¾	C (135 g) packed organic brown sugar
½	C (100 g) organic evaporated cane juice
1	Tbsp pure vanilla extract
1	tsp pure almond extract
2	Tbsp unsweetened organic apple-sauce

Add Ons:

~	Organic evaporated cane juice
~	Raw slivered almonds
1	bag Enjoy Life mini chocolate chips

1. Whisk together dry ingredients.
2. In a small bowl, mix flax meal with hot water and set aside.
3. In a large mixing bowl, cream together butter, brown sugar, and sugar.
4. Add flax meal, applesauce, vanilla, and almond extract. Mix until combined.
5. Slowly add the dry ingredients, about ½ cup at a time to the wet ingredients, until fully incorporated. If for any reason the dough is too dry and doesn't stick together, slowly add in a little water until it comes together and looks like traditional cookie dough. Mix for 1 minute.
6. Stir in chocolate chips.
7. For best results, cover and refrigerate dough for 1 hour. Scoop and roll dough into balls with hands. Roll dough in evaporated cane juice and place on parchment-lined baking sheets.
8. Lightly press 3 slivered almonds into tops of each cookie, flattening dough ball slightly.
9. Bake at 350° for 10 minutes. Do not overbake.
10. Cool on baking sheets for 10 minutes, then move to cooling racks to cool completely. Store in an airtight container for up to 3 days.

Options:

See beginning of the book for tricks on freezing cookie dough or making a dry mix ahead of time!

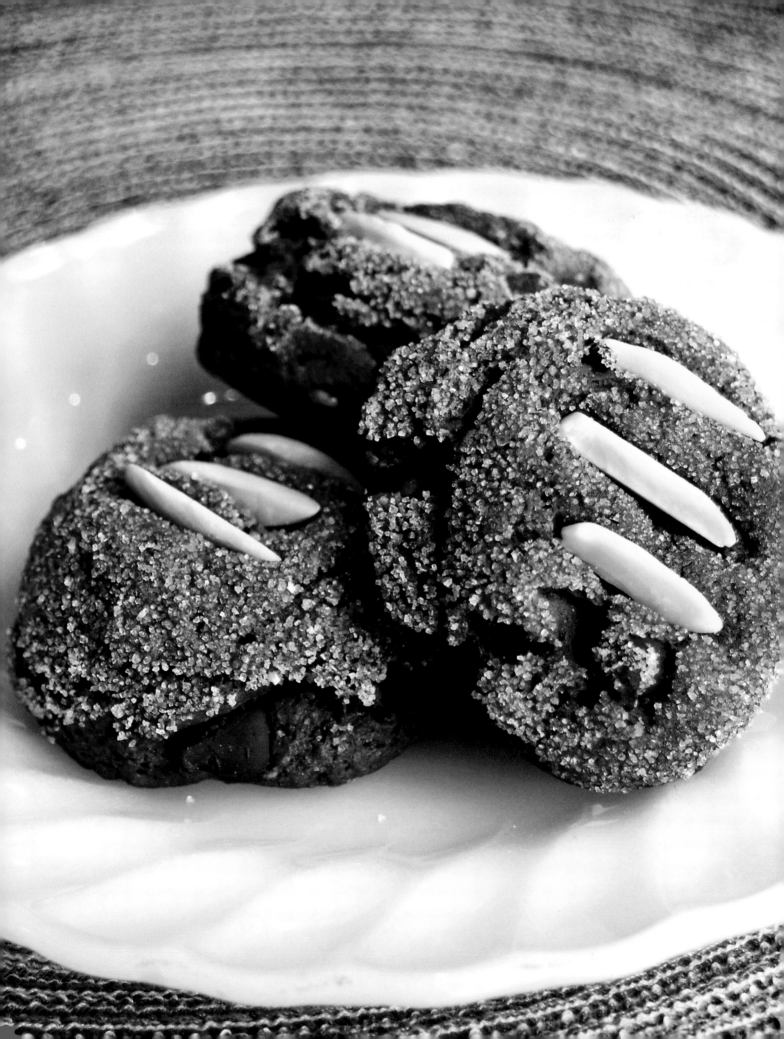

Sweet Potato Spice Cookie

This is a great fall cookie, filled with satisfying spices and sweet potatoes. It's perfect with a cup of coffee or tea if you have a quiet morning or, if you're like me, with a gallon of coffee after the kids are off to school and the morning rush is over.

Dry Ingredients:

1	C (120 g) sorghum flour
½	C (60 g) quinoa flour
¾	C (90 g) potato starch
¾	C (90 g) tapioca starch
2	tsp xanthan gum
1	tsp baking soda
2	tsp baking powder
1	tsp sea salt
2	tsp organic cinnamon
½	tsp nutmeg

Wet Ingredients:

½	C (120 g) nondairy butter or organic vegetable shortening
3	Tbsp pure maple syrup
½	C (90 g) packed organic brown sugar
¾	C (110 g) organic, cooked, mashed sweet potatoes
2	tsp pure vanilla extract
1	Tbsp flax meal mixed with 3 Tbsp hot water

Add Ins:

½	C (75 g) pecans
1	C (150 g) organic raisins
~	Maple Glaze, (p. 383)

1. In a large bowl, whisk dry ingredients together.
2. In a stand mixer, cream butter, maple syrup, and brown sugar together.
3. Add sweet potatoes, vanilla, and flax meal. Mix briefly.
4. Slowly add in dry ingredients. Blend until incorporated. Turn mixer to high and blend for 30 seconds.
5. With the mixer on low, add in raisins and pecans.
6. Scoop by tablespoon onto parchment-lined cookie sheets.
7. Bake in a 350° oven for 10–12 minutes or until set and edges start to brown.
8. Let cool on pans 5 minutes, then transfer cookies to a wire rack to cool completely.
9. Frost with Maple Glaze.

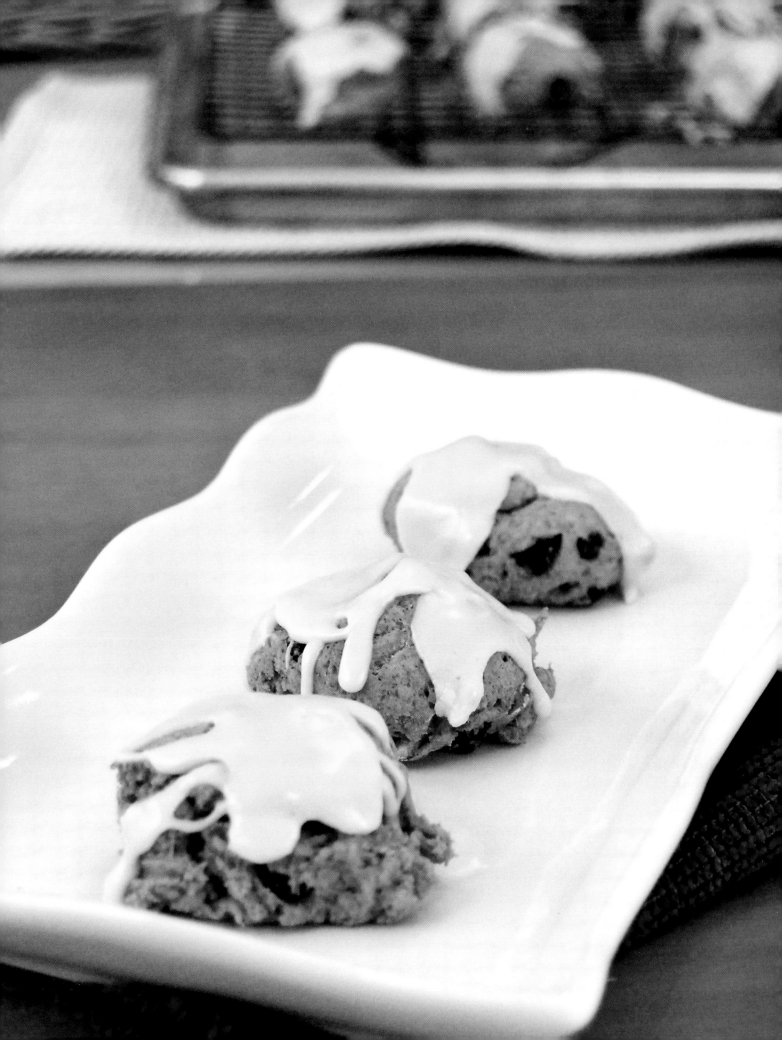

Double Trouble Chocolate Chip Cookies

Another customer favorite here at The Celiac Maniac, these rich, fudgy cookies will leave you wondering why you ever thought brownies were so great! And you can feel a little better with a treat made with powerhouse whole grains like sorghum, teff, and amaranth, not to mention the wonderful antioxidants found in real organic cocoa powder. So go ahead and indulge that chocolate craving! These fudgy treats won't leave you nutritionally bankrupt like those tasteless white rice flour packaged goods do.

Dry Ingredients:

¾	C (90 g) sorghum flour
½	C (60 g) teff flour
¼	C (30 g) amaranth flour
¾	C (90 g) potato starch
¾	C (90 g) tapioca starch
1	C (120 g) organic cocoa powder
1	Tbsp xanthan gum
1½	tsp baking soda
1	tsp baking powder
1	tsp sea salt

Wet Ingredients:

2	Tbsp flax meal mixed with ⅓ C hot water
1	C (240 g) nondairy butter
1	C (180 g) packed organic brown sugar
½	C (100 g) organic evaporated cane juice (or ½ C [120 mL] raw organic honey or ½ C pure maple syrup)
⅓	C (80 mL) unsweetened organic applesauce
1	Tbsp pure vanilla extract

Add Ins:

10	oz bag (about 300 g) GF DF SF chocolate chips (Enjoy Life is our go-to brand)

1. Whisk together dry ingredients.
2. In a small bowl combine flax meal and hot water. Set aside.
3. In a large mixing bowl, cream together butter, brown sugar, and sugar.
4. Add flax meal, applesauce, and vanilla. Mix until combined.
5. Slowly add the dry ingredients, about ½ cup at a time, to the wet ingredients, until fully incorporated. Mix for 1 minute.
6. Stir in chocolate chips.
7. For best results, cover and refrigerate dough for 1 hour or overnight.
8. Drop by teaspoonfuls onto parchment-lined baking sheets.
9. Bake at 350° for about 11–12 minutes. Do not overbake.

Options:

See front of book for freezing cookie dough or making dry mixes ahead of time!

Baking / Desserts / Snacks

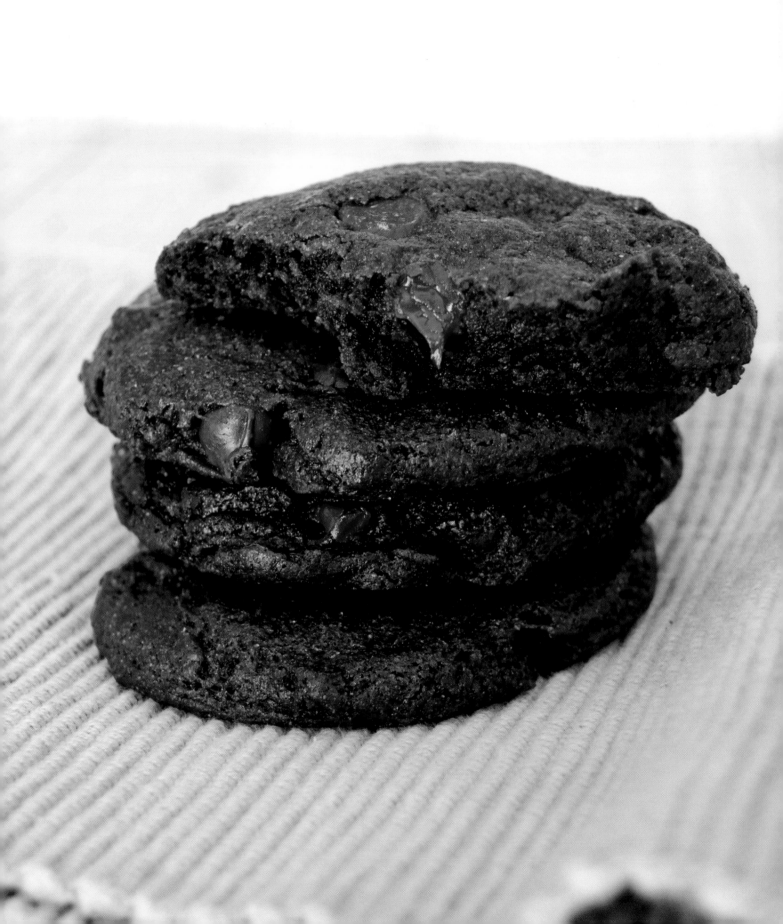

Cranberry Walnut Cookies

If it's any indication of a good cookie, my family polished off a plate of these in about 5 minutes the first time I made them. The tart cranberry plays off of the toasted walnuts nicely, giving a mouth-satisfying, not overly sweet bite. The glaze is optional, of course, but it gives it a little dressed-up feel, perfect for the holidays or special occasions. This cookie and the glaze make a great base for any combination of flavors, so get a little creative with this one! Try adding coconut or dried cherries to the cookie dough, or how about a maple glaze or orange glaze for the tops? The only thing you have to decide is what flavor you're in the mood for!

Dry Ingredients:

1	C (120 g) brown rice flour
¾	C (90 g) sorghum flour
½	C (60 g) potato starch
¾	C (90 g) tapioca starch
2	tsp xanthan gum
1½	tsp baking soda
1	tsp baking powder
1	tsp sea salt
1	tsp cinnamon

Wet Ingredients:

2	Tbsp flax meal mixed with ⅓ C hot water
1	C (240 g) nondairy butter
½	C (90 g) packed organic brown sugar
¾	C (150 g) organic evaporated cane juice (or ½ C [120 mL] raw organic honey or ½ C pure maple syrup)
1	Tbsp pure vanilla extract

Add Ins:

1	C (150 g) toasted walnuts, chopped
1	C (150 g) dried cranberries, coarsely chopped

1. Whisk together dry ingredients.
2. In a small bowl, combine flax meal and hot water. Set aside.
3. In a large mixing bowl, cream together butter, brown sugar, and sugar.
4. Add flax meal and vanilla. Mix until combined.
5. Slowly add the dry ingredients, about ½ cup at a time, to the wet ingredients, until fully incorporated. If for any reason the dough is too dry and doesn't stick together, slowly add in a little water until it comes together and looks like traditional cookie dough. Mix for 1 minute.
6. Stir in walnuts and cranberries.
7. Drop by teaspoonfuls onto parchment-lined baking sheets.
8. Bake at 350° for about 11 minutes. The edges will be slightly browned and they will be soft to the touch in the center. Do not overbake.
9. Cool completely on cooling racks, then drizzle tops with glaze. Recipe follows.

Glaze:

¼	C (25 g) organic powdered sugar
1	tsp softened nondairy butter
2	tsp nondairy milk
¼	tsp pure vanilla extract

1. Whisk together ingredients in a small bowl with a fork until combined and slightly runny in consistency. If it's too thick, add a few drops of water or milk until desired consistency is achieved.
2. Drizzle over cooled cookies.

Baking / Desserts / Snacks

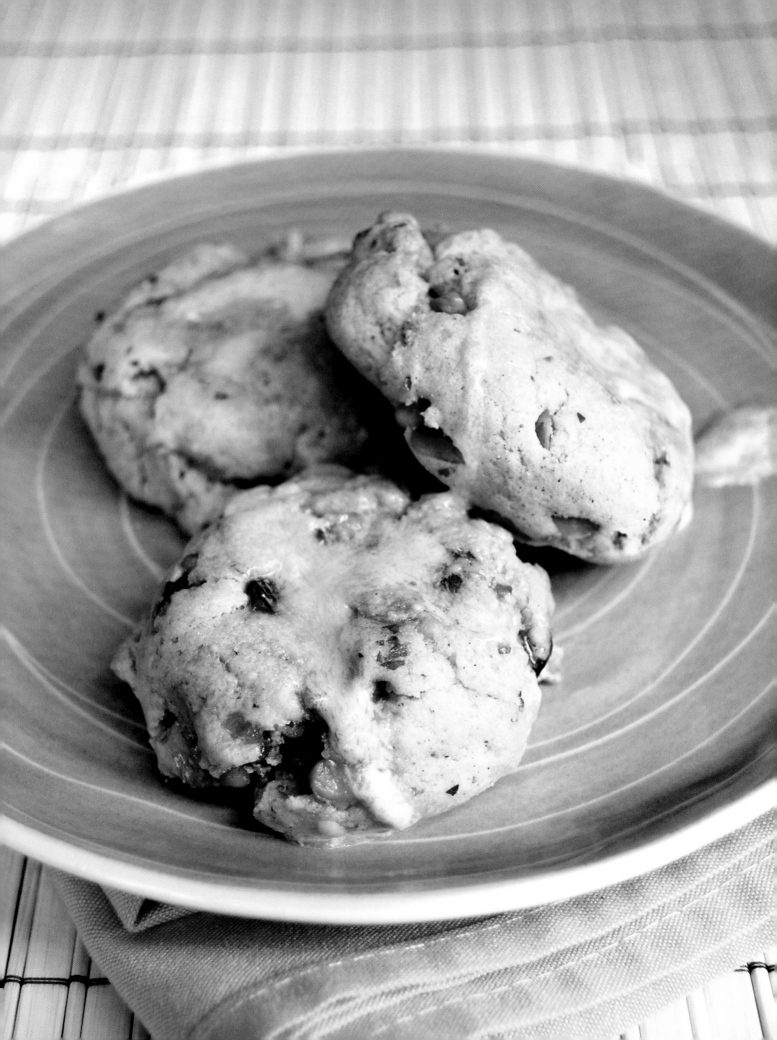

Almond Orange Coconut Cookies

With a delicate balance of nuts, coconut, honey, and orange zest, these cookies are incredibly delicious. Feel free to double the batch, you'll need it!

1	C (120 g) almond meal
¼	C (22 g) organic unsweetened coconut flakes
¼	C (60 mL) raw organic honey
2	Tbsp coconut oil (or nondairy butter)
~	Zest of 1 organic orange

1. In a medium bowl, combine all ingredients and mix well.
2. Place ½-Tbsp scoops of dough on a parchment-lined baking sheet.
3. Pat down each cookie with the palm of your hand.
4. Bake in a 350° oven for 10–11 minutes or until edges are lightly browned and center is set.
5. Let cool on baking sheet for 5 minutes, then transfer to a wire cooling rack to cool completely.

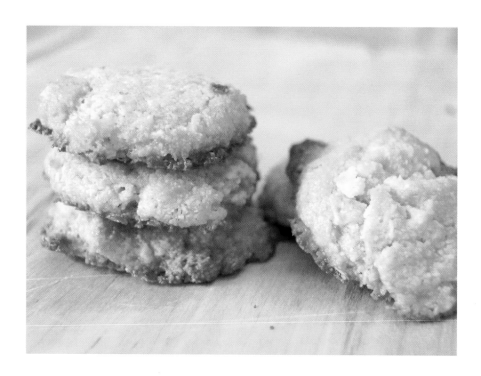

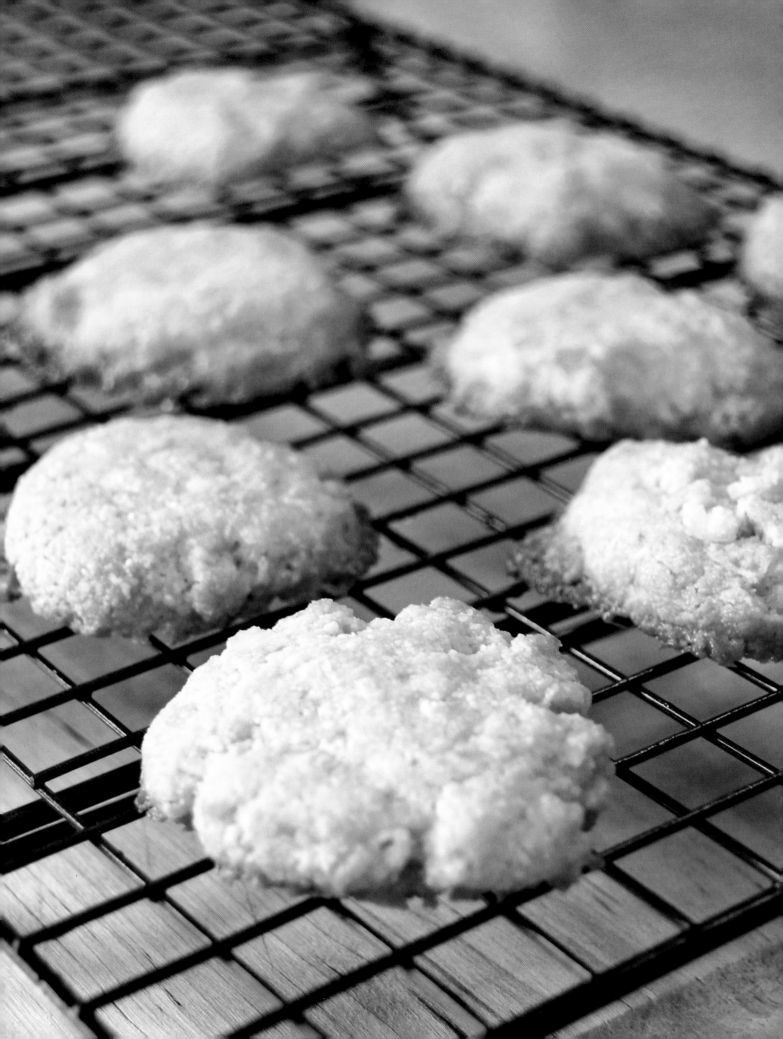

No'Oatmeal Raisin Cookies

Raw seeds make a great flour to use in lots of baked goods. They have a surprisingly neutral flavor, especially sunflower seeds. Plus, they have higher protein, so they help baked goods with lift and texture without having to use nuts, which can be problematic for a lot of folks.

¼	C (40 g) raw pumpkin seeds
¾	C (110 g) raw sunflower seeds
2	Tbsp coconut flour
1	Tbsp tapioca starch
¼	tsp cinnamon
¼	C (60 mL) raw organic honey
2	tsp pure vanilla extract
1	Tbsp unsweetened organic apple-sauce
1	Tbsp coconut oil, melted
2	Tbsp finely shredded unsweetened organic coconut
⅓	C (50 g) organic raisins

1. Place raw pumpkin and sunflower seeds in a food processor and pulse until they are the consistency of a coarse flour.
2. In a large bowl whisk together seed flour, coconut flour, tapioca starch, and cinnamon.
3. Add in honey, vanilla, applesauce, and coconut oil. Mix well with a wooden spoon or in a stand mixer.
4. Fold in coconut and raisins.
5. Scoop 1 Tbsp of dough for each cookie onto a parchment-lined baking sheet.
6. Bake in a 350° oven for 11–12 minutes or until cookies are lightly browned on edges.
7. Allow to cool 5 minutes on baking sheet, then transfer to a wire cooling rack.

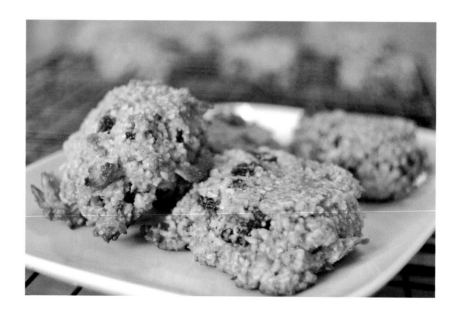

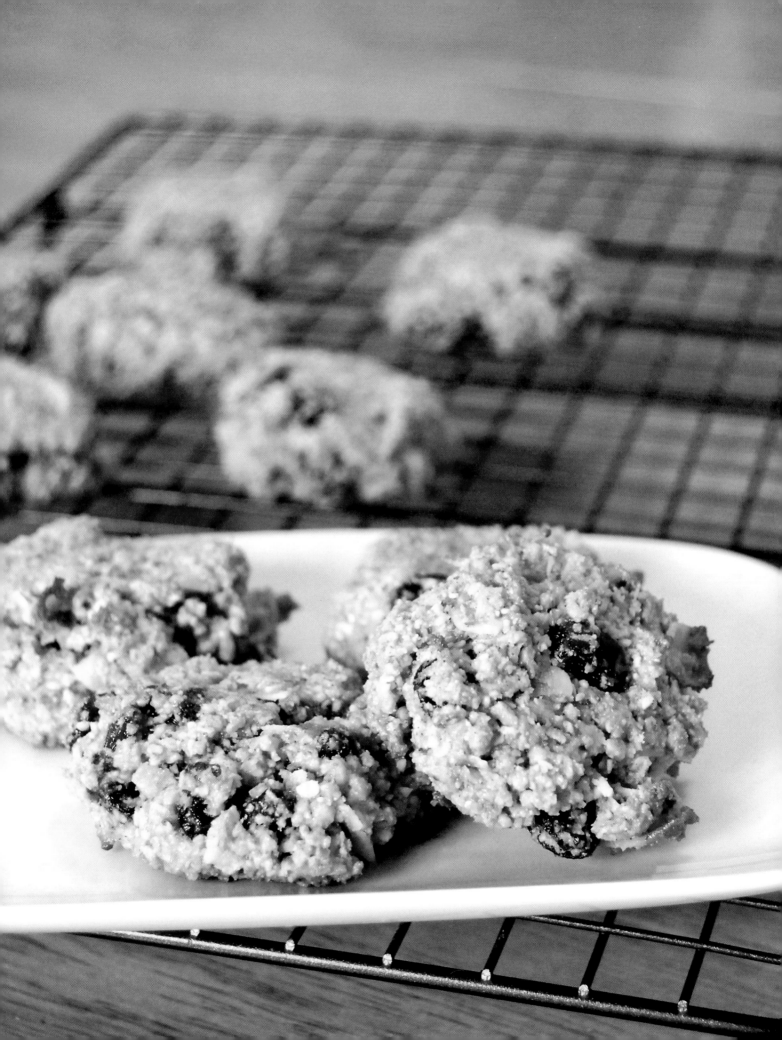

Peanut Butter Cookies

These classic peanut butter cookies remind me of my childhood. You see, while chocolate chip cookies were always my favorite, my mom's favorite was peanut butter. So while I was at school, mom would make a big batch of peanut butter cookies and look innocently at me as I came through the door at 3:30. In time, peanut butter became a close contender in the race for favorite cookie for me. And if you add chocolate chips to this recipe? Well, now it's the best of both worlds! I guess mom really does know best!

Dry Ingredients:

½	C (60 g) sorghum flour
¼	C (30 g) teff flour
⅓	C (40 g) potato starch
⅓	C (40 g) tapioca starch
1	tsp xanthan gum
½	tsp baking soda
½	tsp baking powder
½	tsp sea salt

Wet Ingredients:

¾	C (180 g) nondairy butter
⅓	C (65 g) organic evaporated cane juice
¾	C (135 g) packed organic brown sugar
1 ¼	C (300 mL) GF natural chunky peanut butter
1	Tbsp pure vanilla extract
1	Tbsp flax meal mixed with ¼ C hot water

1. Whisk together dry ingredients.
2. In a large mixing bowl, cream together butter and sugars.
3. Add peanut butter, vanilla, and flax meal mixture water. Mix until combined.
4. Slowly add the dry ingredients, about ½ cup at a time, to the wet ingredients, until fully incorporated. Mix for 1 minute.
5. Chill dough for 1 hour.
6. Roll dough in hands to form balls. Place on parchment-lined baking sheets. Press a fork into tops, then across the other direction to make a checkered pattern on tops.
7. Bake at 350° for about 10–11 minutes or until edges are slightly browned. Do not overbake.
8. Cool completely on wire racks and enjoy. Store in an airtight container for up to 4 days.

Options:

~Be sure to see my options for freezing cookie dough or making the dry mix ahead of time (p. 40).

~Try mixing in chocolate chips to the dough for a chocolate peanut buttery treat!

Baking / Desserts / Snacks

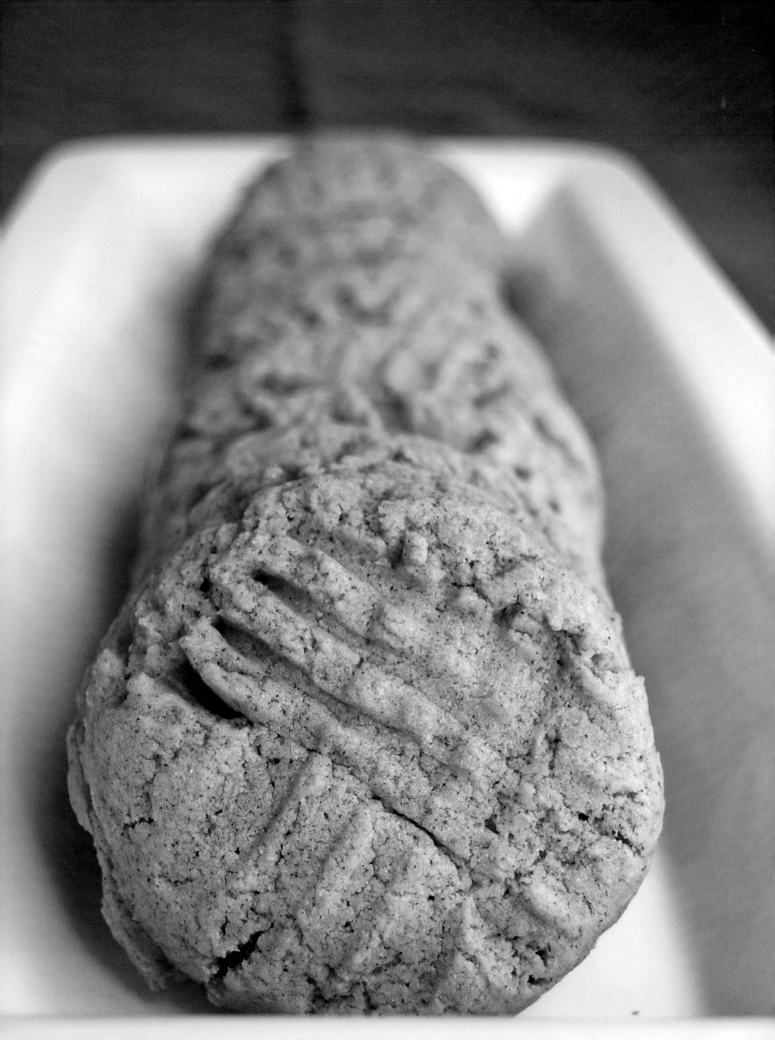

Sugar Cookies

The best-kept secret for sugar cookie cut outs is to roll the dough between two sheets of parchment paper, remove the top sheet, cut out the cookies, remove excess dough, and transfer the paper with cookie shapes to your baking pan. No more trying to scrape up sticky GF dough with a spatula to transfer to your baking sheet. Just be sure to leave some space between your cutouts so cookies have room to spread a little.

Dry Ingredients:

¾	C (90 g) teff flour
½	C (60 g) brown rice flour
¾	C (90 g) sorghum flour
1	C (120 g) potato starch
¾	C (90 g) tapioca starch
2	tsp xanthan gum
1	tsp salt
1½	tsp baking soda

Wet Ingredients:

2	Tbsp flax meal mixed with ⅓ C hot water
1	C (240 g) nondairy butter
1	C (200 g) organic evaporated cane juice
2	Tbsp pure vanilla extract
⅛	tsp pure almond extract
1	Tbsp unsweetened organic apple-sauce

Add On:

~ Sugar Cookie Icing (p. 382)

1. Whisk together dry ingredients.
2. Mix flax meal with hot water. Set aside.
3. In a stand mixer, cream butter and sugar together.
4. Add vanilla, almond extract, applesauce, and flax meal mixture. Mix until combined.
5. Add dry ingredients to wet ingredients a little at a time until fully incorporated. Blend on high for 30 seconds.
6. If dough is too soft, refrigerate for 1 hour before rolling out.
7. Roll dough between sheets of parchment paper (the same size as your baking sheets). When the dough is ¼ inch thick, remove the top sheet of paper. Using cookie cutter, cut shapes into dough. Remove excess dough, leaving cookie shapes on the bottom sheet of parchment. No need to transfer cookies! Place parchment with cookie shapes onto your baking sheet.
8. Bake cookies in a 350° oven for 10 minutes, or until edges start to turn brown.
9. Cool in pan for 3 minutes, then transfer cookies to a wire rack to cool completely.
10. Frost with Sugar Cookie Icing.

Options:

~For chocolate sugar cookies, reduce teff flour by ¼ C and add ⅓ C cocoa powder.

~If you're not in the mood to frost cookies, just sprinkle tops with sugar prior to baking.

~Try cutting out cookies in circle shapes, and then another circle with the middle cut out. After cookies have cooled, spread jelly on the whole circle and top with the second circle that has the hole cut in the middle. Sprinkle with powdered sugar.

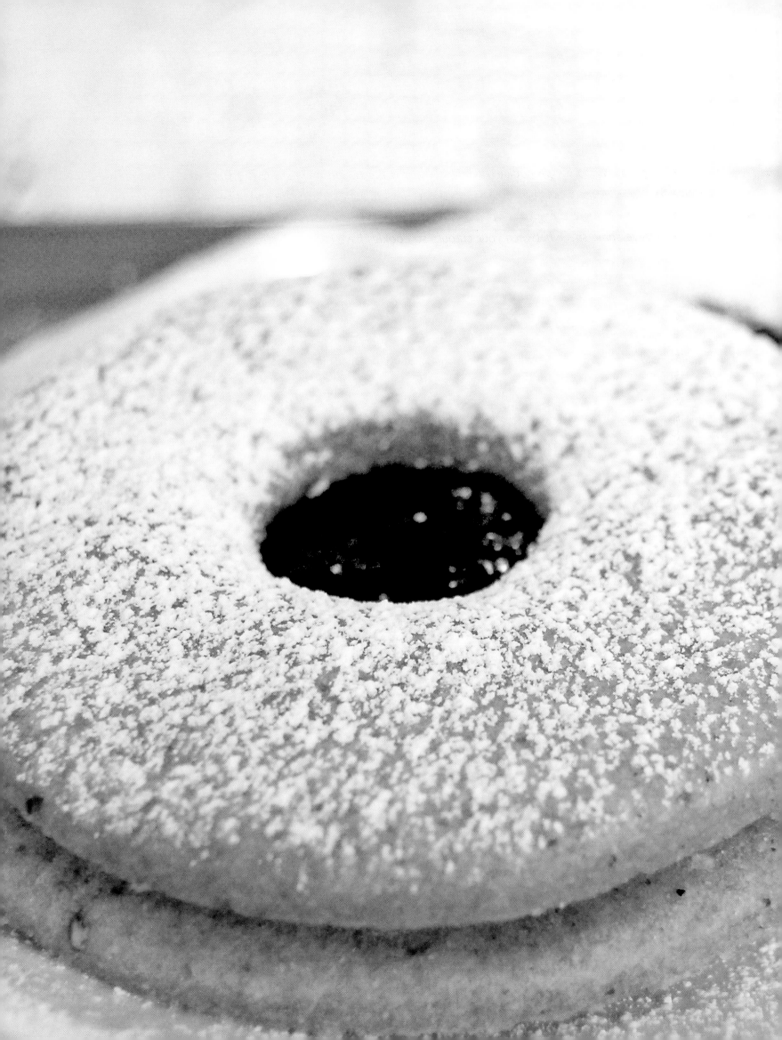

No Bake Cookies

No Bake Cookies are a great way to get your kiddos helping in the kitchen. They get to create a treat and get their hands dirty, and there's very little wait time, unlike baking. You can even let them decide what ingredients to use. Almond butter or sunbutter? Almonds or walnuts? Maybe a few raisins or dried cranberries? Let them decide and see what you can create together!

⅓ C (80 mL) almond butter

1 tsp pure vanilla extract

¼ C (60 mL) coconut oil, softened

2 Tbsp raw organic honey

½ C (45 g) shredded unsweetened organic coconut

½ C (75 g) roasted salted almond slivers

½ C (70 g) GF pretzels, crushed

¼ C (40 g) mini chocolate chips (Enjoy Life brand)

1. Let little hands mix all ingredients in a medium bowl.
2. Roll into balls and place on a parchment-lined baking sheet.
3. Freeze until firm. Store in airtight containers in the fridge or freezer.

Nut-free version

¼ C (60 mL) sunbutter

1½ tsp pure vanilla extract

¼ C (60 mL) coconut oil, softened

2 Tbsp raw organic honey

½ C (45 g) shredded unsweetened organic coconut

1 C (150 g) GF pretzels, crushed

¼ C (40 g) roasted salted sunflower seeds

¼ C (40 g) mini chocolate chips (Enjoy Life brand)

1. See above instructions!

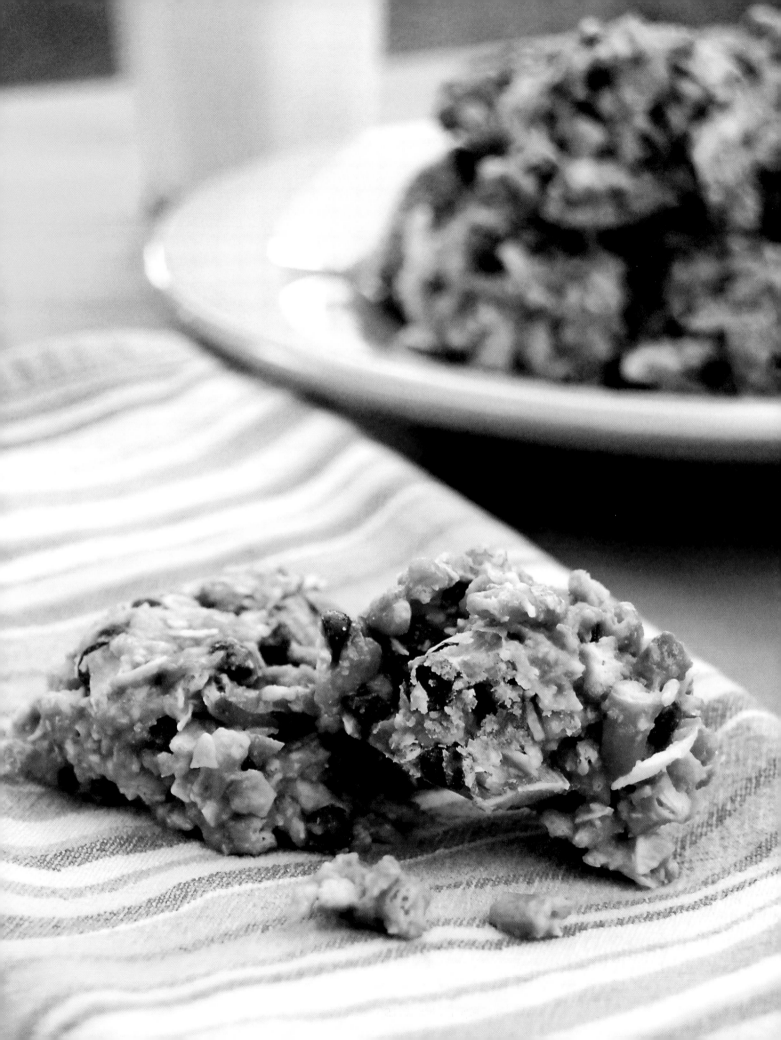

Sunbutter Patty Tagalongs

Girl Scouts have nothing on these cookies! If you've been missing that annual knock at your door since going gluten-free, you will be so excited the first time you make these! The few steps it takes to make these cookies are well worth it, trust me.

2	**dozen Sugar Cookie rounds (recipe p. 294)**
1	**C (150 g) nondairy chocolate chips (Enjoy Life)**
1	**tsp organic shortening (Spectrum brand)**
~	**Organic creamy sunbutter**

1. Roll out sugar cookie dough from recipe. Cut into small 1½-inch circles with a glass or cookie cutter. Bake at 350° for 8–10 minutes or until edges start to turn brown. Cool completely.
2. Turn cookie rounds upside down on a cooling rack placed over a parchment-lined baking sheet.
3. Heat chocolate with shortening in a double boiler until melted.
4. Spoon 1 tsp sunbutter onto each cookie.
5. Spoon chocolate over the tops and sides of each cookie. Tap baking sheet on counter to smooth the chocolate.
6. Place baking sheet in freezer until chocolate is set.
7. Store in an airtight container in the fridge for up to a week.

Options:

~Try using peanut butter or almond butter instead!

~Try adding a few nuts or a sprinkle of sea salt on top of the chocolate before it cools!

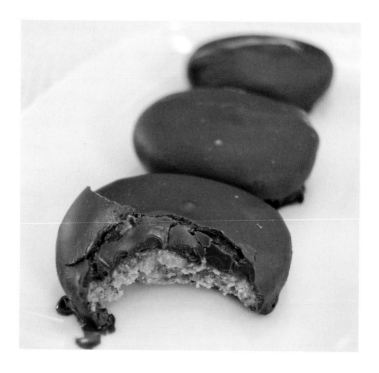

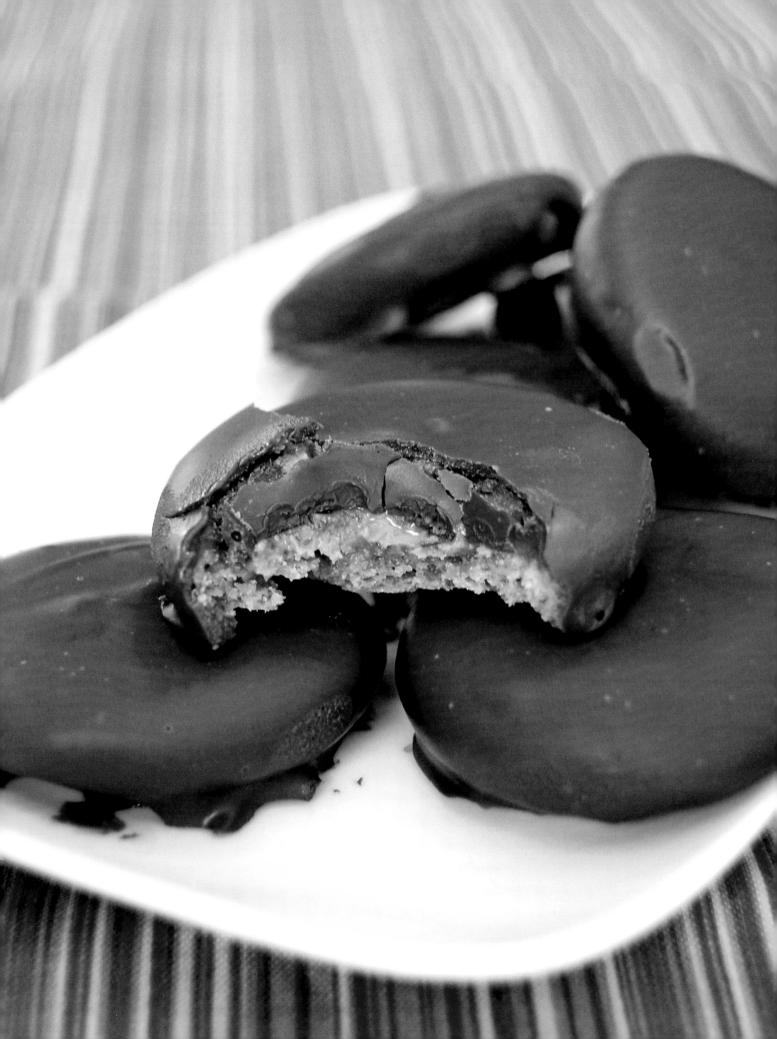

Snickerdoodles

This recipe has been a long time coming. Many, many revisions and versions of this cookie have surfaced over the years, mostly because it has such a particular flavor and texture that it was a little harder to recreate in a gluten-free, dairy-free, egg-free form. But here it is! I cannot tell you how amazing this cookie is! Buttery, crispy edges, tender center, crackly cinnamon and sugar top, and that little zing from the cream of tartar that many snickerdoodle recipes neglect. It's all there. Excuse me for a minute.... I need a tissue. So. Happy!

Dry Ingredients:

1	C (120 g) brown rice flour
½	C (60 g) sorghum flour
½	C (60 g) potato starch
¾	C (90 g) tapioca starch
1	tsp xanthan gum
1	tsp baking soda
2	tsp cream of tartar
½	tsp sea salt

Wet Ingredients:

1	C (240 g) nondairy butter (I like Earth Balance Vegan Buttery Sticks for this one)
1	C (200 g) organic evaporated cane juice
1	Tbsp flax meal mixed with 2 Tbsp hot water
3	Tbsp unsweetened organic apple-sauce

Topping:

~ In a small bowl, mix together 2 Tbsp organic evaporated cane juice and 1 Tbsp cinnamon. Set aside.

1. Whisk together dry ingredients.
2. In a large mixing bowl, cream together butter and sugar.
3. Add flax meal mixture and applesauce. Mix until combined.
4. Slowly add the dry ingredients, about ½ C at a time, to the wet ingredients, until fully incorporated. If for any reason the dough is too dry and doesn't stick together, slowly add in a little water until it comes together and looks like traditional cookie dough. Mix for 1 minute.
5. Chill dough for 1 hour.
6. Roll dough in hands to form balls. Roll tops in cinnamon/sugar topping, pressing down to slightly flatten ball, and place on baking sheets lined with parchment paper.
7. Bake at 350° for about 11–12 minutes or until edges are slightly browned. Do not overbake.
8. Cool completely on wire racks.

Options:

~Be sure to see our options for freezing cookie dough or making the dry mix ahead of time in the front section of the book (p. 40).

Makes about 24 cookies

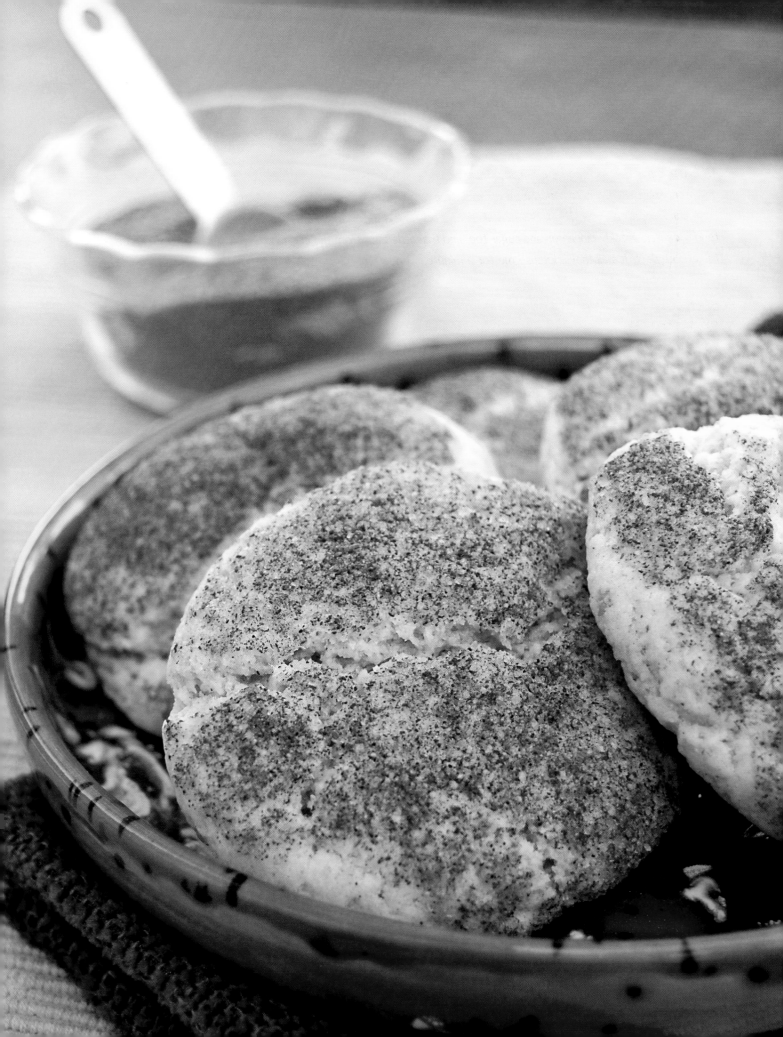

Graham Crackers

If you're craving summertime s'mores and are tired of paying $10 for a box of unflavored cardboard squares pawned off as graham crackers, then this recipe is for you! This is one of my favorite inventions for many reasons. First, it makes a ton of crackers that last for at least a week in a sealed container. Second, the flavor is spot-on to traditional graham crackers so no one will know the difference! And third, they are easily adaptable for many uses, such as the obvious s'mores, pie crusts, ice-cream topping, and even breading for chicken. Go forth and make grahams!

Dry Ingredients:

¾ C (90 g) sorghum flour
½ C (60 g) brown rice flour
¼ C (30 g) amaranth flour
½ C (60 g) potato starch
½ C (60 g) tapioca starch
⅓ C (60 g) packed organic brown sugar
2 tsp cinnamon
1 tsp baking powder
½ tsp xanthan gum
½ tsp baking soda
½ tsp salt

Wet Ingredients:

½ C (95 g) cold organic shortening, cut into pieces (Spectrum brand)
5–6 Tbsp cold water
¼ C (60 mL) raw organic honey
2 tsp pure vanilla extract

1. Whisk together dry ingredients.
2. Using your hands, mix and crumble the shortening into the dry mix until small crumbs form.
3. Add 3 Tbsp cold water, honey, and vanilla. Stir with a spoon until it comes together and forms a ball. If needed, add another Tbsp or two of cold water.
4. Divide dough in half, form into discs, wrap, and refrigerate 1 hour.
5. Using one disc at a time, roll between 2 pieces parchment paper to ⅛ inch thickness. Remove top piece of parchment, place bottom piece with dough on baking sheet.
6. Poke dough all over with fork and score with a knife into squares. Repeat with second disc.
7. Bake at 325° for 15–17 minutes, rotating trays once halfway through baking. Re-cut squares and cool completely. Store in an airtight container for up to a week.

Variation:

~Mix 1 Tbsp cinnamon and 2 Tbsp sugar in a bowl. Sprinkle topping across top of dough before baking for Cinnamon Grahams.

Baking / Desserts / Snacks

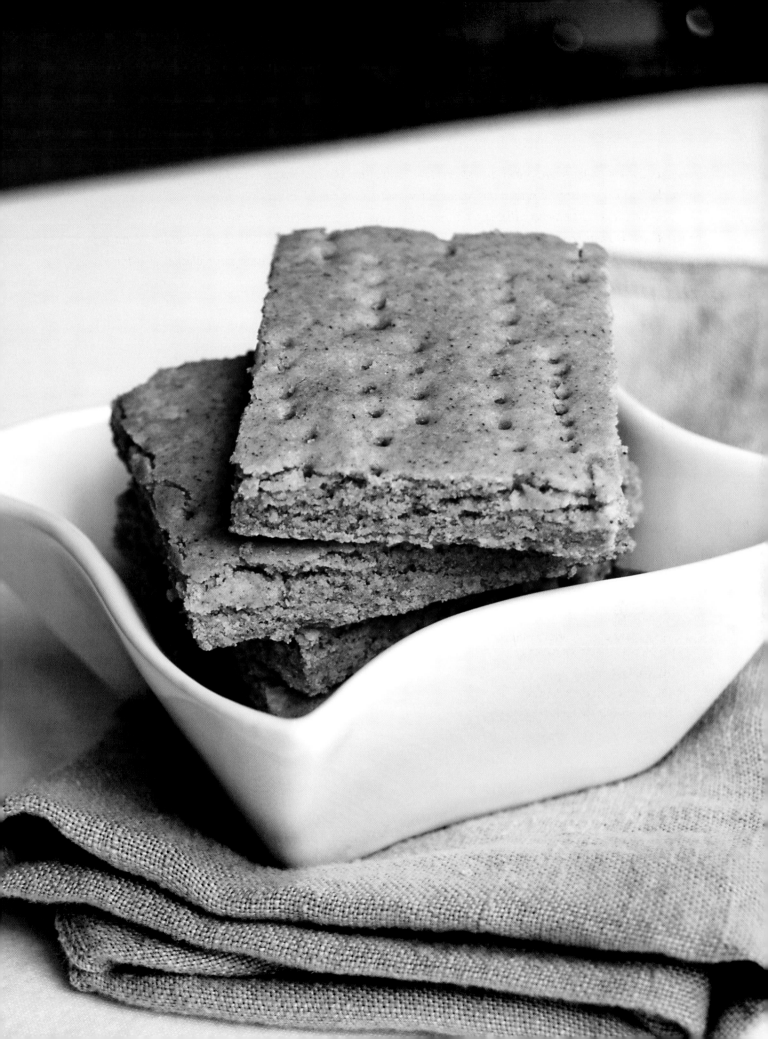

Chocolate Graham Crackers

Here is a recipe for the same yummy graham cracker taste you know and love, with a chocolaty twist! These are very versatile, so use your imagination. Ice cream sandwiches anyone?

Dry Ingredients:

1	C (120 g) brown rice flour
¼	C (30 g) amaranth flour
½	C (60 g) potato starch
½	C (60 g) tapioca starch
½	C (60 g) organic cocoa powder
⅓	C (60 g) packed organic brown sugar
2	tsp cinnamon
1	tsp baking powder
½	tsp xanthan gum
½	tsp baking soda
½	tsp sea salt

Wet Ingredients:

½	C (95 g) cold organic shortening, cut into pieces (Spectrum brand)
5–6	Tbsp cold water
¼	C (60 mL) raw organic honey
~	2 tsp pure vanilla extract

1. Whisk together dry ingredients.
2. Using your hands, mix and crumble the shortening into the dry mix until small crumbs form.
3. Add 3 Tbsp cold water, honey, and vanilla. Stir with a spoon until it comes together and forms a ball. If needed, add another Tbsp or two of cold water.
4. Divide dough in half, form into discs, wrap, and refrigerate 1 hour.
5. Using one disc at a time, roll between 2 pieces parchment paper to ⅛ inch thickness. Remove top piece of parchment, place bottom piece with dough on baking sheet.
6. Poke dough all over with fork and score with a knife into squares. Sprinkle top of dough with sugar, if desired. Repeat with second disc.
7. Bake at 325° for 15–17 minutes, rotating trays once halfway through baking.
8. Re-cut squares and cool completely.
9. Store in an airtight container for up to a week.

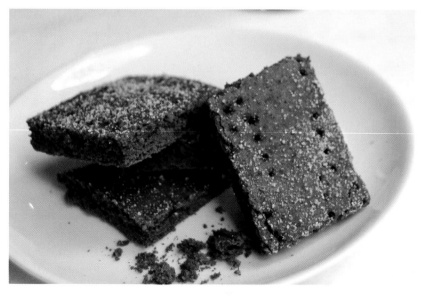

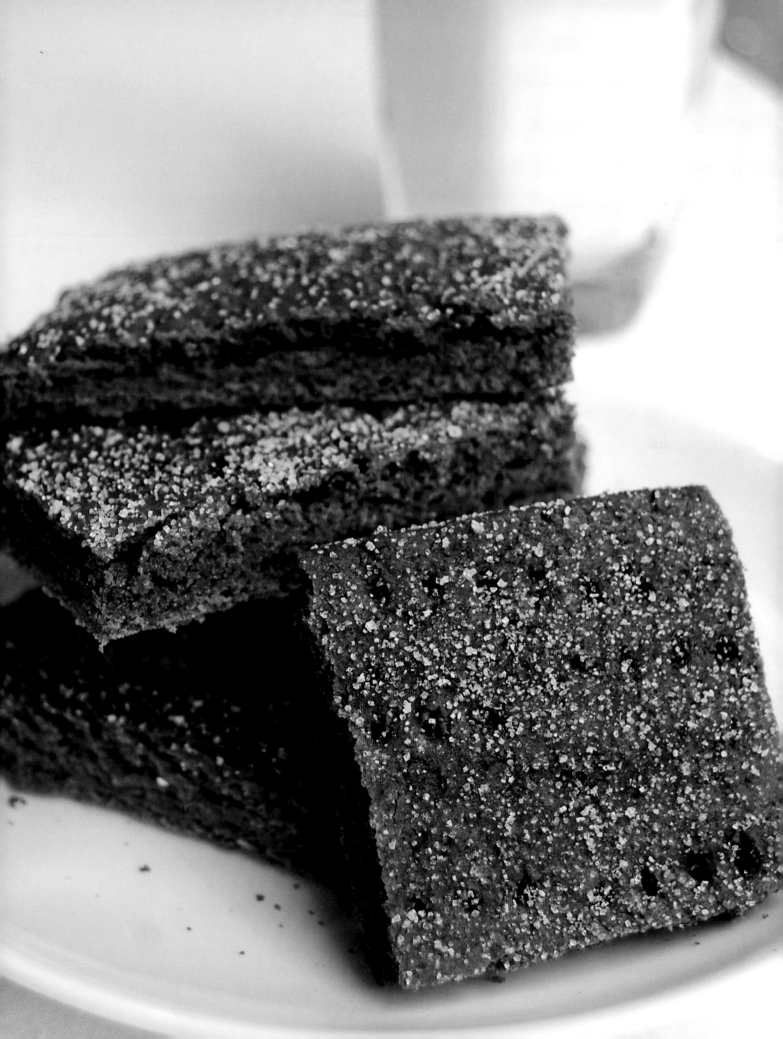

Fudgy Brownies

When I was growing up, every once in a great while my mom would splurge on a box of name-brand brownies. She would mix them up, bake them, and then set them in the garage on a shelf to cool faster than they would in the warm house. It was never fast enough! I remember opening the door to the garage a million times in a 15-minute span just willing those brownies to cool enough to be cut. Oh the agony! But luckily, my impatience was always rewarded with warm, gooey, chocolaty goodness. Of course, now I really know what was in those boxed brownies (It's OK mom! We didn't know what we were doing back then!) and this version will give you the same heart palpitations in the wait for coolness that those nasty, preservative- and wheat-laden boxed brownies gave you, but without the tummy aches. This version is a must have for our bakery customers.... I think they might be on to something!

Dry Ingredients:

⅓	C (40 g) sorghum flour
½	C (60 g) teff flour
¼	C (30 g) potato starch
⅓	C (40 g) tapioca starch
½	C (60 g) organic cocoa powder
1	tsp xanthan gum
½	tsp baking soda
½	tsp sea salt

Wet Ingredients:

⅓	C (80 g) nondairy butter, very soft
⅓	C (80 mL) coconut oil, melted
1¼	C (250 g) organic evaporated cane juice
2	tsp pure vanilla extract
1	C (240 mL) warm water

Add Ins:

¾	C (110 g) nondairy, soy free, chocolate chips or chunks of your favorite nondairy dark chocolate

1. Preheat oven to 350°.
2. Grease 9" by 13" baking pan.
3. In a stand mixer, blend softened butter, oil, and sugar until combined. Add vanilla.
4. Alternate adding dry ingredients and warm water to mixing bowl until both are used. Batter should be very thick (a bit thicker than a traditional brownie batter). If it's too wet it will still be delicious, it just won't have the crusty top. Mix on high speed for 1 minute.
5. Stir in chocolate chips/dark chocolate pieces.
6. Spread batter with a rubber spatula into prepared pan.
7. Bake for 25 minutes.
8. Cool completely in pan before cutting. Or if desperate, pile in a bowl with a spoon while still warm and eat it like there's no tomorrow! Um . . . I mean, eat slowly and chew completely to enjoy each and every bite of this occasional treat.

Baking Time Notes:

Glass pan—25 minutes

Dark nonstick pan—25 minutes

Light aluminum pan—30–35 minutes

Or until a toothpick inserted in the middle comes out clean

Sugar note:

If you don't mind a cakier brownie, you can cut the sugar by ¼–½ C depending on how sweet you like it. If you like a fudgier, crispy top brownie, add another ¼–½ C sugar. This recipe meets in the middle, where the sugar has been reduced to the point that you still get a slightly crusty top but without the sugar coma. You can replace the sugar altogether with 1 C maple syrup or ¾ C honey, but the texture and flavor will not be quite as good as the brownie you remember as a kid.

Variations:

~Add ½ C chopped walnuts or pecans when you add the chocolate chips.

~After spreading the batter into the pan, take spoonfuls of peanut butter and swirl them into the batter.

~Mix in nuts and mini GF marshmallow to the batter prior to baking for a rocky road-like treat.

~Frost with chocolate or vanilla Buttercream Frosting (p. 326) for an extra decadent dessert.

Baking / Desserts / Snacks

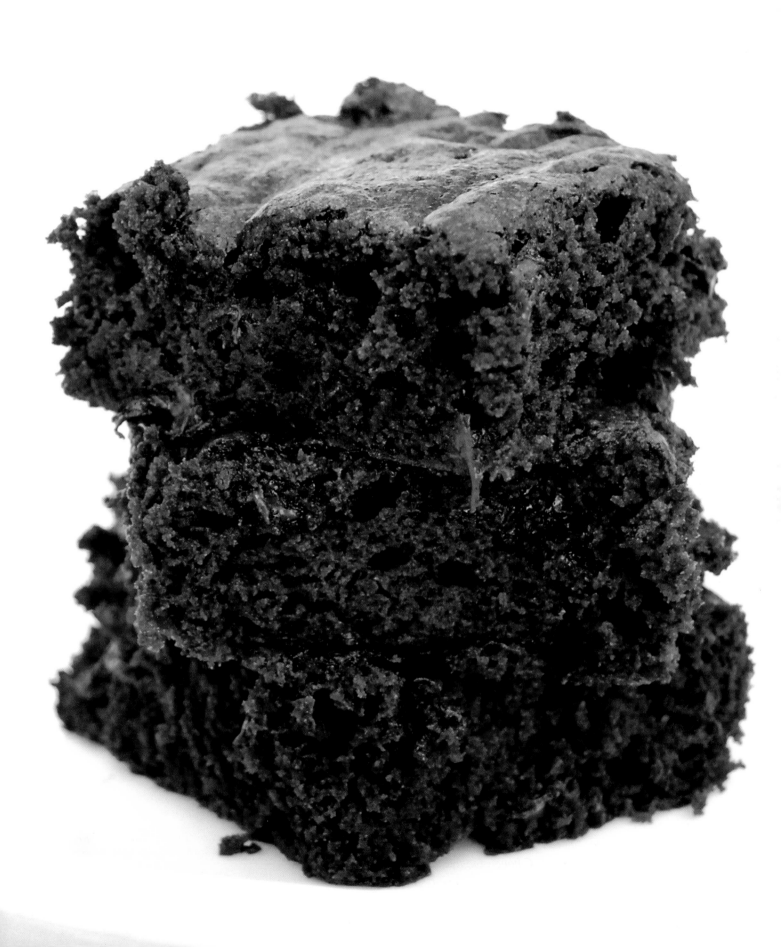

Cocoa Rice Crisp Squares

A chocolaty twist on an original classic! So happy there are options for crisp rice cereal that are gluten-free! And if you're craving the original, feel free to swap out the chocolate cereal for plain, crisp rice cereal.

¼	C (60 g) nondairy butter (Earth Balance brand)
5	C (about 950 g) GF mini marshmallows (I like Elyon natural marshmallows—takes 2 bags)
5	C (950 g) chocolate crisp rice cereal (EnviroKids brand is tasty)
1	tsp pure vanilla extract
2	Tbsp raw organic honey

1. In a large saucepan melt butter over low heat.
2. Add marshmallows and stir until they are all melted. Remove from heat.
3. Add chocolate crisp rice cereal, vanilla, and honey. Stir until they are well combined with the melted marshmallows.
4. Using a piece of wax paper, press the mixture into a greased 9" by 13" pan. Cool.
5. Cut into squares. Much better the same day you make them!

Option:

~I love adding about 1 C organic crunchy peanut butter or almond butter to the nondairy butter and marshmallows to melt!

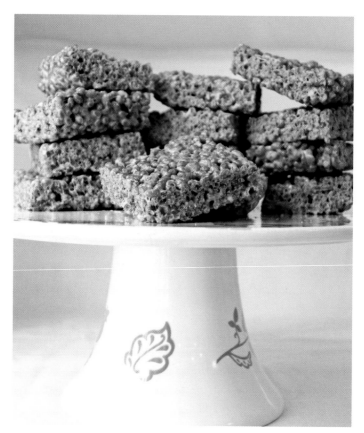

Baking / Desserts / Snacks

Chunky Cocoa Crisp Snack Bars

Be careful with this one! It's so chocolaty and decadent, it's hard to eat just one. Almost along the lines of a great piece of fudge, it satisfies that chocolate craving like nobody's business.

5	oz (140 g) GF DF chocolate chips (Enjoy Life brand)
8	oz (240 mL) sun butter
⅓	C (80 g) nondairy butter (Earth Balance brand)
¾	C (110 g) roasted salted sunflower seed kernels
¾	C (65 g) unsweetened organic finely shredded coconut
¼	C (45 g) sesame seeds
¾	C (135 g) ground flax seeds
1	C (150 g) raw pumpkin seeds
1	C (90 g) GF puffed rice cereal
½	C (75 g) organic raisins

1. In a small saucepan melt together chocolate chips, sunbutter, and butter.
2. In a large bowl combine remaining ingredients.
3. Pour chocolate mixture over seed mixture and mix well.
4. Press into a greased 9" by 13" pan.
5. Refrigerate until firm and cut to serve.

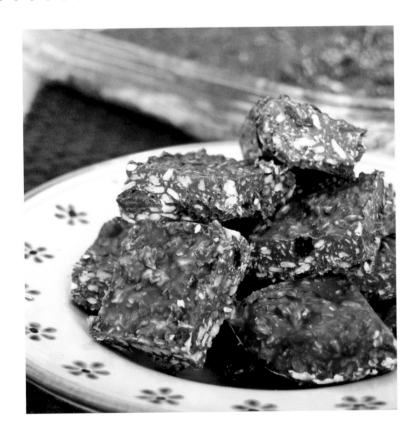

Almond Butter Nut Balls

These tasty little snacks are packed with great ingredients and they're so much fun for the kids to make! You can also freeze leftovers and take out a few at a time when needed, which works great for school lunches and after-school snacks.

Nut Balls:

8	Medjool dates, pits removed
½	C (120 mL) almond butter
¾	C (90 g) almond meal
3	Tbsp coconut flour
¼	C (60 g) nondairy butter (Earth Balance brand)
½	C (45 g) unsweetened organic coconut flakes
2	Tbsp unsweetened coconut butter (also called coconut cream)
1	tsp pure vanilla extract
2	Tbsp raw organic honey

Add Ins:

¼	C (40 g) GF DF mini chocolate chips (Enjoy Life brand)

Toppers:

~	Finely shredded unsweetened organic coconut
~	Organic Cocoa powder

1. Place all ingredients in a food processor. Pulse until ingredients are pureed and soft.
2. Remove mixture to a bowl and hand mix in chocolate chips.
3. Take 1-Tbsp scoops of mixture and roll into balls. Little hands do this very well!
4. Roll balls in the shredded coconut or cocoa powder and place on wax-paper lined plates or a small baking sheet.
5. Freeze until firm, about 1 hour.
6. Store in an airtight container in the fridge for up to 2 weeks, or store in the freezer for up to 3 months. To use, refrigerate until soft enough to eat.

Option:

-Try adding ½ C (45 g) GF puffed rice cereal as an add-in!

-Get creative and try different nut or seed butters.

-Try using maple syrup instead of honey.

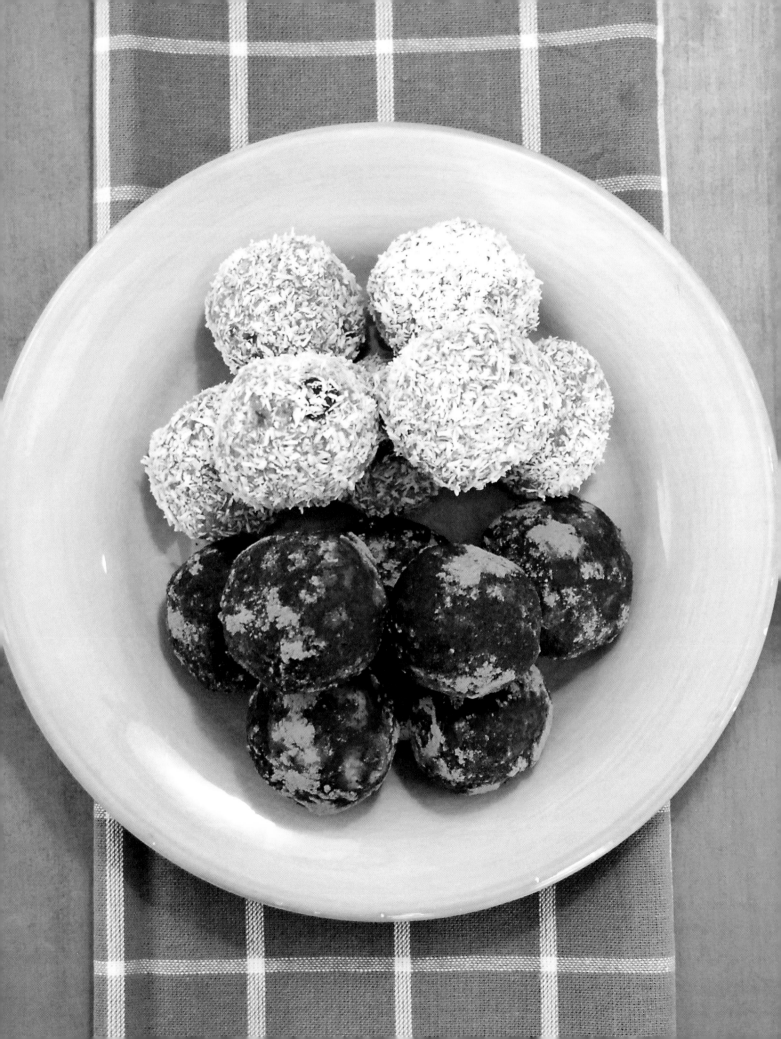

Macadamia Bars

When you have food intolerances, traveling or running errands all day can turn ugly real fast with a car full of hungry kids and a famished spouse. And when stopping at the corner market for a quick snack is impossible due to the fact that everything either has gluten in it or it will cost you your first-born child, then one must be prepared ahead of time. So I created these delicious, and portable, macadamia bars to take along for the ride and still have some spending money in my pocket! And like a lot of recipes in this book, there is flexibility in the ingredients. Don't like macadamias? Try walnuts, pecans, or almonds. Not a fan of dried cherries? Dried cranberries work great as well. Be creative and see what flavor combinations you like! I've even included a nut-free version as well.

8	Medjool dates, sliced in half, pits removed
¾	C (65 g) unsweetened organic coconut flakes (or ½ C [45 g] finely shredded unsweetened organic coconut)
½	C (75 g) organic raisins
¾	C (110 g) macadamia nuts
¾	C (110 g) sunflower seeds (raw or roasted)
½	C (75 g) dried cherries
¼	tsp cinnamon
½	tsp pure vanilla extract
1	tsp raw organic honey

1. Add all ingredients to a food processor and blend for about 1 minute or until everything is chopped into small pieces and starts to stick together. If you have a small food processor, you can mix ingredients in a bowl and process it in batches until it is all combined.

2. Place mixture on a large piece of plastic wrap. With your hands, shape into a rectangle, pressing and patting it until very dense and sticks together nicely.

3. Wrap tightly and refrigerate for a few hours, until very firm. Slice into bars and enjoy!

4. Store at room temperature for up to 1 week, in the fridge for up to 2 weeks, or wrap bars individually and freeze until needed. To thaw, simply set on counter for about 30 minutes to bring to room temperature before eating.

Nut-Free Version (Seeded Bars)

9	Medjool dates, cut in half, pits removed
¾	C (65 g) unsweetened organic coconut flakes (or ½ C [45 g] finely shredded unsweetened organic coconut)
⅓	C (50 g) organic raisins
¾	C (110 g) raw pumpkin seeds
¾	C (110 g) sunflower seeds (roasted and salted)
¼	C (40 g) dried cherries (or cranberries)
¼	tsp cinnamon
½	tsp pure vanilla extract
2	tsp raw organic honey

1. Follow instructions above for Macadamia Bars.

Makes about 14 bars

Baking / Desserts / Snacks

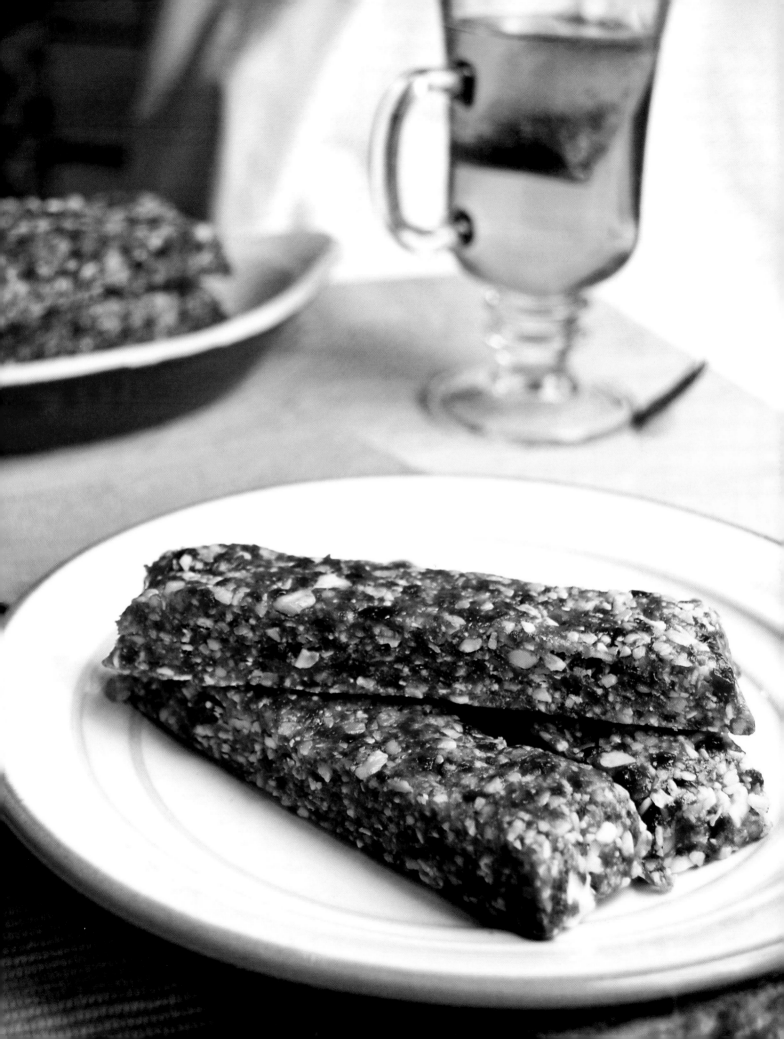

Pumpkin Bread

Baking pumpkin bread has been a holiday tradition in my family for years. I'm not quite sure where the recipe originally came from, but my mom perfected it into this delectable, comforting, loaf of goodness that we would devour each Christmas season. When I went off to college, this was one of the recipes that got packed to join me in my new life... a little slice of home that I couldn't be without. I continued the tradition with my kids, baking this bread each Christmas, as well as dozens more to give to friends and family. Needless to say, the first Christmas after the Maniac was diagnosed with CD, I was determined, and a little desperate, to have this bread be a part of our holidays. And even though it was the first time I'd tried to convert an actual family recipe to GF, somehow, after only one attempt, it was perfect. I was destined to have my pumpkin bread that Christmas! This was by far one of the most sought-after products in our frozen retail line of baked goods, and now I share the goodness with you. So maybe, just maybe, you will feel inspired enough to start a little holiday tradition with your own family.

Dry Ingredients:

½	C (60 g) brown rice flour
1	C (120 g) sorghum flour
¾	C (90 g) teff flour
¾	C (90 g) potato starch
½	C (60 g) tapioca starch
2	tsp xanthan gum
1½	tsp cinnamon
½	tsp nutmeg
2	tsp baking soda
1½	tsp baking powder
1½	tsp sea salt
1½	C organic evaporated cane juice

Wet Ingredients:

1	tsp baking powder (to be used w/applesauce)
½	C (120 mL) organic unsweetened applesauce, room temperature
1	C (240 mL) coconut oil, melted
¾	C (180 mL) warm water
2	C (475 mL) organic canned pumpkin

Makes 2 loaves

1. Whisk together dry ingredients in the bowl of a stand mixer. Create a well in the center of the ingredients.
2. Mix 1 tsp baking powder into applesauce.
3. Add oil, warm water, pumpkin, and applesauce mixture to the well of the dry ingredients.
4. Mix together on low until ingredients are fully incorporated. Turn mixer to medium-high and mix for 1 minute.
5. Spray 2 nonstick loaf pans with a cooking spray. Pour batter into both loaf pans, making sure to divide batter evenly.
6. Bake in a 350° oven for 55 minutes. Turn loaves part way through to ensure even baking. Remove from oven and let cool, in pans, on a wire rack, for 10 minutes. Remove loaves from pans and let cool completely on wire rack before slicing.
7. Store in an airtight container for up to 3 days.

Options:

~See freezing instructions at the beginning of the book to keep this delicious bread even longer.

~For a special holiday treat, slice the bread lengthwise into 3 sections. Then spread vegan cream cheese across each layer. Sprinkle cream cheese with a very slight amount of curry powder. Put slices back together, wrap and store loaf in the fridge, or you can freeze as discussed in the front of the book. To eat, simply cut into regular slices and enjoy the extra pretty and tasty layers of cream cheese!

~Every so often I like to add about 1 C dairy-free chocolate chips to this bread. The chocolate really enhances the pumpkin flavor.

~Try adding 1½ C roughly chopped pecans to the batter before baking. Yum-merific!

Baking / Desserts / Snacks

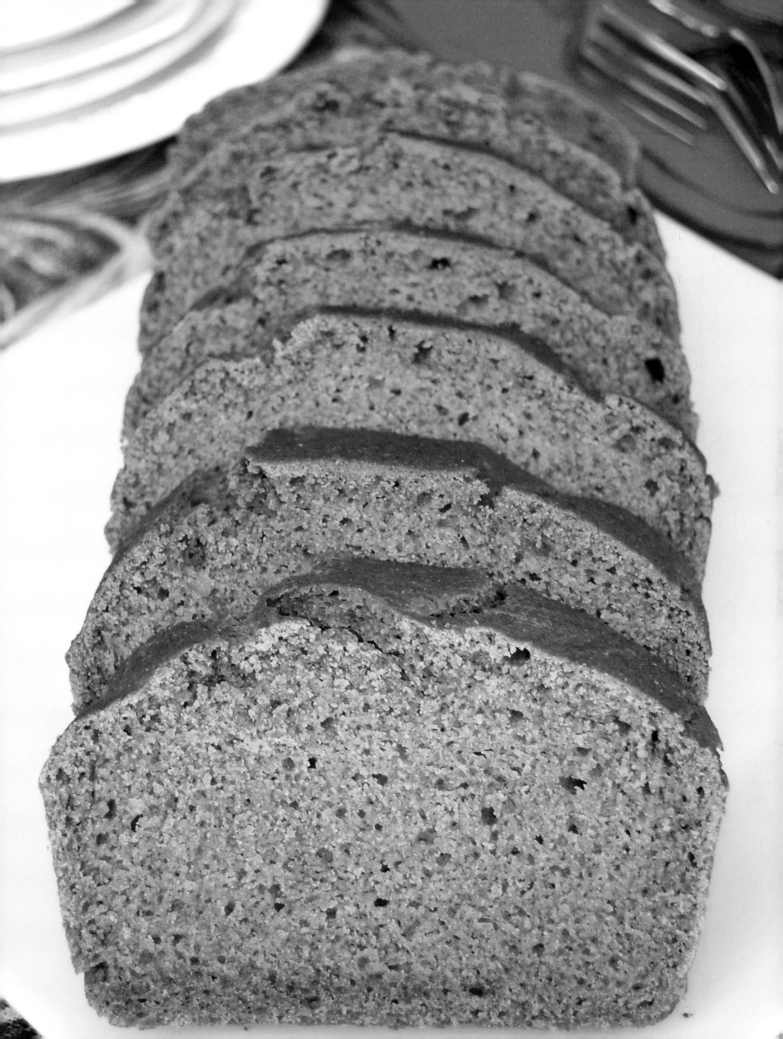

Banana Bread

I love quick breads because you can throw all of the ingredients into one bowl and mix. No creaming this and fully incorporating that. Just dump and mix well. Yay for recipes that let me be a little lazy! I like to let my overripe bananas get very, very ripe. Almost black. Disgusting, I know, but the riper the better for banana bread. This provides lots of great banana flavor and extra moisture for the bread. And who doesn't love that? For quick breads, also make sure your ingredients are at least room temperature, maybe even a touch warmer thanks to the microwave. Nice warm ingredients make for a much higher rise while baking. Eggs? We don't need no stinkin' eggs!

Dry Ingredients:

½	C (60 g)	millet flour
1¼	C (150 g)	sorghum flour
1	C (120 g)	teff flour
1¼	C (150 g)	potato starch
¾	C (90 g)	tapioca starch
2	tsp	xanthan gum
1	tsp	cinnamon
1¼	C (250 g)	organic evaporated cane juice
2	tsp	baking soda
2	tsp	baking powder
1½	tsp	sea salt

Wet Ingredients:

1	tsp	baking powder (to be used with applesauce)
½	C (120 mL)	organic unsweetened applesauce, room temperature
1	C (240 mL)	coconut oil, melted
¾	C (180 mL)	warm water
2	C (480 g)	ripe bananas (about 7–8 bananas) (see tip below if using frozen bananas)
1	tsp	pure vanilla extract

1. Whisk together dry ingredients in the bowl of a stand mixer. Create a well in the center of the ingredients.
2. Mix 1 tsp baking powder into applesauce. Add oil, warm water, bananas, vanilla, and applesauce mixture to the well of the dry ingredients.
3. Mix together on low until ingredients are fully incorporated. Turn mixer to medium-high and mix for 1 minute.
4. Spray 2 nonstick loaf pans with a cooking spray. Pour batter into both loaf pans, making sure to divide batter evenly.
5. Bake in a 350° oven for 55 minutes. Turn loaves part way through to ensure even baking. Remove from oven and let cool, in pans, on a wire rack, for 10 minutes. Remove loaves from pans and let cool completely on wire rack before slicing.
6. Store in an airtight container for up to 3 days. Or see front of book for freezing instructions.

Options:

~Try adding 1 C dairy-free chocolate chips to the batter before baking.

~Try adding 1½ C roughly chopped pecans or walnuts to the batter before baking. Yummerific!

Tip:

~Frozen bananas: let thaw overnight in the fridge. To use, add applesauce and warm in microwave until room temperature. Add baking powder then add to mixing bowl.

Makes 2 loaves

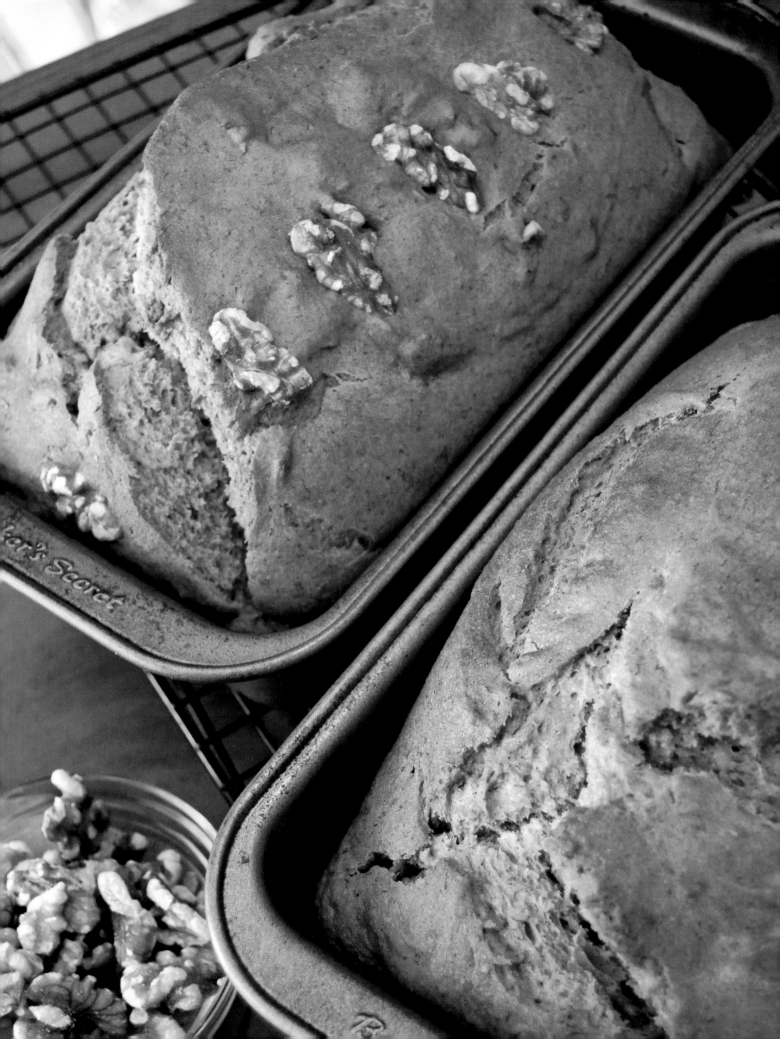

Cranberry Walnut Bread

Again, my mom was the inspiration behind this delicious quick bread recipe. She always made cranberry nut bread during the holidays and gave them away as gifts to friends and neighbors. Of course, we had to keep a few loaves in the freezer to enjoy long past the New Year! And you should too, since this bread freezes so incredibly well. And like the pumpkin and banana bread, pre-slicing before freezing makes it so much easier to enjoy a slice at a time when you want it. Or need it.

Dry Ingredients:

½	C (60 g) brown rice flour
¾	C (90 g) sorghum flour
½	C (60 g) teff flour
¼	C (30 g) almond meal
¾	C (90 g) potato starch
¾	C (90 g) tapioca starch
2	tsp xanthan gum
1½	tsp cinnamon
2	tsp baking soda
1½	tsp baking powder
1½	tsp sea salt
1¼	C (250 g) organic evaporated cane juice

Wet Ingredients:

1	tsp baking powder (to be used with applesauce)
1½	C (350 mL) organic unsweetened applesauce, room temperature
1	C (240 ml) coconut oil, melted
¾	C (180 ml) warm water
1	Tbsp pure vanilla extract

Add Ins:

1	(12 oz) bag (340 g) fresh or frozen organic cranberries (thawed if frozen), coarsely chopped
1	C (150 g) chopped walnuts

1. Whisk together dry ingredients in the bowl of a stand mixer. Create a well in the center of the ingredients.
2. Mix 1 tsp baking powder into applesauce. Add oil, warm water, vanilla, and applesauce mixture to the well of the dry ingredients.
3. Mix together on low until ingredients are fully incorporated. Turn mixer to medium-high and mix for 1 minute.
4. Fold in walnuts and cranberries.
5. Spray 2 nonstick loaf pans with a cooking spray. Pour batter into both loaf pans, making sure to divide batter evenly.
6. Bake in a 350° oven for 55–65 minutes. Turn loaves part way through to ensure even baking. Remove from oven and let cool, in pans, on a wire rack, for 10 minutes. Remove loaves from pans and let cool completely on wire rack before slicing.
7. Store in an airtight container for up to 3 days.

Options:

~See freezing instructions in the front of the book to freeze and enjoy this bread long through the holidays.

~To make this bread nut free, simply eliminate the walnuts and almond meal. No need to adjust the dry ingredients.

~For a cranberry-orange treat, I like to add in the zest of 1 orange and replace the warm water with orange juice. It's amazing!

Makes 2 loaves

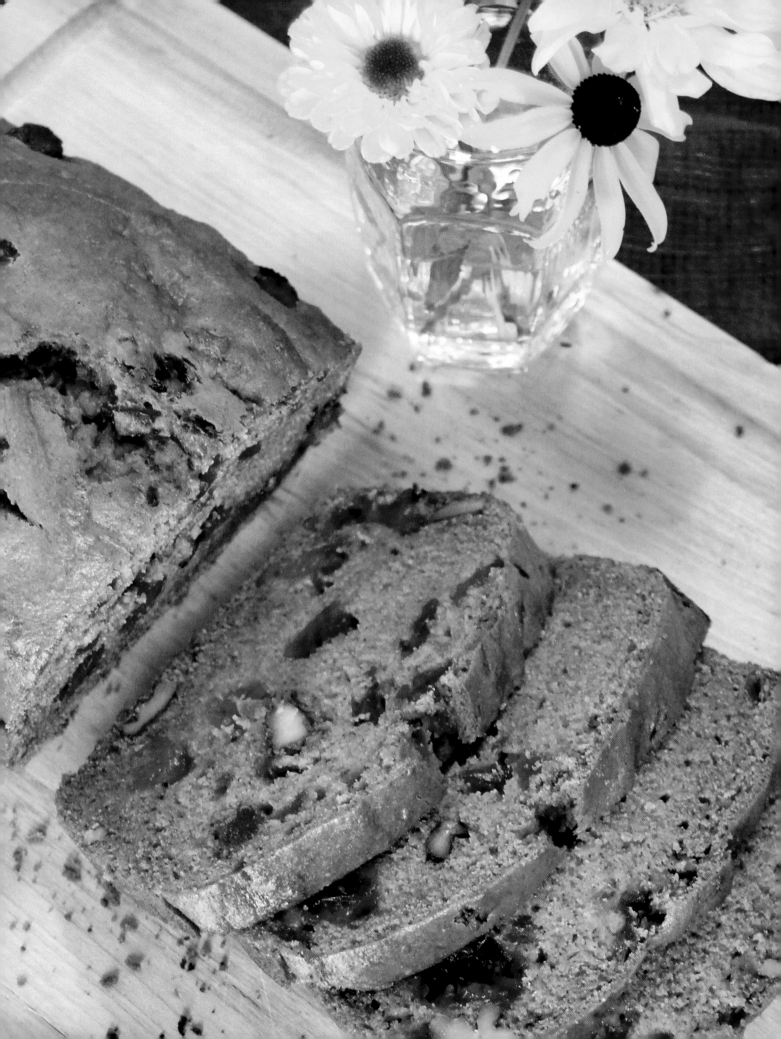

Orange Olive Oil Bread

I'd heard of a quick bread being made with olive oil but I couldn't get my head around the concept. Heavy, fragrant olive oil? In a sweet bread? It took a few years, but I finally came around. And I'm oh so glad I did! This bread is my new favorite, but don't tell the pumpkin, OK? It's so moist and surprisingly not overly dense. It's amazing, let's just leave it at that.

Dry Ingredients:

¼	C (30 g) brown rice flour
½	C (60 g) sorghum flour
¼	C (30 g) teff flour
½	C (60 g) potato starch
½	C (60 g) tapioca starch
1½	tsp xanthan gum
½	tsp baking soda
2	tsp baking powder
½	tsp sea salt
⅔	C (130 g) organic evaporated cane juice
½	C (45 g) unsweetened finely shredded organic coconut
~	Zest of 1 small organic orange

Wet Ingredients:

1	tsp baking powder (to be used with the applesauce)
½	C (120 mL) organic unsweetened applesauce, room temperature
1	Tbsp pure vanilla extract
¾	C (180 mL) canned lite coconut milk
⅓	C (80 mL) olive oil
~	Juice from 1 organic orange

For the Glaze:

½	C (50 g) gluten-free organic powdered sugar
2	Tbsp fresh squeezed organic orange juice

1. In a large bowl, whisk together dry ingredients until combined.
2. In a small bowl, add baking powder to applesauce and stir.
3. In a stand mixer, combine remaining wet ingredients and mix briefly. Add applesauce mixture and mix again briefly to combine.
4. With mixer on low, add dry ingredients to the mixing bowl slowly until fully incorporated.
5. Blend on high 30 seconds.
6. Pour batter into a greased loaf pan. Bake in a 350° oven for 55–60 minutes, or until top is browned and toothpick inserted in the center comes out clean.
7. Remove pan from oven. With a toothpick poke some holes across the top of the loaf. Spoon the glaze over the top of the loaf. Cool for 10 minutes in the pan.
8. Remove loaf from pan and cool completely on a wire rack before slicing.
9. Wrap and store in an airtight container for up to 3 days.

Tip:

~See freezing instructions at the front of the book to enjoy this loaf of bread even longer!

Makes 1 loaf

Baking / Desserts / Snacks

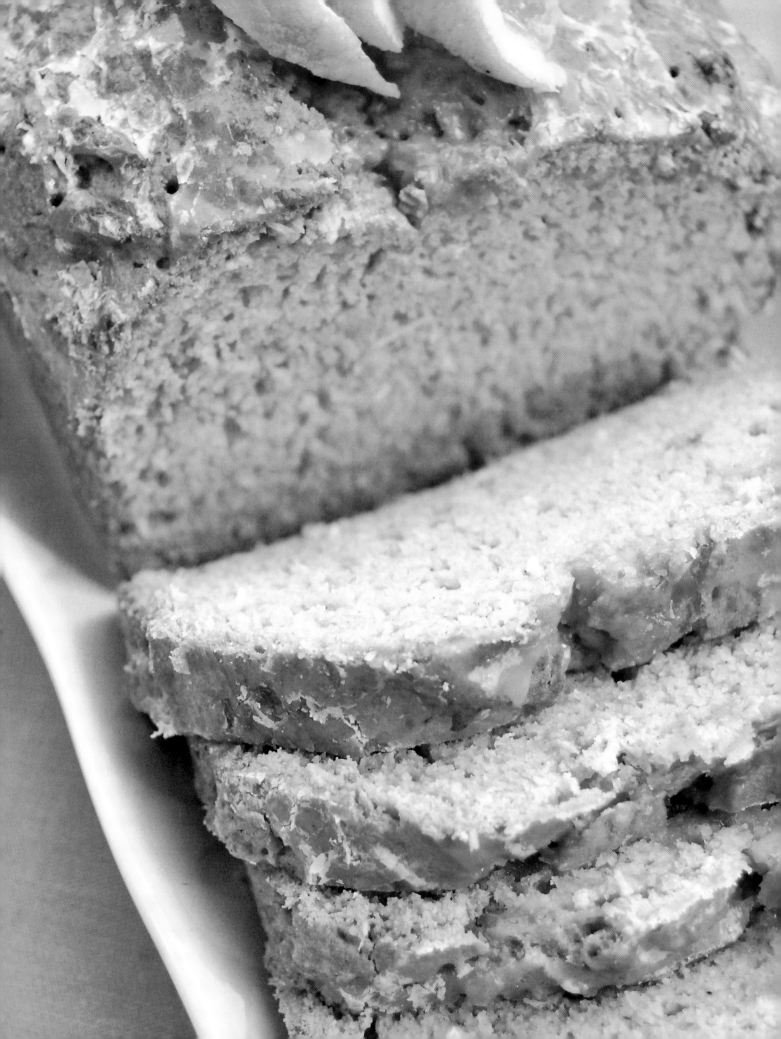

Vanilla Cupcakes

These aren't your traditional vanilla cupcakes. They aren't bland or forgettable. The vanilla shines through, but you can really taste that you're enjoying a hearty, healthy cake. And topped with vanilla or chocolate buttercream? Well now you're just talking crazy delicious!

Dry Ingredients:

⅓	C (40 g)	teff flour
⅓	C (40 g)	millet flour
⅓	C (40 g)	sorghum flour
⅓	C (40 g)	potato starch
3	Tbsp	tapioca starch
¾	tsp	xanthan gum
1½	tsp	baking powder
½	tsp	baking soda
¾	tsp	salt

Wet Ingredients:

⅓	C (80 g)	nondairy butter (Earth Balance brand)
¾	C (150 g)	organic evaporated cane juice
½	C (120 mL)	coconut oil, melted
2	Tbsp	pure vanilla extract
1	tsp	baking powder (to mix with applesauce)
⅓	C (80 mL)	unsweetened organic applesauce, room temperature
½	C (120 mL)	warm water

1. Whisk together dry ingredients.
2. In a stand mixer, cream together butter, sugar, and coconut oil.
3. Add vanilla.
4. Mix baking powder with applesauce and add to mixer. Blend until combined.
5. Slowly mix in dry ingredients, a little at a time, until incorporated.
6. Add in warm water until the batter is the consistency of traditional cake batter. If it's too dry, add a little more water.
7. Mix on high for 1 minute.
8. Line a muffin pan with cupcake liners. Scoop cake batter into the liners, ¾ full.
9. Bake in a 350° oven for 14–15 minutes or until tops are golden and spring back when touched.
10. Frost with vanilla or chocolate buttercream frosting (p.326).

Makes about 12

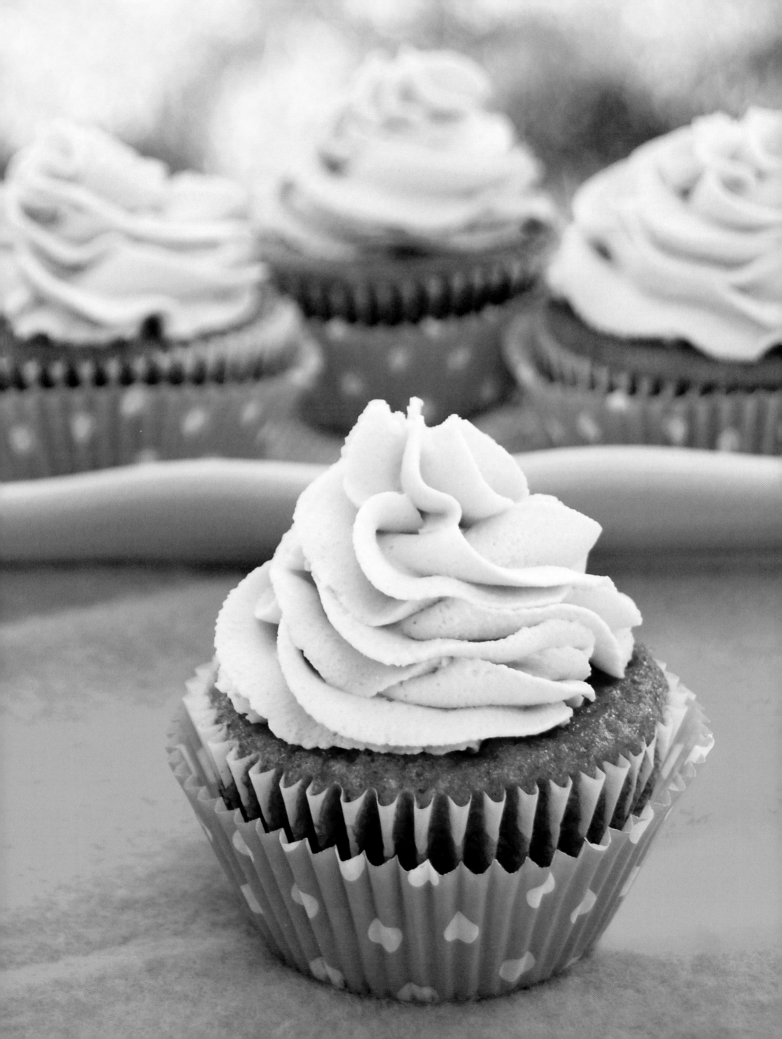

Chocolate Cupcakes

There is nothing, and I mean NOTHING "alternative" about these amazing cupcakes. Rich, chocolaty, and extremely satisfying, they can go head-to-head with any conventional chocolate cake. Pair with rich, fudgy chocolate or vanilla buttercream (p. 326). And for even more indulgence? Add in some GF DF chocolate chips for some extra-chocolaty goodness!

Dry Ingredients

¼	C (30 g) millet flour
⅓	C (40 g) sorghum flour
⅓	C (40 g) teff flour
⅓	C (40 g) potato starch
¼	C (30 g) tapioca starch
¾	tsp xanthan gum
1½	tsp baking powder
½	tsp baking soda
¾	tsp sea salt
⅓	C (40 g) organic cocoa powder

Wet Ingredients:

¼	C (60 g) nondairy butter (Earth Balance)
¾	C (150 g) organic evaporated cane juice
½	C (120 mL) coconut oil, melted
1	Tbsp pure vanilla extract
½	tsp baking powder (to mix with the applesauce)
⅓	C (80 mL) room temperature unsweetened organic applesauce
⅔	C (160 mL) warm water

1. Whisk together dry ingredients.
2. In a stand mixer, cream together butter, evaporated cane juice, and coconut oil.
3. Add vanilla.
4. Mix baking powder with applesauce and add to mixer. Blend until combined.
5. Slowly mix in dry ingredients, a little at a time, until incorporated.
6. Add in warm water until the batter is the consistency of traditional cake batter. If it's too dry, add a little more water.
7. Mix on high for 1 minute.
8. Line a muffin pan with cupcake liners. Scoop cake batter into the liners, ¾ full.
9. Bake in a 350° oven for 14–15 minutes or until tops are golden and spring back when touched.
10. Frost with chocolate or vanilla buttercream frosting, next page.

Makes 12

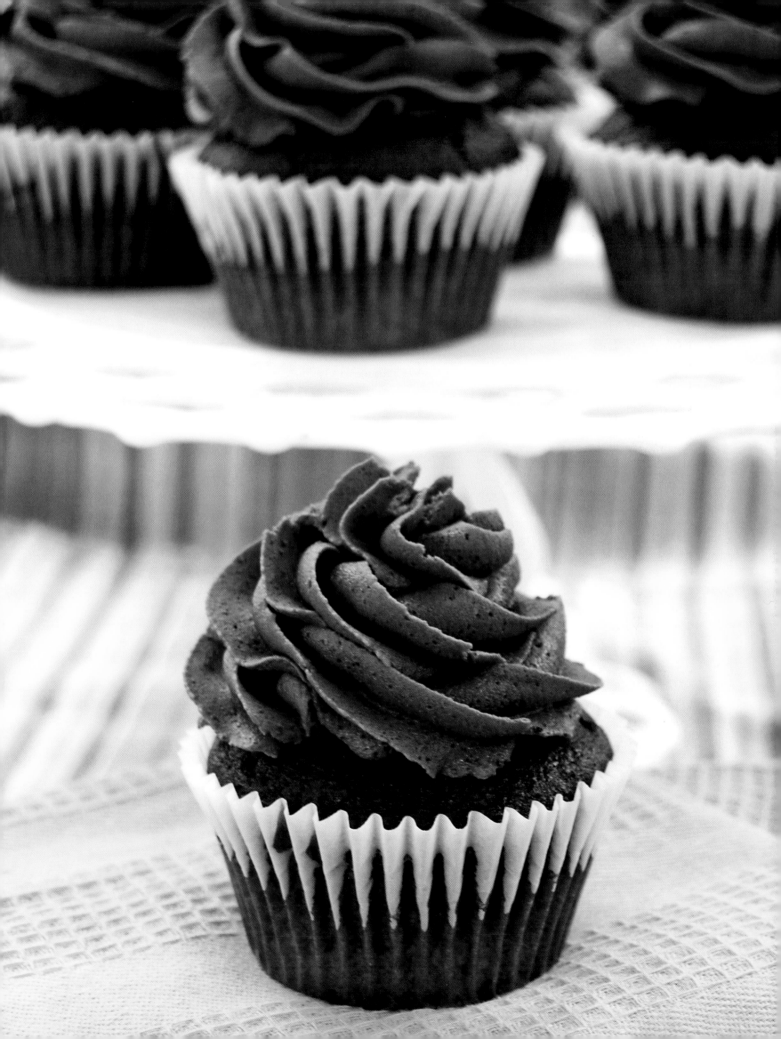

Vanilla Buttercream Frosting

This delectable buttercream will satisfy any craving you ever had for the real thing. By far the best non-allergenic version, this frosting is a hit with absolutely everyone young and old, gluten-free, dairy-free, or not. We love it on cupcakes, brownies, and even my Morning Glory Muffins (p. 62)!

1	C (240 g) nondairy butter (or ½ C [120g] butter ½ C [95g] shortening)
2	Tbsp pure vanilla extract
1	lb (450 g) organic powdered sugar

1. Blend butter and vanilla.
2. Add powdered sugar, a little at a time, until fully incorporated. If too thick, add water, 1 Tbsp at a time, until desired consistency.

Tip:

If you can, add the scraped inside of 1 vanilla bean. It takes this frosting to a whole new level!

Chocolate Buttercream Frosting

Really, do I need to say anything about rich, buttery (but without the dairy) chocolate frosting? You know you love it.

1	C (240 g) nondairy butter (or ½ C [120 g] butter ½ C [95 g] shortening)
2	Tbsp pure vanilla extract
½	C (60 g) organic cocoa powder
1	lb (450 g) organic powdered sugar (reserve 1 C/100 g)

1. Blend butter and vanilla.
2. Add in cocoa powder, mix well.
3. Add powdered sugar, a little at a time, until fully incorporated. If too thick, add water, 1 Tbsp at a time, until desired consistency.

Baking / Desserts / Snacks

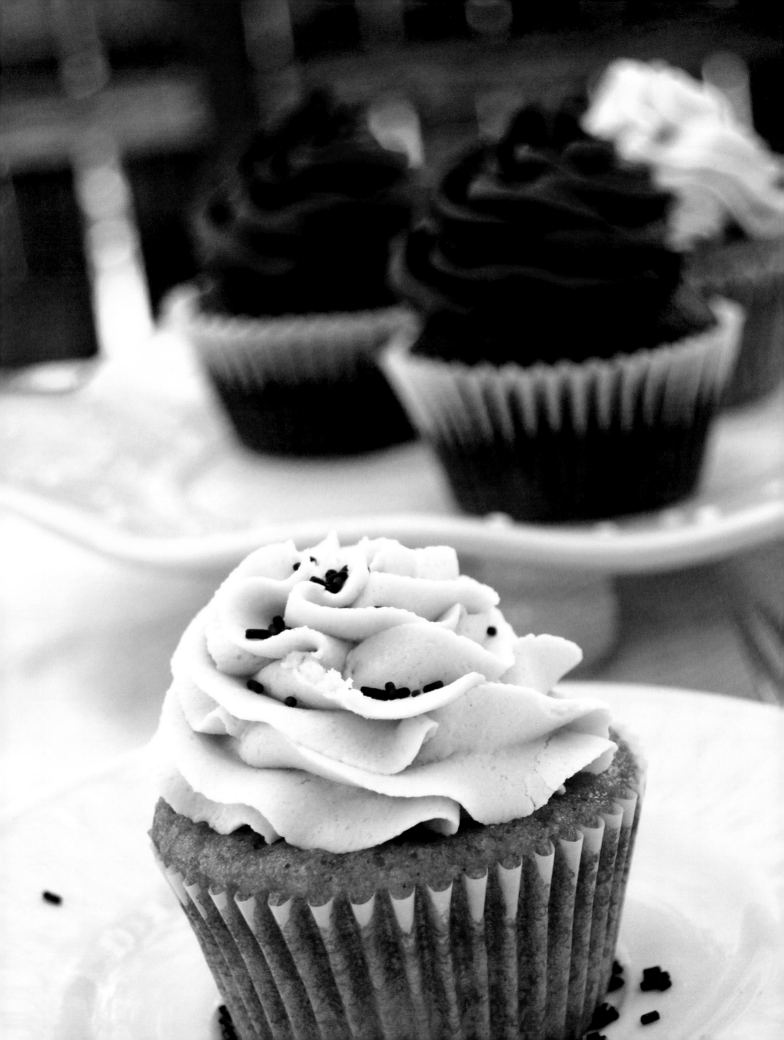

Easy-Bake Oven Mix Vanilla Cake

My kids were elated when I created this recipe. There's nothing that breaks a mama's heart more than seeing her little girl sad and dejected at Christmas because she wants an Easy-Bake Oven but knows she won't get one because she can't eat anything it bakes. Uh-uh. Not on my watch. So here is a nice little mix you can throw together and have on hand when the baking mood strikes your little one! And no worries, since they are allergy friendly! (I should add that these were developed and made for a traditional kids' baking oven, with the light bulb. This recipe was created far before the new high-tech ones that have a heating element and not a light bulb.)

For the Mix:

2	Tbsp sorghum flour
2	tsp brown rice flour
3	Tbsp teff flour
1	tsp millet flour
¼	C (30 g) potato starch
⅛	tsp xanthan gum
1	tsp baking powder
¼	tsp baking soda
⅛	tsp sea salt
2	Tbsp organic evaporated cane juice (feel free to eliminate the sugar and add 1 tsp honey or maple syrup when making a cake)

To Make Cake:

3	level Tbsp cake mix
1–2	Tbsp water
1	tsp pure vanilla extract

1. Preheat oven 10 minutes.
2. In a small bowl, mix 3 level Tbsp cake mix with 1 tsp pure vanilla extract and 1 Tbsp warm water. If batter is too thick, add a little more water until batter is consistency of regular cake batter.
3. Bake 11–12 minutes. Cool 5 minutes in pan. Remove cake to cooling rack to cool completely.
4. Frost cake with vanilla frosting recipe, below.

Vanilla Frosting (for 1 cake)

¼	C (25 g) organic powdered sugar
⅛	tsp pure vanilla extract
~	Pinch of sea salt
2	tsp soft nondairy butter
~	A few drops of water

1. In a small bowl combine all frosting ingredients. Stir with a fork until combined.
2. Spread over cooled cake and enjoy!

Options:

~For chocolate cake, add 2 Tbsp organic cocoa powder to the cake mix.

~For chocolate frosting, add 2 tsp organic cocoa powder to the frosting ingredients.

Makes about 5 cake mixes

Baking / Desserts / Snacks

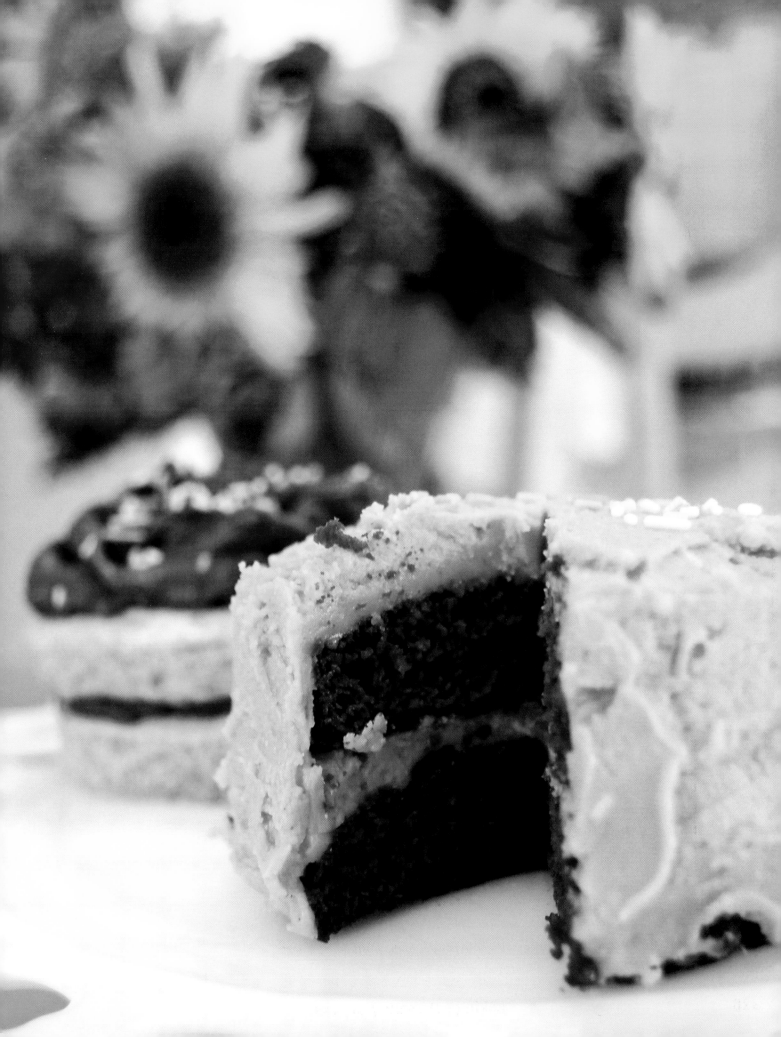

Birthday Bundts

I call these birthday Bundts, and not just chocolate cake, because my oldest daughter asks for these every year for her birthday. She doesn't want a sheet cake. Doesn't want a layer cake. And a big "no thanks" to cupcakes. Being able to have her own "fancy" little chocolate Bundt on her special day makes it that much more special. And while they look like they'd be complicated and time-consuming, they are really very easy to make, but have a big visual impact. Give it a try for your special someone's special day.

Dry Ingredients:

¼	C (30 g) brown rice flour
⅓	C (40 g) sorghum flour
⅓	C (40 g) teff flour
½	C (60 g) potato starch
⅓	C (40 g) tapioca starch
1	tsp xanthan gum
1½	tsp baking powder
½	tsp baking soda
⅓	C (40 g) organic cocoa powder

Wet Ingredients:

¼	C (60 g) nondairy butter (Earth Balance brand)
⅔	C (130 g) organic evaporated cane juice
⅓	C (80 mL) coconut oil, melted
1	Tbsp pure vanilla extract
⅓	C (80 mL) unsweetened organic applesauce mixed with ½ tsp baking powder
⅔	C (160 mL) warm water

1. In a medium bowl whisk together dry ingredients.
2. In a stand mixer cream together butter and sugar.
3. Add coconut oil, vanilla, applesauce mixed with baking powder, and warm water. Mix until combined.
4. Slowly add dry ingredients to the wet ingredients and mix on low until fully incorporated. Turn mixer to high and mix for 1 minute.
5. Scoop dough into a greased mini Bundt pan.
6. Bake in a 350° oven for 14–16 minutes or until cake springs back to the touch.
7. Cool in pan for 10 minutes, then remove cakes carefully by placing a cooling rack on top the pan, inverting, tapping pan, and then removing pan.
8. Cool cakes on wire rack.
9. Frost with Chocolate Ganache (p. 332) or Buttercream Frosting (p. 326), or heck, why not both?

Options:

~I like to add chocolate chips to the batter prior to baking for an extra chocolate touch!

Tip:

~When storing frosted cupcakes and cakes, leave the lid of your container slightly askew. This allows for just enough airflow to keep the frosting from turning watery and creating too much moisture.

Makes 10–11

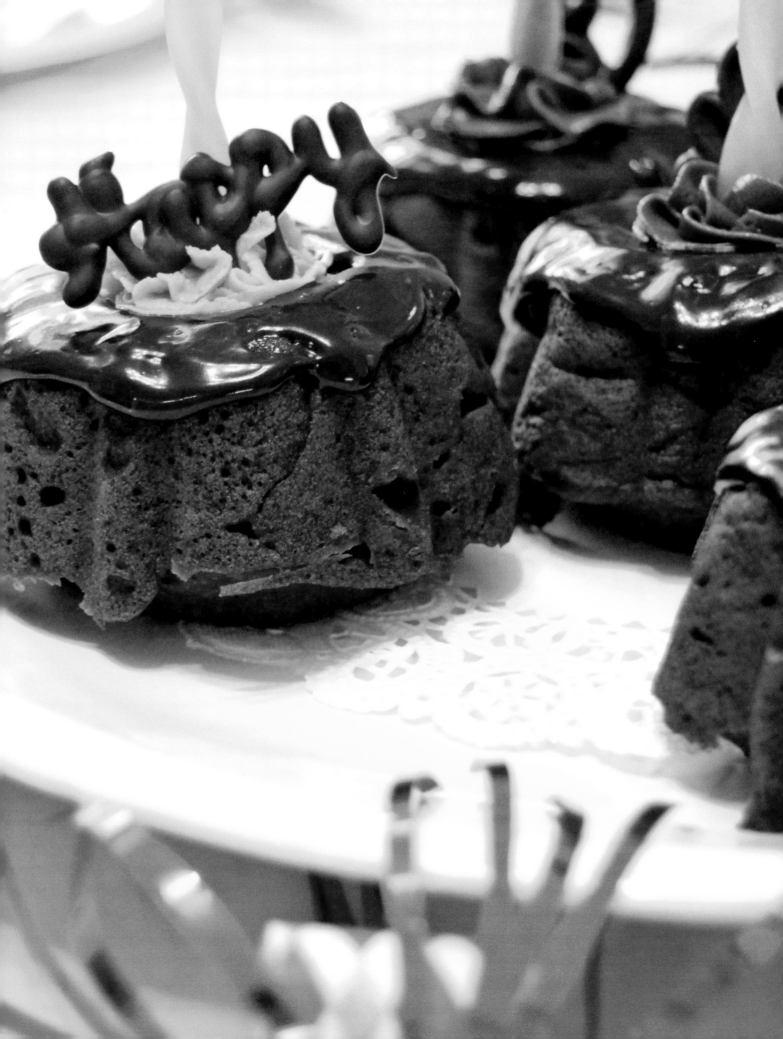

Chocolate Ganache

Chocolate Ganache is one of those elegant toppings that seem difficult to make, until someone teaches you, and then you realize it's easier than boiling water! The original, made with dark chocolate and heavy cream, is spectacular, but using full-fat canned coconut milk gives you the same indulgent flavor without the allergic reaction. This sauce is wonderful drizzled on just about anything you can imagine, plus it's great as a quick frosting for a cake. Everyone will think you went all out, but you'll know it was as easy as simmering some coconut milk and stirring!

½ **C (120 mL) canned lite coconut milk**

1 **C (150 g) GF DF semisweet chocolate chips (Enjoy Life works well)**

1. In a small saucepan heat milk until it starts to bubble around the edges.
2. Add in chocolate chips, remove from heat.
3. Whisk chocolate and milk until smooth and combined. Use immediately to frost cakes, cookies, etcetera, or store in a jar with a tight-fitting lid in the fridge or freezer. Heat in microwave to use.

Options:

~Makes a great dip for strawberries. Just reheat with a small amount of coconut milk and dip away!

~Drizzle over ice cream for an "almost hot fudge."

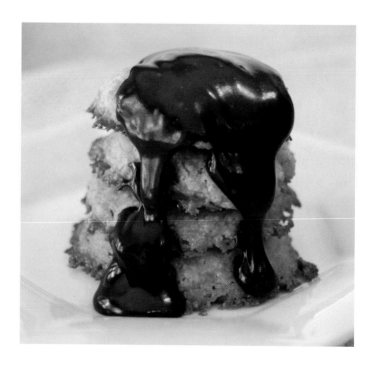

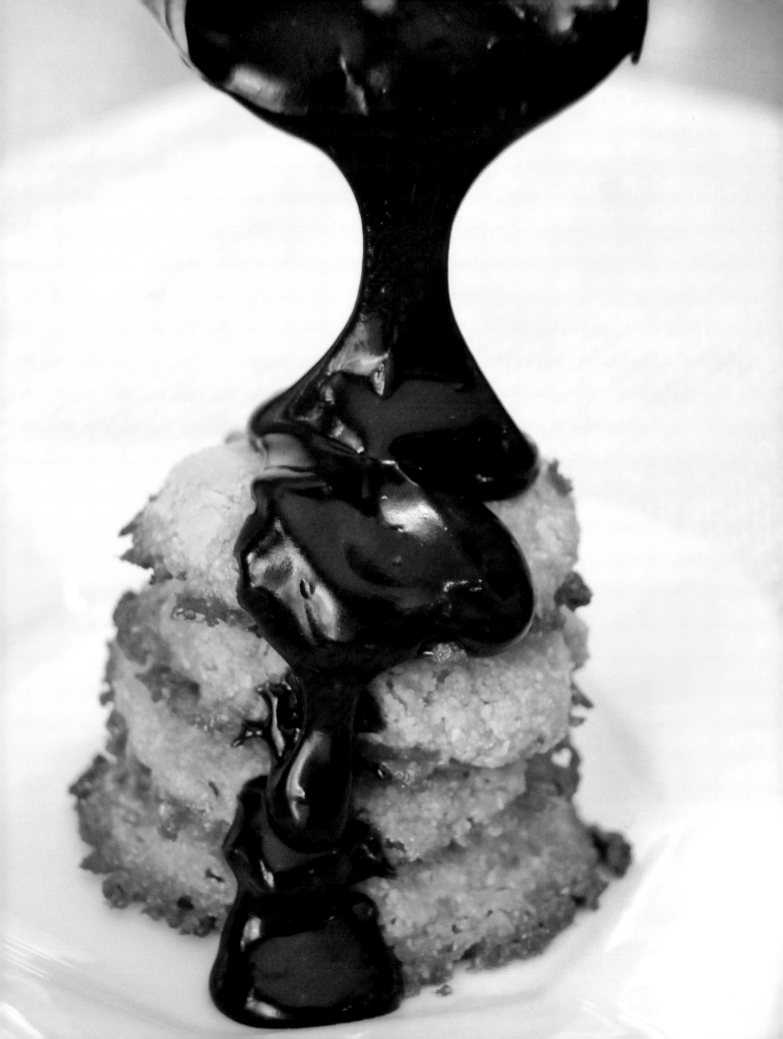

Flower Pot Cakes

I originally saw this recipe on a popular blog, The Pioneer Woman, *but never thought I could make it. But when my daughter saw them and begged for them at her next birthday party, I knew I needed to get creative. It is possible, and they are actually so easy to make! The best part is you can make them a day ahead so you're not trying to assemble the day of the party. OK, that's not the best part... the really best part is that they're absolutely delicious!*

~ **Chocolate Cupcakes (p. 324)**

~ **Vanilla Ice Cream (p. 346) or your favorite nondairy store brand, softened (I like So Delicious Vanilla Coconut Milk Ice Cream)**

~ **GF Chocolate sandwich cookies (Glutino or Kinnikinnick)**

~ **Cleaned and washed 3-inch terra cotta pots**

~ **Clear drinking straws**

~ **Flowers**

1. Place cupcake in the bottom of a cleaned terra cotta pot.
2. Push a straw into the center of each cupcake and cut the straw so that it's level with the top of the pot.
3. Scoop some softened ice cream on top of cupcake and around the straw. You want it to come about ½ inch below the rim of the pot.
4. Place sandwich cookies in a food processor and pulse until they become crumbs.
5. Spoon cookie crumbs over ice cream so that it comes to the top of the pot.
6. Store in freezer and take out at least 1 hour before serving to soften. Terra cotta is a great insulator so it takes awhile for them to soften.
7. Cut flowers to desired height and place one or two stems into each straw. Move crumbs around so they cover the straw and serve!

Makes as many as you need

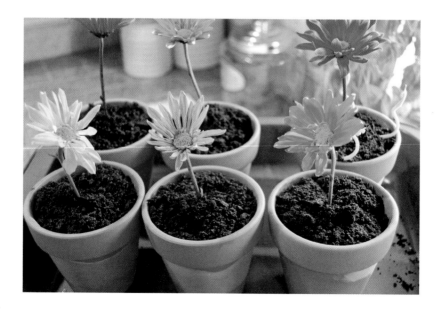

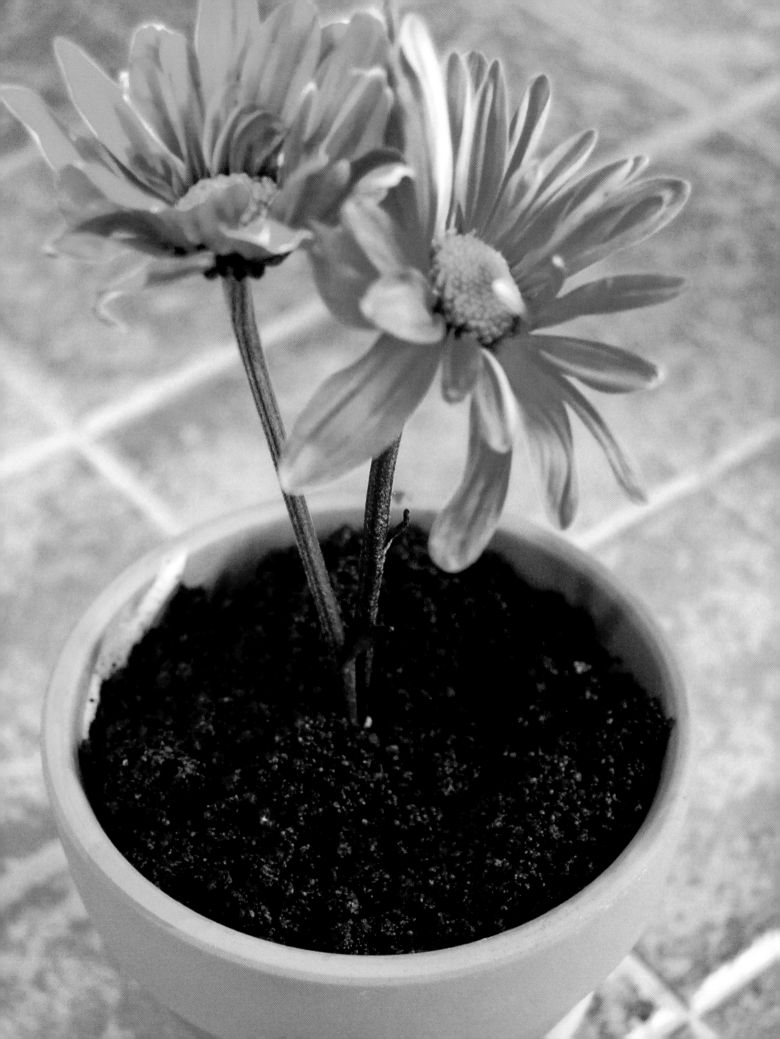

Java Chip Bundt

Chocolate, coffee, cake. Now that's my kind of splurge! This decadent, rich cake really hits the spot, and then some. To make the extra-strong coffee, simply brew coffee normally, except add twice as much coffee grounds. Let it cool to room temperature before using.

Dry Ingredients:

2	Tbsp brown rice flour
2	Tbsp sorghum flour
3	Tbsp teff flour
3	Tbsp potato starch
3	Tbsp tapioca starch
½	tsp xanthan gum
¾	tsp baking powder
¼	tsp baking soda
¼	tsp sea salt
3	Tbsp organic cocoa powder

Wet Ingredients:

2	Tbsp nondairy butter or organic shortening
¼	C (50 g) organic evaporated cane juice
¼	C (60 mL) coconut oil, melted
2	tsp pure vanilla extract
¼	C (60 mL) unsweetened organic applesauce mixed with ¼ tsp baking powder
⅓	C (80 mL) warm water
¼	C (60 mL) extra-extra-strong coffee

Add Ins:

¼	C (40 g) mini chocolate chips (Enjoy Life)

1. In a medium bowl whisk together dry ingredients.
2. In a stand mixer cream together butter and sugar.
3. Add coconut oil, vanilla, applesauce mixed with baking powder, warm water, and coffee. Mix until combined.
4. Slowly add dry ingredients to the wet ingredients and mix on low until fully incorporated. Turn mixer to high and mix for 1 minute. Fold in chocolate chips.
5. Scoop dough into a greased mini Bundt pan.
6. Bake in a 350° oven for 14–16 minutes or until cake springs back to the touch.
7. Cool in pan for 10 minutes, then remove cakes carefully by placing a cooling rack on top the pan, inverting, tapping pan, and then removing pan.
8. Cool cakes on wire rack.
9. Frost with Mocha Java Glaze on the following page.

Makes 6

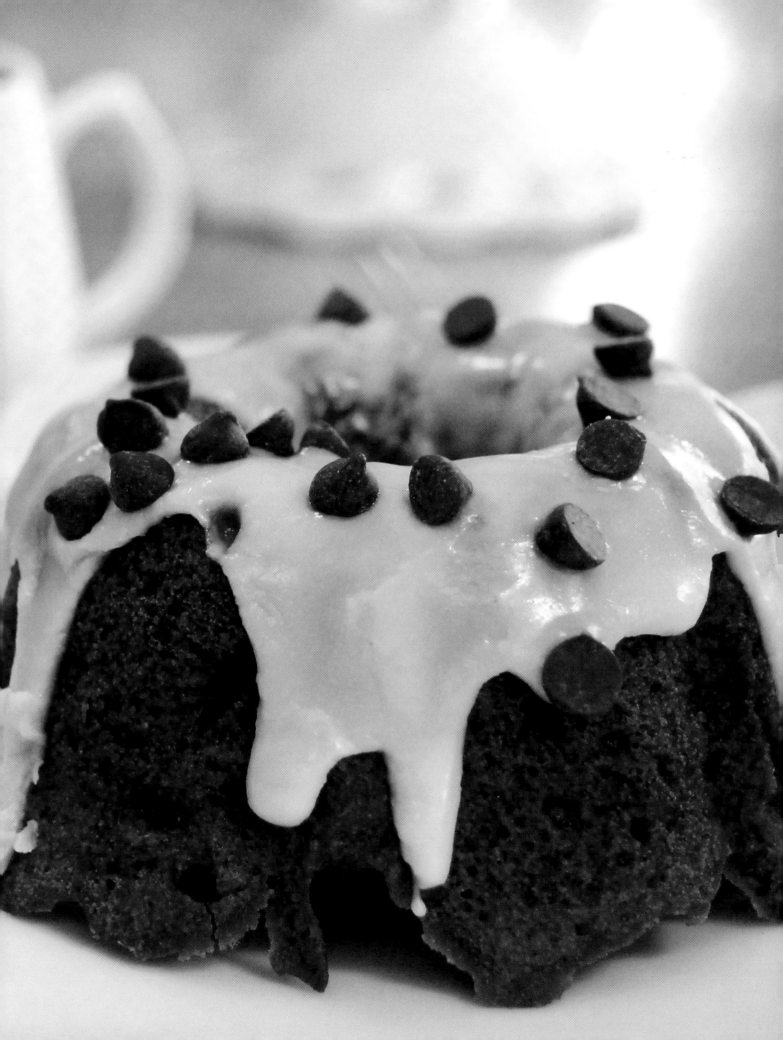

Mocha Java Glaze

While I know it will be difficult, try not to drink this glaze like a cup of coffee. You will not be happy with yourself. It is still delicious drizzled over Java Chip Bundts (p.336), or Double Trouble Cookies (p. 284), or maybe a new scone recipe you adapt from one in this book!

2　C (200 g) organic powdered sugar

1　tsp softened nondairy butter

2–3　Tbsp strong coffee (double-strength, cooled)

1. In a medium bowl, whisk together ingredients until smooth.
2. Spoon over Mocha Java Bundts on the previous page.

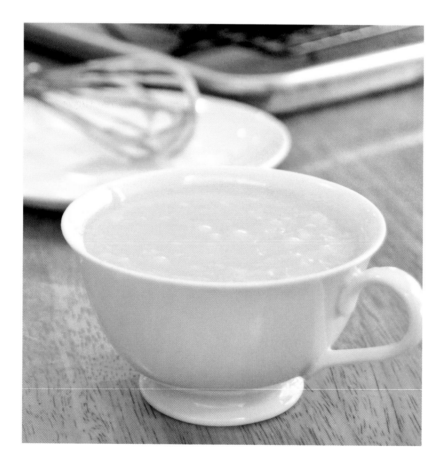

Lemon Icing

The fresh juice and lemon zest really make this icing pop, so don't rely on a lemon extract for this one. Fresh lemons are the way to go to capture that amazing flavor and tanginess that only fresh lemon juice can deliver. Drizzle over Lemon Poppy Seed Bundt Cakes (p. 340), Vanilla Cupcakes (p. 322), or try a drizzle over warm Blueberry Muffins (p. 58) instead of the crumb topping. Delicious anyway you spoon it!

2	**C (200 g) organic powdered sugar**
~	**Juice of ½ organic lemon**
1	**tsp nondairy butter, melted**
1–2	**Tbsp nondairy milk**
~	**Zest of ½ lemon**

1. In a medium bowl whisk together powdered sugar, lemon juice, butter, lemon zest, and 1 Tbsp of milk until combined and smooth.
2. If icing is too thick, add milk, a few drops at a time, until desired consistency.

Tip:

~If you add too much liquid and the icing is too runny, simply add more powdered sugar, a Tbsp at a time, until it thickens.

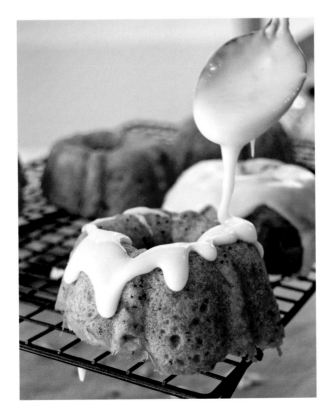

Lemon Poppy Seed Bundt

This little bundle of deliciousness was first introduced at a farmers market in our hometown one summer. We sold out in 15 minutes. I was pretty sure at that point I had a winner—but you'll know it when you take your first bite. The cake is so soft and spongy, so lemony, so absolutely perfect! We love it as is, but we especially love it with a few sliced strawberries on top. Any fresh summer berry would be a great accompaniment to this lovely little cake though, so have a fun with it!

Dry Ingredients:

3	Tbsp teff flour
3	Tbsp brown rice flour
1 ½	Tbsp sorghum flour
¼	C (30 g) potato starch
2	Tbsp tapioca starch
½	tsp xanthan gum
¾	tsp baking powder
¼	tsp baking soda
¼	rounded tsp sea salt

Wet Ingredients:

3	Tbsp nondairy butter (Earth Balance brand)
¼	C (60 mL) coconut oil, melted
⅓	C (65 g) organic evaporated cane juice
1	Tbsp pure vanilla extract
¼	C (60 mL) organic unswseetened applesauce mixed with ½ tsp baking powder
~	Juice of ½ organic lemon (reserve the juice of the other half for the icing)
1	tsp pure lemon extract
~	Zest of ½ lemon
¼	C (60 mL) warm water (if needed)
2	tsp poppy seeds

1. Whisk together dry ingredients. Set aside.
2. In a stand mixer blend together butter, oil, and sugar until combined.
3. Add vanilla, applesauce mixture, lemon juice, lemon extract, and lemon zest.
4. Slowly add dry ingredients to the wet, mixing until fully incorporated. Add small amounts of warm water if the batter is too thick. Batter should be a litter thicker than traditional cake batter.
5. Mix in Poppy Seeds.
6. Fill a greased or sprayed mini Bundt pan with batter, about ¾ full. Smooth the tops with a spoon.
7. Bake in a 350° oven for 14–15 minutes, or until a toothpick inserted in the center comes out clean and cake springs back to the touch.
8. Cool in pans for 5 minutes, then invert onto a cooling rack. Tap the pan gently to release the cakes. Let cakes cool completely before icing with Lemon Icing recipe on the previous page.

Tip:

~Zest lemon first, then cut in half and juice. Much easier to zest a full lemon than one that has already been juiced!

Makes 6 mini Bundt cakes

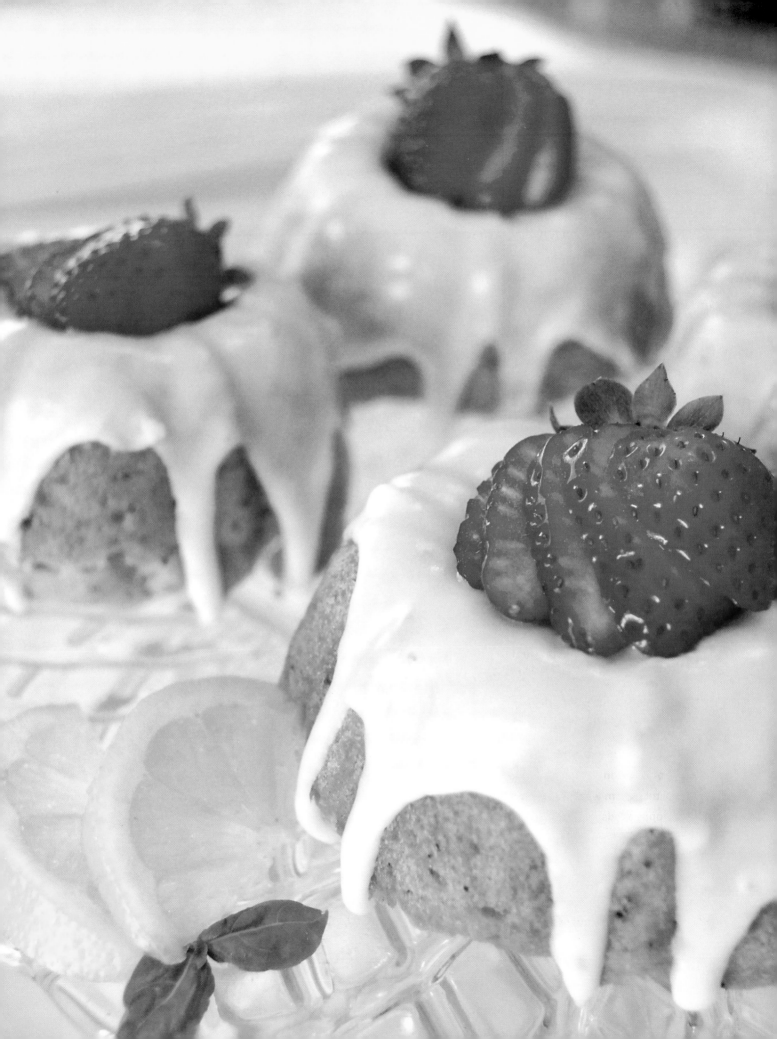

Cookies 'n' Cream Coconut Milk Ice Cream

This is my daughter's favorite ice cream, and she thought she'd never have it again after learning she had food allergies. And then along came a wonderful company who finally and thankfully brought us a gluten-free version of the famous chocolate sandwich cookie we all loved as kids! So for her birthday one year I surprised her with homemade cookies 'n' cream ice cream to have with her cake. She was so excited I don't think she remembers any of her presents that year... but she remembers the ice cream! And by making it with honey and coconut nectar there is no sugar added (except for those in the cookies, which is plenty) so enjoy each blissful bite!

Ice Cream:

2	**cans (about 900 mL) lite coconut milk, chilled (I like Trader Joes brand)**
1½	**Tbsp pure vanilla extract (plus adding the scraped inside of a vanilla bean really sends this ice cream over the top, but it's not essential for the recipe if you don't have one)**
~	**Pinch of sea salt**
¼	**C (60 mL) organic raw honey**
¼	**C (60 mL) coconut nectar (if you have to use sugar, you can use it in place of the nectar)**

Add In:

1	**C (150 g) crushed GF chocolate sandwich cookies (I used Glutino)**

1. Whisk together all ingredients, except cookie crumbs, until well blended. Pour into your prepared ice cream maker bowl and follow manufacturer instructions.
2. After about 25 minutes, add in cookie crumbs. Let machine go for about another 10 minutes or until desired consistency. Serve immediately and enjoy the goodness!

Note:

~We've tried a lot of ice cream makers over the years, and our current machine is a Cuisinart stainless steel and it's amazing! It actually makes ice cream so firm you can scoop it onto cones. Really!

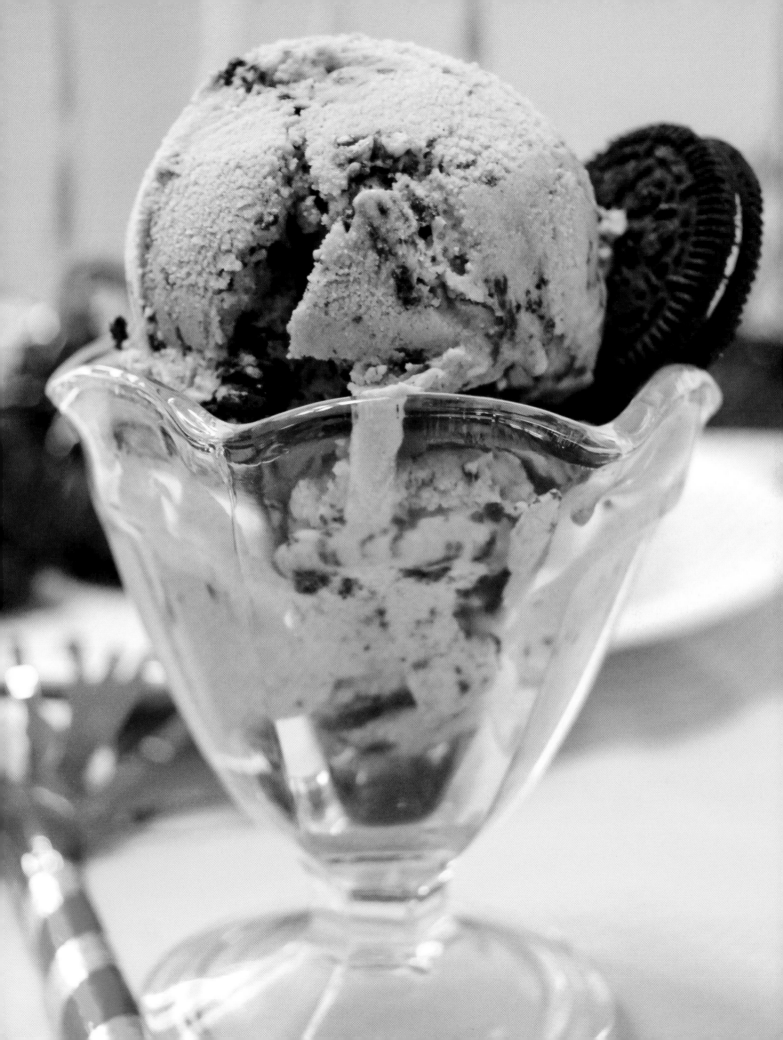

Chocolate Cherry Almond Ice Cream

The combination of cherries, chocolate, and almonds is absolute perfection in a bowl. The cherries turn the ice cream pink during the process, which I believe adds to its deliciousness. Garnish with a few toasted almonds for even more flavor.

Ice Cream:

2	cans (about 900 mL) lite coconut milk, chilled
1½	Tbsp pure vanilla extract (plus adding the scraped inside of a vanilla bean really sends this ice cream over the top, but it's not essential for the recipe if you don't have one)
1	tsp pure almond extract
~	Pinch of sea salt
¼	C (60 mL) organic raw honey
¼	C (60 mL) coconut nectar (if you have to use sugar, you can use it in place of the nectar)

Add In:

¼	C (40 g) mini GF DF chocolate chips (Enjoy Life)
1	C (150 g) chopped frozen or fresh pitted cherries

1. Whisk together all ingredients, except chocolate chips and cherries, until well blended.

2. Pour into your prepared ice cream maker bowl and follow manufacturer instructions.

3. After about 25 minutes, add in chocolate chips and cherries. Let machine go for about another 10 minutes or until desired consistency. Serve immediately and enjoy the goodness!

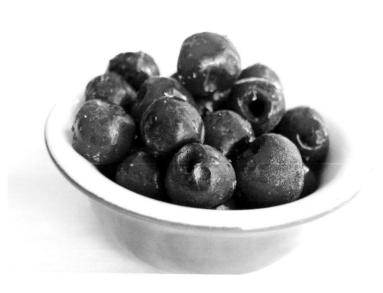

Baking / Desserts / Snacks

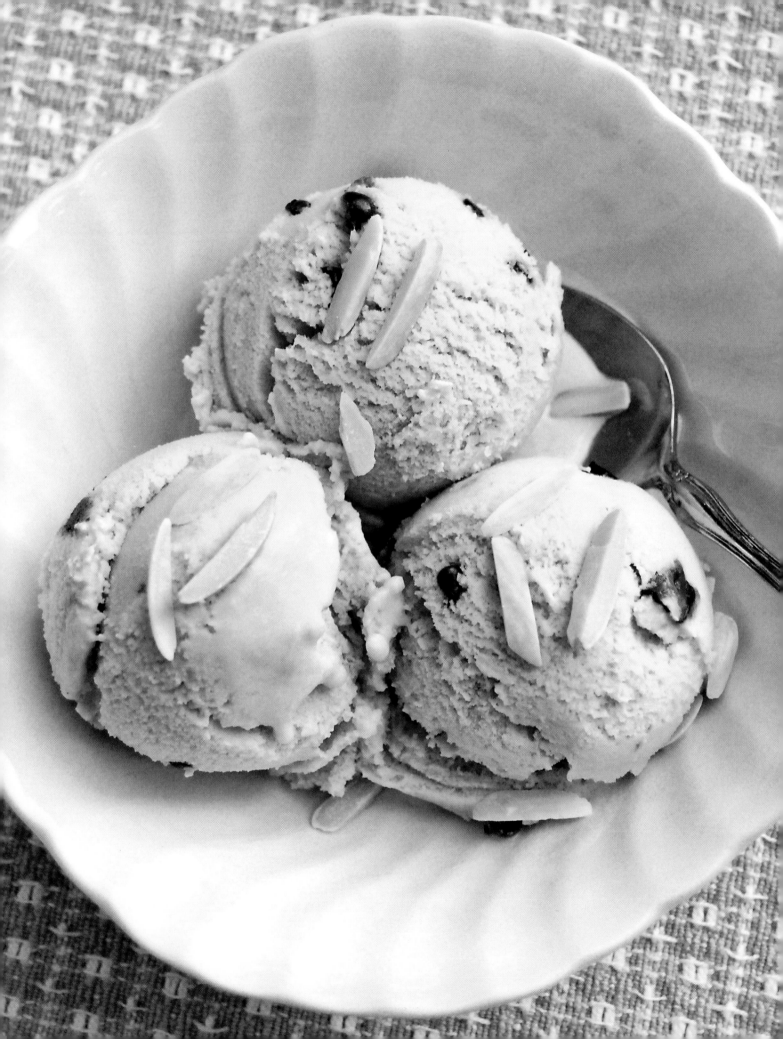

Vanilla Ice Cream

A wonderful basic vanilla ice cream, that's anything but basic. Delicious and made without dairy, it is perfect to pair with Peach Cobbler (p. 350), Berry Crisp (p. 348), or scooped into cookies for Ice Cream Sandwiches (p. 360).

2	**cans (about 900 mL) lite coconut milk, chilled**
1½	**Tbsp pure vanilla extract**
2	**vanilla beans, split and insides scraped out, discard outside bean and use inner scrapings**
~	**Pinch of sea salt**
¼	**C (60 mL) organic raw honey**
¼	**C (60 mL) coconut nectar (if you have to use sugar, you can use it in place of the nectar)**

1. Whisk together all ingredients until well blended.
2. Pour into your prepared ice cream maker bowl and follow manufacturer instructions.

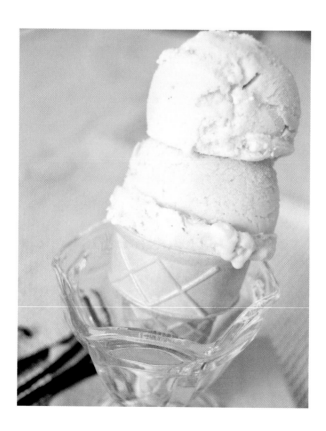

Frozen Banana Splits

Summer treats are great, but if you have a family member that cannot tolerate dairy, summer can be long and deprived. While there are some great dairy-free ice cream choices at the market these days, sometimes I like to not have to leverage the house to buy a pint or two for the family. This frugal sundae option is healthy, refreshing, and budget friendly. So go ahead and indulge, with no worries about your next mortgage payment!

4	ripe organic bananas, peeled, sliced lengthwise, then cut in half
1½	C (225 g) frozen organic strawberries, thawed slightly, and coarsely chopped
1	can (about 400 g) organic pineapple chunks, in juice
~	Chocolate Ganache (p. 332)
4	fresh cherries

1. Line a cookie sheet with wax paper. Place bananas on wax paper and place in the freezer. Freeze for about 1 hour, or until the bananas are firm and almost frozen through, but not hard.
2. Place bananas in serving bowls.
3. Spoon strawberries, pineapple, and chocolate over bananas.
4. Top with a fresh cherry and serve immediately.

Serves 4

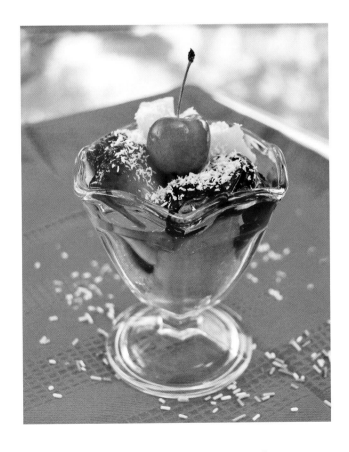

The Healthy Gluten-Free Life

Berry Crisp

This makes a wonderful, easy dessert in the summer when berries are at their peak! Although sometimes, in the dead of winter when I can't stand the white stuff anymore (a.k.a. snow), I pull out the frozen berries that we picked fresh the previous summer and whip up a little Berry Crisp to warm our tummies. It helps, if only but a little.

Filling:

5	C (750 g) fresh or frozen organic berries
2	Tbsp raw organic honey
1	Tbsp arrowroot starch
1	Tbsp brown rice flour
~	Squeeze of lemon juice
½	tsp cinnamon

Topping:

1	Tbsp flax meal mixed with 2 Tbsp hot water
¼	C (30 g) almond meal
½	C (75 g) chopped pecans
¼	C (40 g) raw sunflower seed kernels
2	Tbsp organic brown sugar (you can use honey or coconut nectar here, but I really love the flavor of the brown sugar for this crisp)
1	tsp cinnamon
3	Tbsp organic shortening (Spectrum), melted

1. Mix flax meal and hot water, set aside to thicken.
2. In a large bowl, mix the filling ingredients together until berries are all coated.
3. In medium bowl, mix together the topping ingredients until combined and crumbly.
4. Grease a small casserole dish (I use a 7" by 8" or so). Pour coated berries into the dish until it's just about level with the top of the dish.
5. Spoon topping over berries and spread around to cover evenly.
6. Bake in a 350° oven for 45–55 minutes or until bubbly and top is browned.

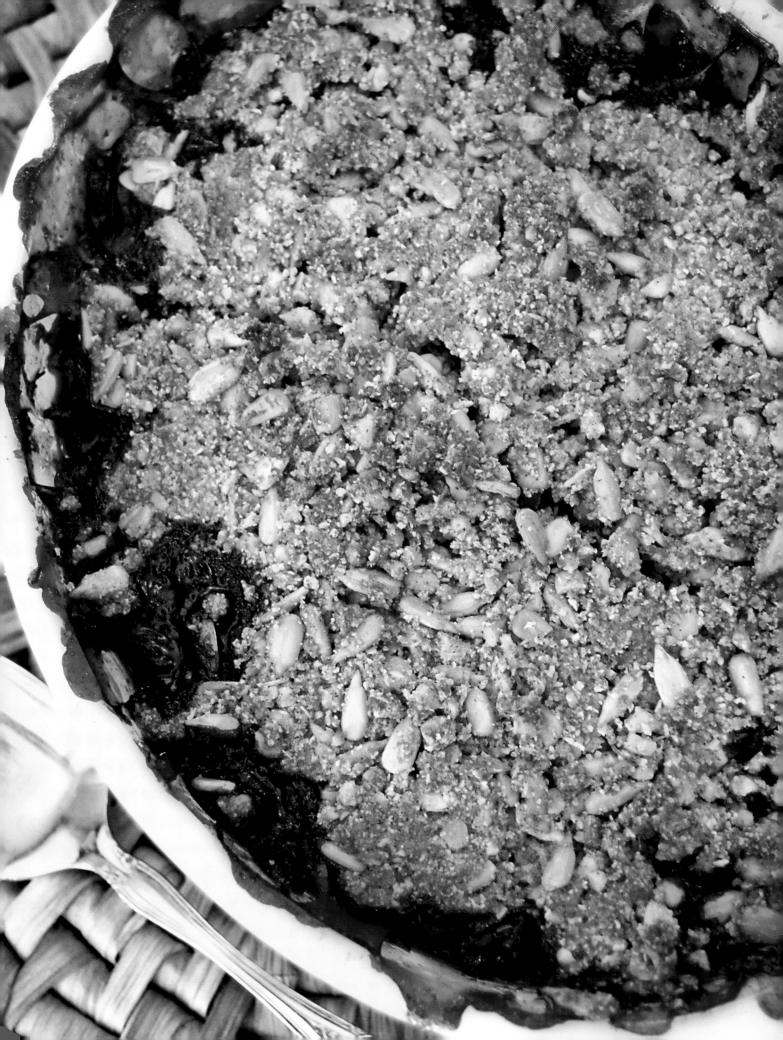

Peach Cobbler

This one's for my Mama! Her original recipe, converted to gluten-free, and still just as wonderful. With each bite I'm taken back to ten years old and summertime peaches from our backyard tree. This makes a nice size dish for the family, but feel free to double for a larger 9" by 13" baking dish to serve company. And since the sugar is minimal, we even eat leftovers for breakfast!

Dry Ingredients:

¼	C (30 g) teff flour
3	Tbsp brown rice flour
¼	C (30 g) sorghum flour
¼	C (30 g) potato starch
3	Tbsp tapioca starch
½	tsp xanthan gum
1	tsp baking powder
¼	tsp baking soda
½	tsp sea salt

Wet Ingredients:

¼	C (60 g) nondairy butter (Earth Balance brand)
¼	C (60 ml) coconut oil, melted
⅓	C (60 g) packed organic brown sugar
1½	tsp pure vanilla extract
3	Tbsp unsweetened organic applesauce with ½ tsp baking powder
¾	C (180 mL) warm water

Add in:

4	C (600 g) sliced organic peaches (You can peel them, or be lazy like me and just slice them. Either way it will be yummy.)

1. Preheat oven to 350°.
2. Melt butter in a 9" by 9" baking dish in the preheating oven.
3. In a medium bowl whisk together dry ingredients.
4. In a stand mixer combine wet ingredients and blend together.
5. Slowly add dry ingredients to the wet ingredients until fully incorporated. Blend on high for 30 seconds.
6. Pour half of batter into baking dish with the butter. Spoon peaches evenly over the batter. Top with remaining batter.
7. Bake 45–55 minutes or until top is browned, peaches are bubbling, and dough in the center is cooked.

Options:

~Try replacing peaches with fresh blackberries!

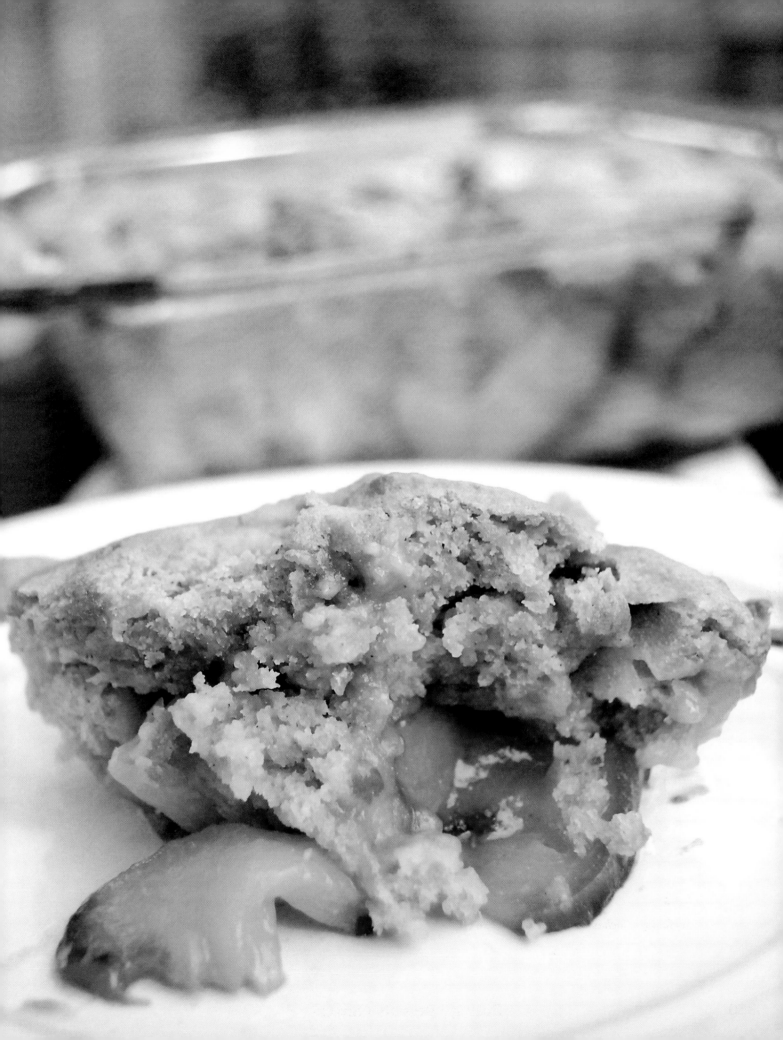

Shortcakes

There's no time like summertime to enjoy a heaping helping of strawberry shortcake. Or how about blackberry shortcake? It's beautiful, it's delicious, it screams summer. Oh heck, why not make both? With a hearty, healthy shortcake recipe like this one, you can even have it for breakfast without any remorse. Strawberry shortcake for dessert, blackberry shortcake for breakfast.... Sounds good to me!

Dry Ingredients:

¾	C (90 g) sorghum flour
¾	C (90 g) teff flour
½	C (60 g) potato starch
½	C (60 g) tapioca starch
1	tsp xanthan gum
1	tsp baking powder
½	tsp baking soda
½	tsp sea salt

Wet Ingredients:

½	C (120 ml) coconut oil, melted
⅓	C (65 g) organic evaporated cane juice
2	tsp pure vanilla extract
1	Tbsp organic unsweetened applesauce
¾	C (180 ml) coconut milk (or other nondairy milk)

1. In a medium bowl, whisk together dry ingredients.
2. In a stand mixer blend coconut oil and sugar.
3. Add vanilla and applesauce, mix to combine.
4. Add dry ingredients and milk alternately until a stiff dough forms and both are used.
5. Drop by large spoonfuls onto a parchment-lined cookie sheet.
6. Sprinkle with sugar and bake at 350° for 25–30 minutes until golden and firm. Remove to a wire rack to cool completely.
7. When cool, cut cakes in half. Spoon blackberries (or your favorite berries) over middle, cover with tops, spoon on more berries, and top with Coconut Whipped Cream (recipe p. 380). Enjoy your summer evening!

Makes 6

Baking / Desserts / Snacks

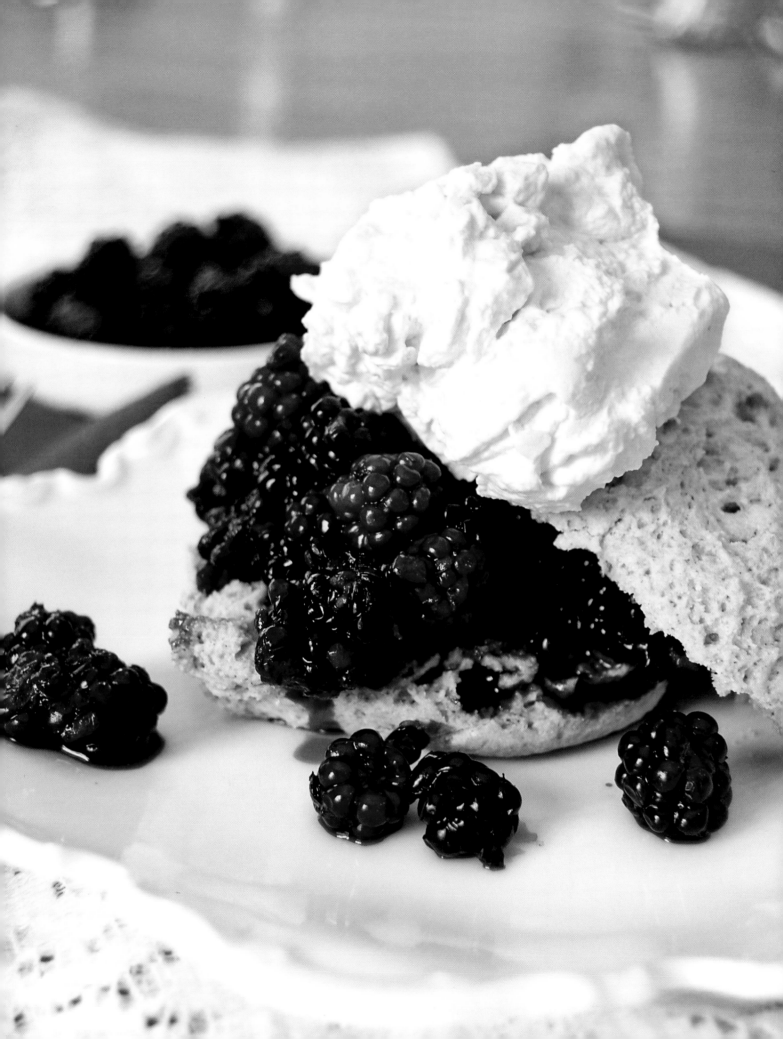

Pecan Praline Bananas

Who knew that real maple syrup, when reduced, could taste so heavenly, gooey, caramely? Oh how I love this dessert! Any recipe that uses such simple, healthy ingredients to create such a satisfying dessert is a keeper in my book.

Sauce:

⅓	C (80 mL) pure maple syrup
1	Tbsp nondairy butter
¼	C (60 mL) canned lite coconut milk
3	Tbsp chopped pecans

Bananas:

1	Tbsp coconut oil
4	bananas, peeled, cut in half, then sliced in half lengthwise

1. In a small saucepan, over medium-high heat, combine maple syrup, butter, milk and pecans. Bring to a boil then reduce heat to medium-low and simmer until the mixture thickens and reduces a bit. About 10 minutes.

2. While sauce cooks, heat oil in a large nonstick skillet over medium-high heat. Add bananas and brown on both sides, about 1 minute per side.

3. Place cooked bananas on plates and spoon pecan praline mixture over each banana.

Serves 4

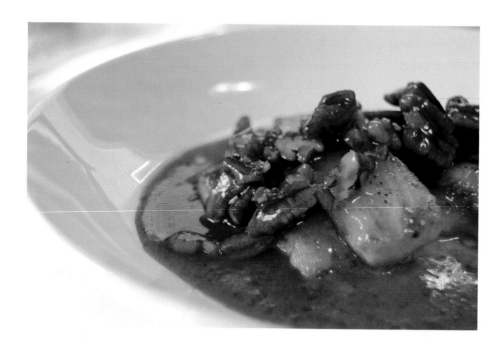

Baking / Desserts / Snacks

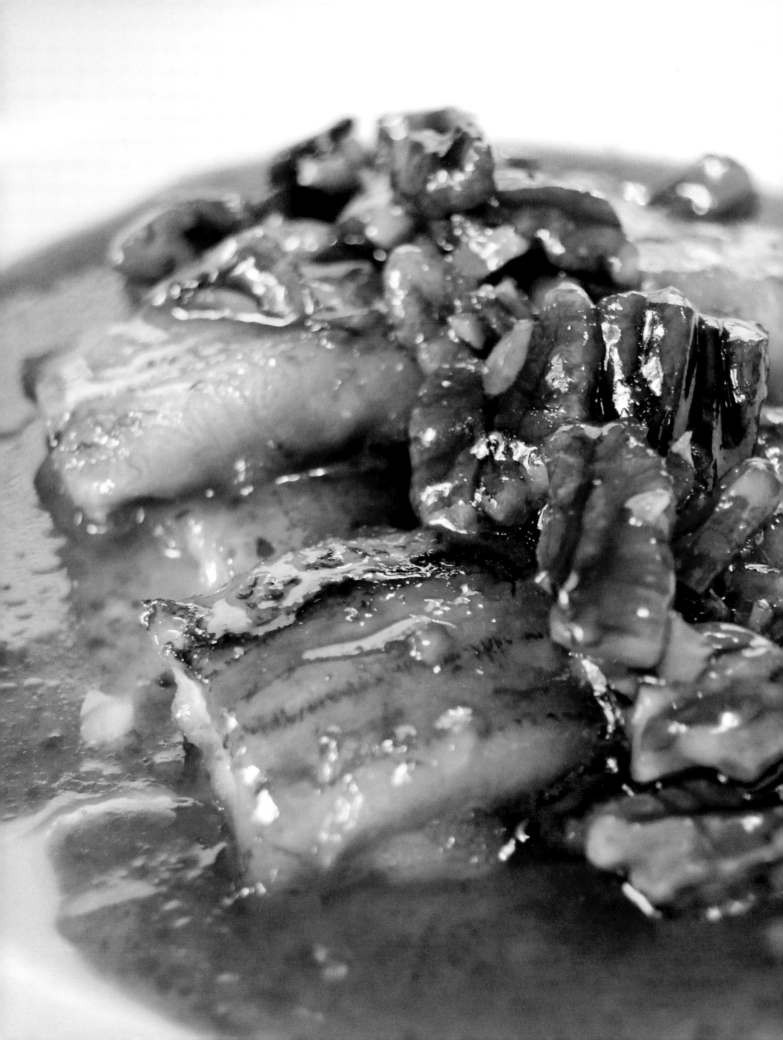

Pie Crust

This pie crust and I have a love-hate relationship. I'm not gonna lie, it's a difficult dough to work with. Don't expect a Martha-esque looking pie from the get-go, it will take some practice. I've said a few choice words to this crust in those first days. But I'll be darned if it isn't perfectly flaky and delicious each time I eat it! So I have pushed through and gotten past the realization that I can't manipulate this dough very well and that it will only be capable of basic pie-dom. I'm OK with it now. Because with each flaky bite I accept that I am easy. Easy for pie! I'd say easy as pie, but this dough really does take a little getting used to, but it's worth it!

Dry Ingredients:

¼ C (30 g) pea flour (look for Bob's Red Mill brand at your local health food store)

⅔ C (80 g) teff flour

¾ C (90 g) brown rice flour

⅔ C (80 g) potato starch

⅔ C (80 g) tapioca starch

1 tsp sea salt

2 tsp xanthan gum

2 Tbsp organic evaporated cane juice

Wet Ingredients:

1¼ C (238 g) Spectrum organic shortening, chilled until firm

1 Tbsp raw apple cider vinegar

1 Tbsp flax meal mixed with 3 Tbsp hot water (let sit for 5 minutes)

5 Tbsp ice cold water (may need more or less depending on dough consistency as you mix)

1. Whisk together dry ingredients.

2. Cut cold shortening into dry ingredients with a pastry blender until pea-size crumbs form.

3. Add vinegar, flax meal mixture, and some of the ice water, stirring with a fork, just until dough comes together and makes a ball. If the dough is still too dry, keep adding water, a tablespoon at a time until the dough comes together.

4. Divide dough in half, and shape each into a disk. Wrap each disk in plastic wrap and chill for 1 hour or freeze for 30 minutes if you're in a hurry for pie, which I always am, so just skip the chilling part and freeze it!

5. To prepare crust, place 1 disk between 2 sheets of wax paper. Roll evenly in all directions until it is a large enough circle to cover the bottom of your pie pan. Or in my case, we love little individual pies, so at this point use a large circle cutter to cut out multiple pie bottoms for whatever pan you are using. I like to use a "Texas"-size muffin pan for these.

6. Place bottom crust in a greased pan, pressing lightly with your fingers to fit the shape of the pan.

7. Fill pie shell with desired fruit.

8. Roll out your top crust the same way, between wax paper. Place on top of pie and crimp edges with your fingers.

9. Cut slits in top of crust to allow steam to escape while baking. If desired, brush crust with some oil and sprinkle with a touch of sugar.

10. Bake 1 large pie in 350° oven for about 1 hour or until fruit is bubbling and crust is browned. If your crust starts turning too brown, feel free to cover loosely with a piece of foil while it finishes baking.

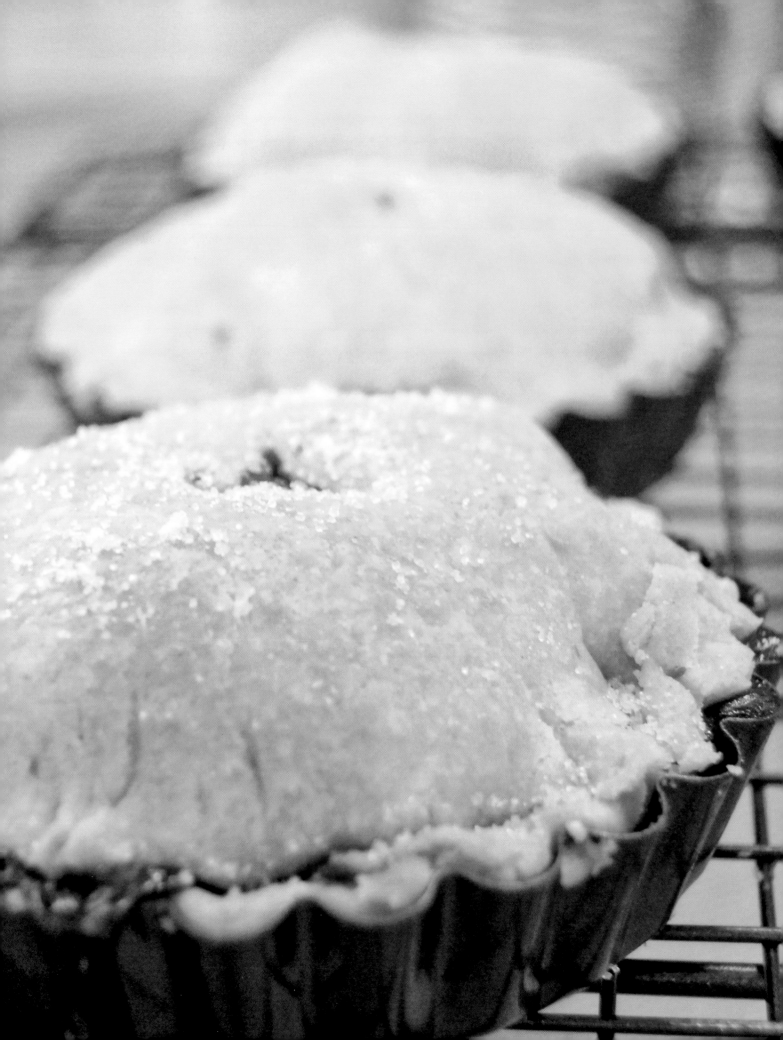

Pie Apples
(a.k.a. Cooked Apples)

This recipe started out as a quick weeknight dessert that would appease the family without the sugar rush before bedtime. Over time, it morphed into a great, make-ahead blend that worked well in quick mini-pies, muffins, pancakes, and over ice cream. Anything that is this easy, flavorful, and versatile is a keeper in my household. As a side note, we just called this cooked apples for awhile, but my astute six-year-old one day asked me to make "those pie apples." I couldn't call them anything but pie apples ever since.

4	**organic apples, peeled, cored and diced (Granny Smith or Pink Lady apples work well)**
¼	**C (60 mL) organic 100% apple juice**
2	**tsp organic cinnamon**
~	**Pinch of nutmeg**

1. Add all ingredients to a medium pot. Heat over medium heat until it starts to simmer.

2. Turn heat to low and simmer, uncovered, until apples are tender, about 15 minutes.

3. Eat as is, drizzle over ice cream, or let cool and freeze in an airtight container until needed. Makes a great pie filling for mini pies, which cook quickly.

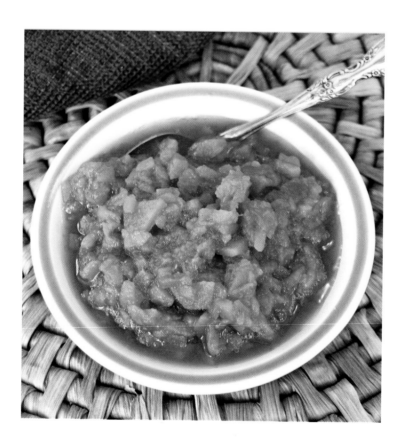

Baking / Desserts / Snacks

Frozen Chocolate Dipped Bananas

This recipe is so simple, I almost feel bad including it in a cookbook. However, each time my kids bring these for snacks to after-school clubs, the plate is clean in minutes and the moms track me down afterward to get the recipe. So, here it is for everyone! Bananas are packed with magnesium and are a superb replacement for ice cream for those who cannot do dairy. Plus, the dark chocolate contains antioxidants! No guilt dessert? Feel free to go bananas!

6	**large organic bananas, peeled and cut in half**
12	**Popsicle sticks**
9	**oz (about 250 g) dark chocolate (or about 1½ C semisweet chocolate chips, such as Enjoy Life)**
1	**Tbsp organic palm shortening (Spectrum brand)**

Toppings:

~ **Chopped nuts**

~ **GF sprinkles**

~ **Toasted coconut**

1. Push popsicle sticks into bottom of bananas, about halfway up. Place bananas on a wax paper–lined cookie sheet. Cover with plastic wrap and freeze for 2 hours, or until hard.

2. In a double boiler, heat chocolate with shortening, just until melted. Remove from heat.

3. Dip bananas into chocolate, place back onto the wax paper, and quickly top with your favorite topping. Chocolate cools fast so you need to work quickly.

4. Repeat for all frozen bananas. Place tray in freezer until chocolate is fully set. Once set, store bananas in an air tight container in the freezer for up to 2 weeks.

Makes 12 bananas

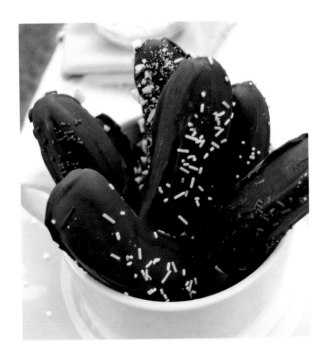

The Healthy Gluten-Free Life

Ice Cream Sandwiches

Just about everyone I know loves a good ice cream sandwich. Especially one made with soft chocolate chip cookies! Next time you bake a batch of cookies, make a few of these incredible sandwiches, wrap them tightly, and freeze. Then anytime the craving strikes, you have a rich, soft-baked, ice cream sandwich at your fingertips! On second thought, maybe that's not such a good idea.... I'll let you decide the strength of your will power for these beauties.

~ **Double Trouble Cookies (p. 284) or Chocolate Chips Cookies (p. 274)**

~ **Vanilla Ice Cream (p. 346) or your favorite nondairy vanilla ice cream (such as Turtle Mountain's So Delicious)**

~ **GF DF mini chocolate chips (I use Enjoy Life)**

1. Place a small scoop of ice cream on the bottom of one cookie.
2. Press another cookie (bottom side to the ice cream) on the other side and press lightly to stick together.
3. Place chocolate chips in a shallow dish. Roll ice cream edges of sandwiches in chips, pressing with your fingers to help them stick.
4. Wrap sandwiches in plastic wrap and freeze until firm. Serve or place wrapped sandwiches in an airtight container to enjoy later. Simply let cookies sit at room temperature for 10 minutes or so to soften.

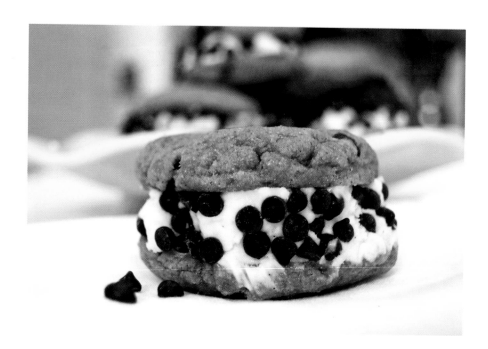

Baking / Desserts / Snacks

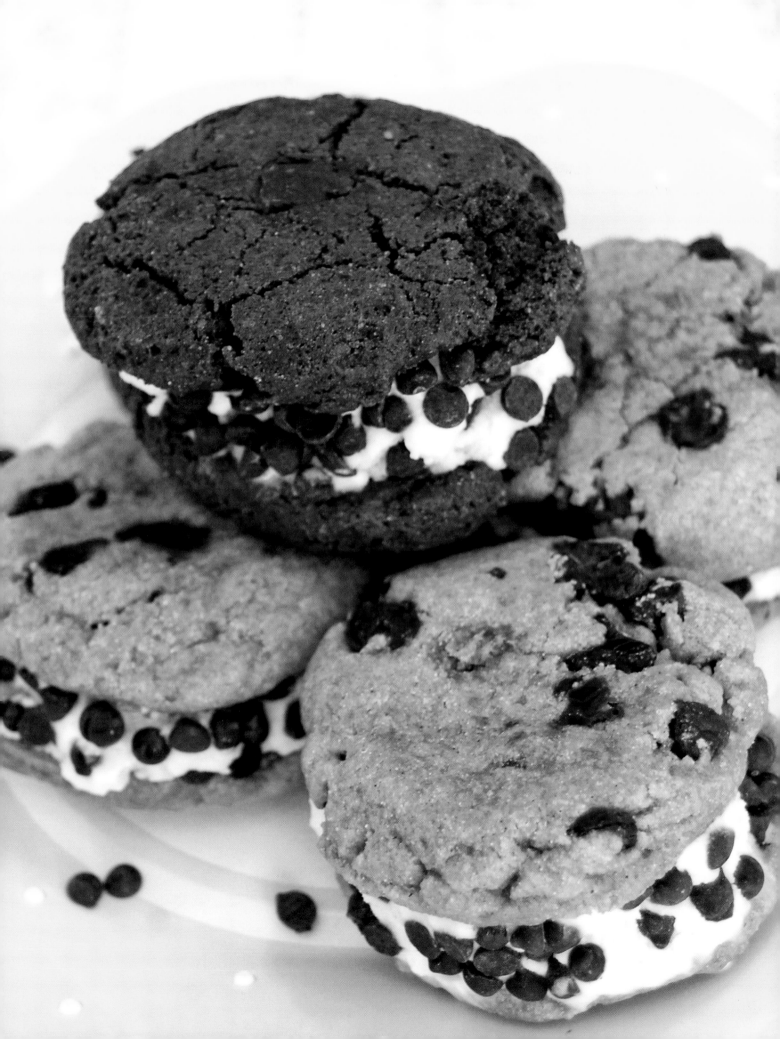

Butter Cups

I call these "butter cups" because they are great with any nut or seed butter. We usually use almond or sunflower butters. They are fun for the kids to help make and even more fun to eat! The taste combination of chocolate and sunbutter (or almond butter) is classic and satisfying, and these don't disappoint. The only disappointing thing would be not making these yummy treats right now!

2	C (300 g) GF DF chocolate chips (Enjoy Life)
2	tsp organic palm shortening (Spectrum)
~	Sunbutter or almond butter of choice
~	Mini baking cups

1. In a double boiler, heat chocolate chips with the shortening. Stir occasionally until almost all the chips are melted. Remove from heat and stir until all chocolate is melted.

2. Carefully spoon the melted chocolate into baking cups, and using the spoon, spread it up the sides until the inside of the cups are covered in chocolate.

3. Place coated baking cups on a sheet pan. Place pan in the freezer until chocolate hardens.

4. With a teaspoon, scoop sunbutter into each chocolate cup.

5. Cover each filled cup with more chocolate, covering the sunbutter.

6. Place tray of filled cups back in the freezer until chocolate hardens.

7. Enjoy! Or store cups in an airtight container in the fridge for up to a week.

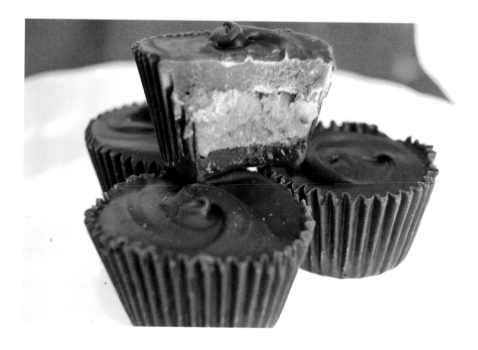

Baking / Desserts / Snacks

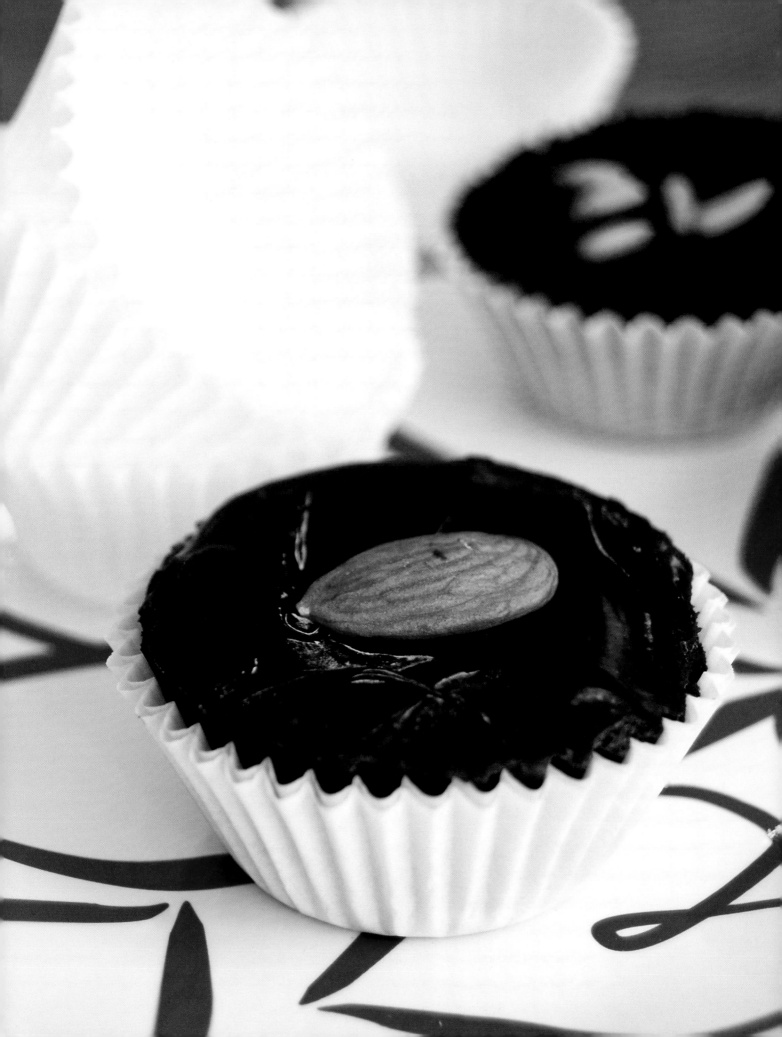

Homemade 'Shmallows

Store bought "traditional" marshmallows are full of high fructose corn syrup, artificial flavors and colors, and a few things I can't pronounce. So every once in a while my kids and I like to whip up a batch of homemade 'shmallows, as we call them, for a special treat. And while, yes, there is a lot of sugar in these (really that's all a marshmallow is), for me it's about controlling what ingredients I use and providing a safe indulgence for my kids. Sometimes the life of a food-intolerant family is the opposite of spontaneous. Everything is always planned in order to maintain morale and safety. With treats like this, we can feel a little footloose and fancy-free without the freedom of getting sick.

For the 'Shmallows:

⅓	C water
1½	packages (10 grams or 1½ Tbsp) unflavored gelatin
¼	C (60 mL) room temperature water
⅛	tsp sea salt
¾	C (150 g) organic evaporated cane juice
½	C (120 mL) golden syrup (I use Lyle's Golden Syrup, or you can use organic corn syrup if desired)
1	Tbsp pure vanilla extract

For Dusting:

¼	C (25 g) organic powdered sugar
¼	C (30 g) GF cornstarch

1. Add ⅓ C (80 mL) cold water to the bowl of a stand mixer fit with a whisk attachment.
2. Sprinkle 1½ packages of gelatin evenly over cold water, let sit.
3. Meanwhile, in a medium saucepan over medium-low heat, combine ¼ C room temperature water, salt, sugar, and golden syrup. Heat, stirring occasionally until sugar is dissolved.
4. Turn heat up to medium-high. Using a candy thermometer, heat to boiling. Let simmer until it reaches exactly 240°.
5. Immediately remove from heat.
6. Turn mixer to low. Slowly stream the hot sugar mixture into the gelatin mixture, being very careful! Mix on medium for 1 minute.
7. Add vanilla, mix on low to incorporate.
8. Turn mixer to high and whip for about 10 minutes, until mixture is very thick and sticking to the whisk.
9. Lightly spray an 8" by 8" glass pan with cooking spray. Mix powdered sugar and cornstarch to combine in a small bowl. Dust the glass pan with the mixture—this is easiest with a sifter. Make sure all of the spray and pan are dusted, and tap out any excess to use later.
10. Spread the 'shmallow mixture evenly into pan. Using a rubber spatula, spread as evenly as possible. You may want to rinse spatula often with hot water or spray with cooking spray to prevent sticking.
11. Dust top lightly with powdered sugar mixture.
12. Let sit for at least 5 hours to set.
13. Remove to a cutting board, dusted with powdered sugar mixture. Cut with a pizza cutter, sprayed with cooking spray, to desired sizes. Dust each side of each 'shmallows with powdered sugar mixture to prevent sticking.
14. Store loosely in an airtight container for up to 2 weeks!

Option:

~*Recipe is easily doubled for a 9" by 13" pan!*

~*For chocolate 'shmallows, in step 7 add vanilla plus 3 Tbsp organic cocoa powder. Continue with remaining steps. Add 1 Tbsp cocoa powder to the powder sugar/cornstarch mixture for dusting.*

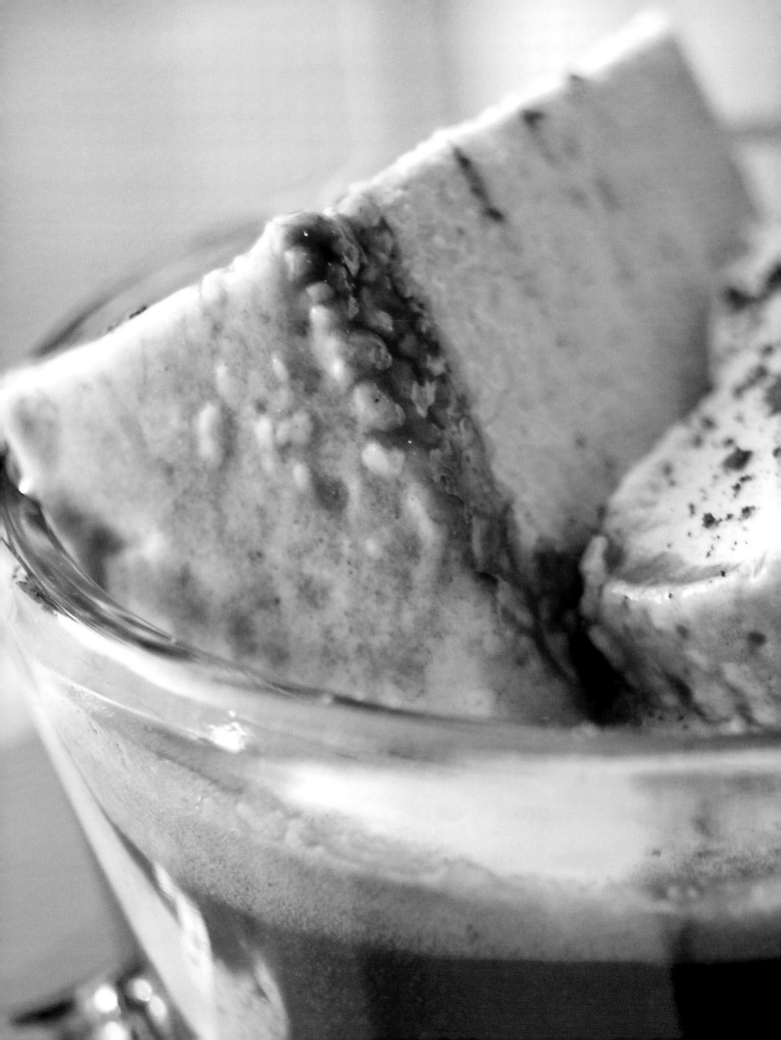

Cookie Doh Bites
(I'm sorry)

These are so good. So incredibly wonderful. So hard to stop eating! I'm sorry for even putting the thought in your head to make something this sinfully wrong. Please only make a few at a time, and only on special occasions, like Christmas, school parties, etcetera. Please? It will be the only way I can live with myself for unleashing this kind of goodness onto the world.

1	C GF DF chocolate chips (Enjoy Life)
1	Tbsp organic palm shortening (Spectrum)
~	Frozen Chocolate Chip Cookie Doh Balls (see recipe p. 274) or Peanut Butter Cookie Doh Balls (p. 292)

1. In a double boiler, heat chocolate chips with the shortening. Stir occasionally until almost all the chips are melted. Remove from heat and stir until all chocolate is melted.

2. With a fork, dip frozen cookie doh balls into chocolate. Tap the fork on the side of the bowl, getting as much excess chocolate (if there is such a thing!) off as possible. Place covered doh ball onto a wax paper–lined cookie sheet.

3. Repeat with all cookie doh balls . . . but you're only doing a few, right?

4. Refrigerate until chocolate is hard. Store in an airtight container in the fridge for up to a week. But they won't last that long, will they?

5. If you have leftover melted chocolate, why not add some of your favorite nuts to it to make Nut Clusters? See the next page for instructions.

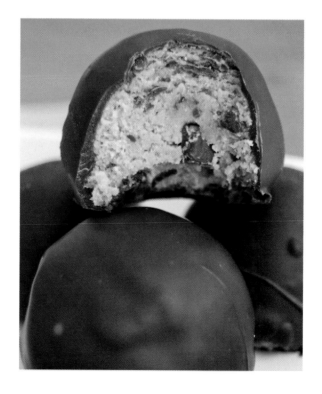

Baking / Desserts / Snacks

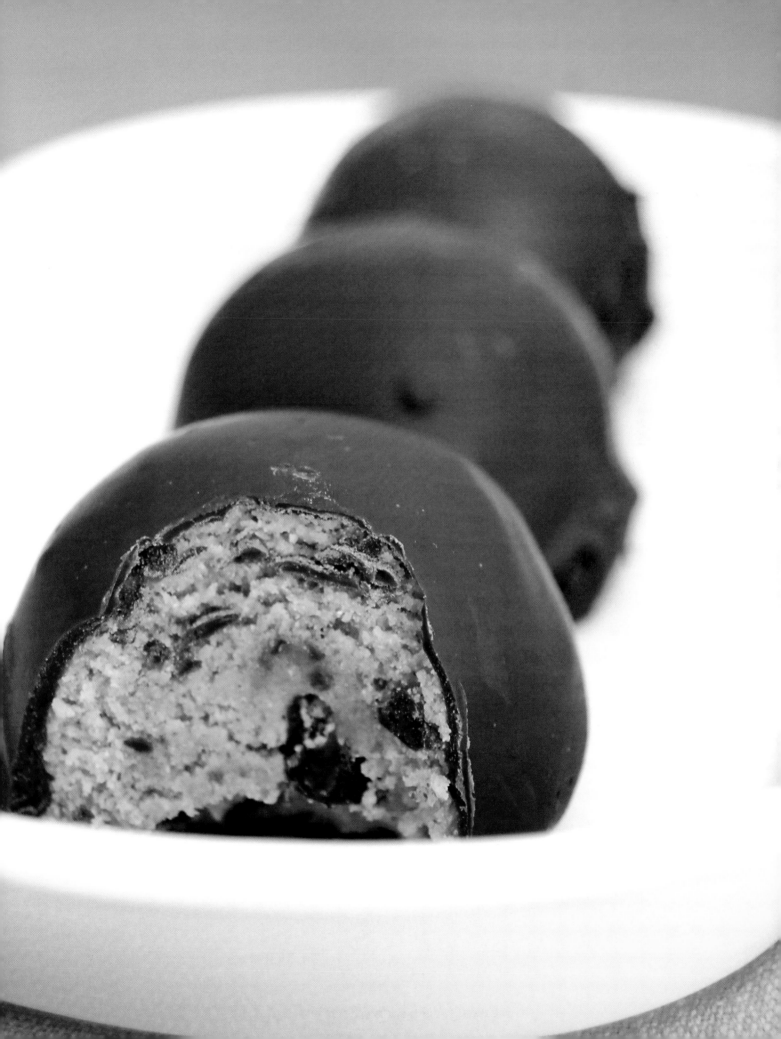

Nut Clusters

One of my favorite indulgences is a small chocolate almond cluster with a pinch of sea salt. They are so easy to make, and you won't believe how much cheaper it is to make them than buy them by the pound at the supermarket. They last for a couple of weeks in a sealed container, and it really hits the spot when you want a something a little sweet and salty.

1	C (150 g) GF DF chocolate chips (Enjoy Life)
1	Tbsp organic palm shortening (Spectrum)
1	C (150 g) chopped, toasted nuts of choice (I love using almonds or macadamias)
~	Sea salt

1. In a double boiler, heat chocolate chips with the shortening. Stir occasionally until almost all the chips are melted. Remove from heat and stir until all chocolate is melted.
2. Add nuts to chocolate and stir to combine. There should be a ratio of a lot of nuts to chocolate. If it looks too thin, add some more nuts.
3. With a teaspoon, scoop clusters and place onto a wax paper–lined cookie sheet.
4. Sprinkle each cluster with a tiny amount of sea salt.
5. Repeat until all of the mixture is used.
6. Refrigerate until chocolate is hard. Store in an airtight container for up to 2 weeks.

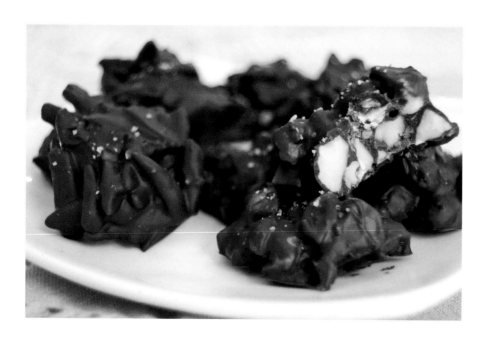

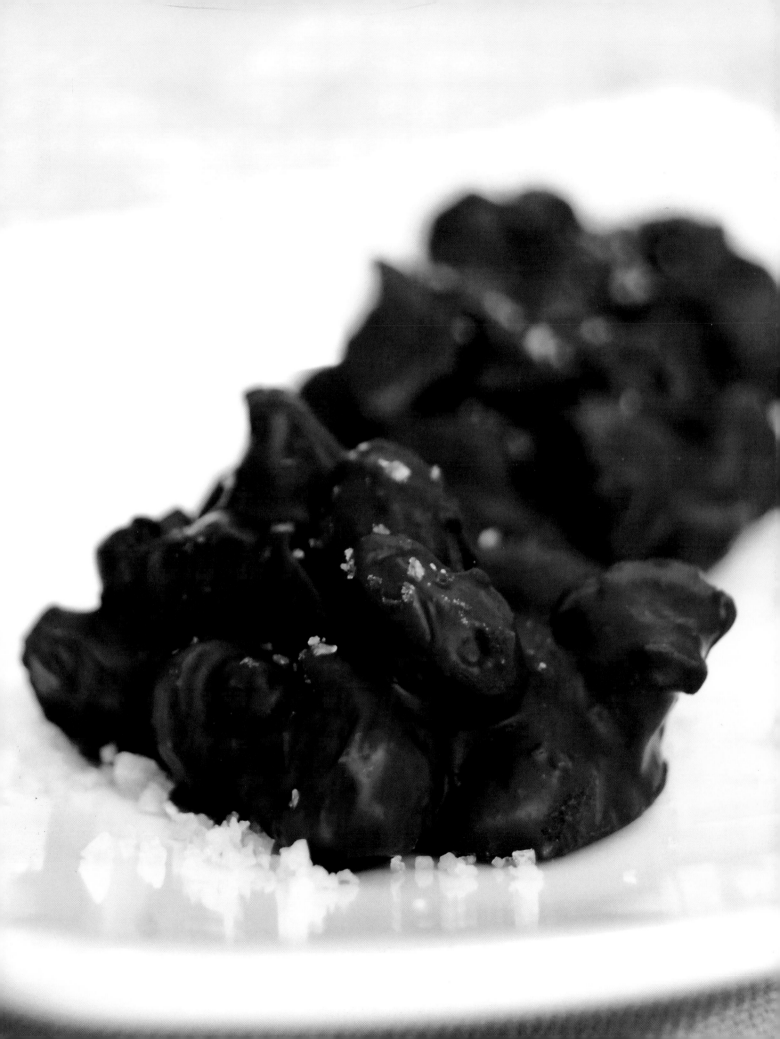

Spiced Maple Pecans

Fast, easy, healthy, almost addicting—these nuts make a great after-school snack, hostess gift, or holiday exchange gift. This recipe is easily doubled, and you will need it! They go fast with little hands around.

¼	tsp cinnamon
¼	tsp ground ginger
1	tsp sea salt
~	Pinch of freshly ground pepper
3	Tbsp pure maple syrup
2	C (300 g) raw pecans

1. In a small bowl, mix together cinnamon, ginger, salt, and pepper. Set aside.
2. Place maple syrup in a medium bowl, set aside.
3. In a large skillet, toast the pecans over medium-high heat, stirring almost constantly, until nuts are slightly toasted and hot (about 5 minutes).
4. Add nuts to the maple syrup bowl and toss to coat.
5. Sprinkle spice mixture over nuts and stir to evenly coat.
6. Spread nuts in a single layer on a parchment-lined baking sheet. Cool completely.

Options:

~Try adding ¼ tsp pumpkin pie spice to the spice mixture for a fall treat!

Makes 2 cups

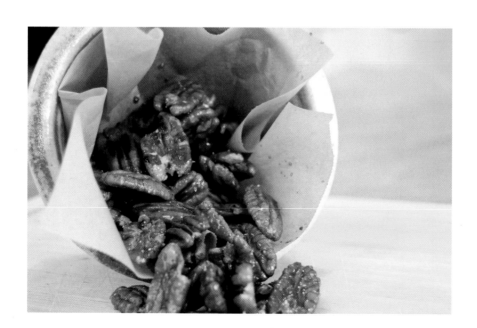

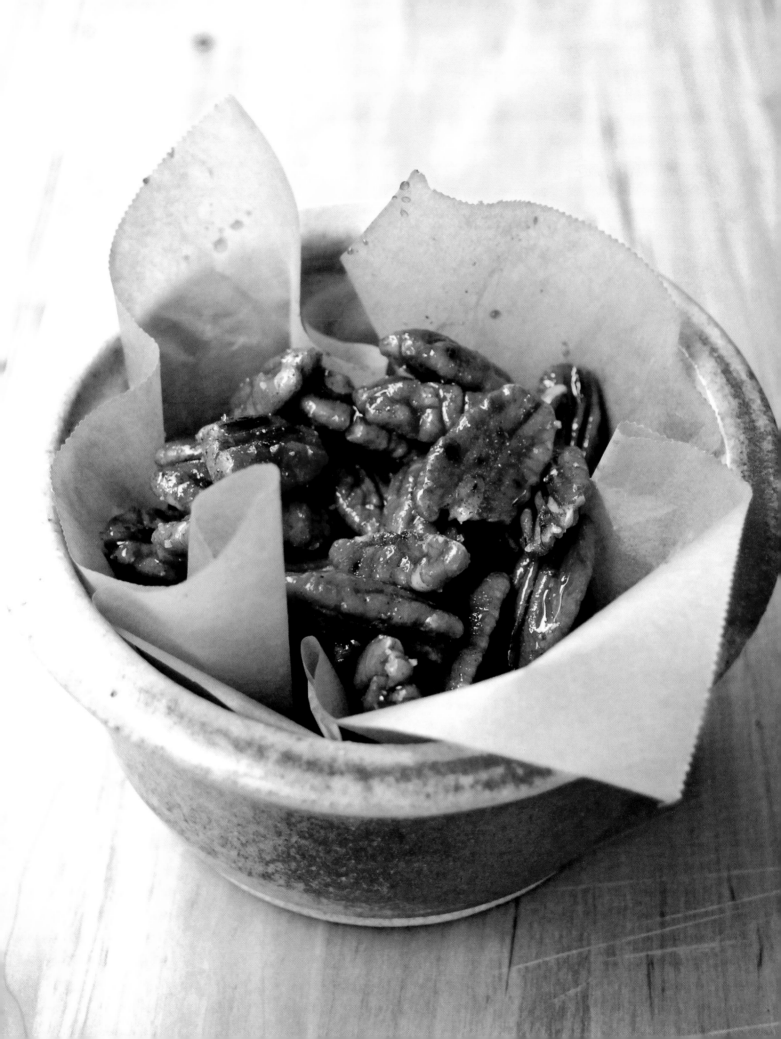

Cinnamon Sugar Popcorn

This popcorn was voted, unofficially, the "best snack ever!" at preschool and elementary school three years running by the kids, teachers, and moms. Well, who can argue with that kind of rock-solid scientific research? With its crunchy, salty sweetness you will quickly see why it consistently gets straight A's in my family's book. Feel free to adjust the sugar and oil to your liking.

For the Popcorn:

⅓	C (about 50 g) organic popping corn
2	tsp coconut oil
~	Brown paper bag (lunch size)
~	Tape

Topping:

~	About 2 Tbsp coconut oil
2	tsp cinnamon
2	tsp sugar
¼	C organic raisins

1. Add popcorn kernels to the paper bag.
2. Drizzle coconut oil over kernels in the bag.
3. Fold top of bag over twice and seal with a strip of tape.
4. Pop in microwave about 2 min 24 sec, or use the Popcorn 1.75 oz bag setting if your microwave has it.
5. Pour popped corn into a large bowl and drizzle with 2 Tbsp coconut oil. Sprinkle with cinnamon, sugar, and raisins and toss to combine. If desired, you can add a small sprinkle of sea salt.

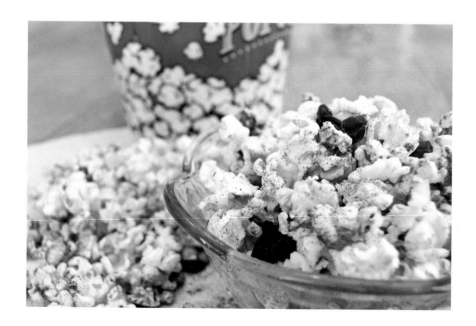

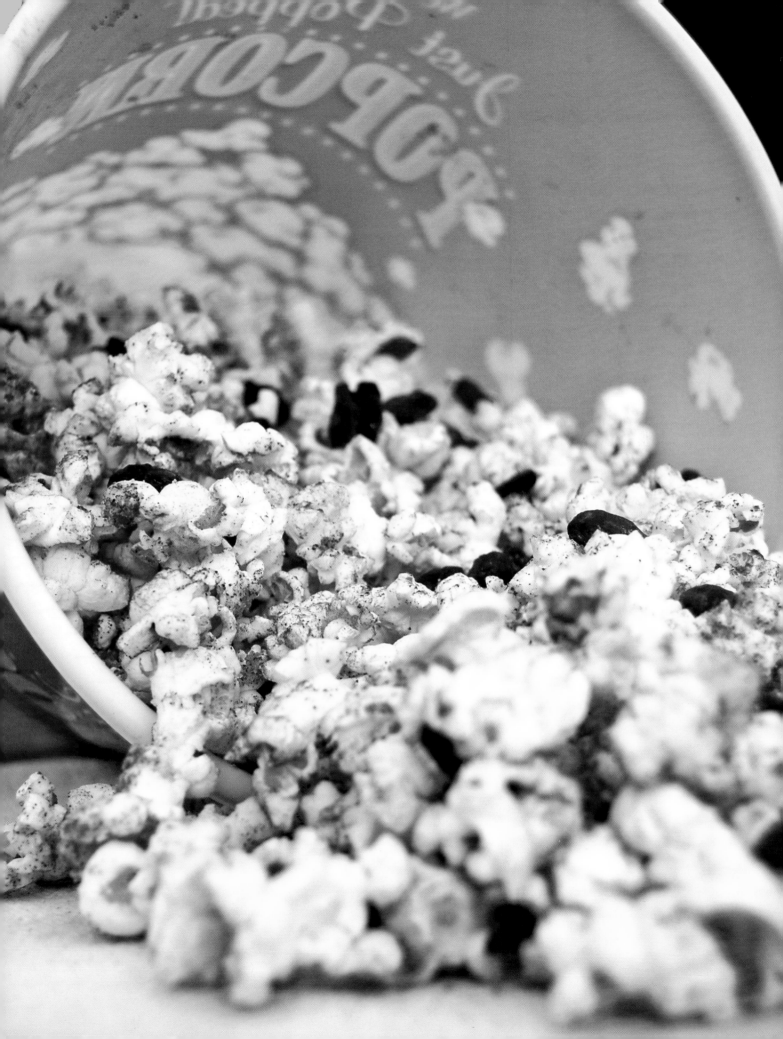

Makenna's Mix

I'm always surprised how many people ask me for recipes for trail mix. Trail mix to me is always a hodge-podge of whatever I like or whatever I have in my pantry at that moment. Over time, though, my kids have picked their favorite ingredients and we tend to make the same combo over and over again. This is my older daughter's favorite, which she can and sometimes does eat each and every day. After the initial cost of buying all of the ingredients, it is so much cheaper than buying premade trail mixes. And again, you control the ingredients so you control their safety.

¼	C (40 g) raw almonds
¼	C (40 g) raw pecans
¼	C (40 g) roasted salted sunflower seeds kernels
¼	C (22 g) unsweetened organic coconut flakes
¼	C (40 g) organic raisins
¼	C (40 g) organic dried cranberries
¼	C (35 g) GF pretzels
1	Tbsp mini chocolate chips (Enjoy Life)

1. Mix all ingredients in a large zip-top bag to combine.
2. Store in an airtight container for up to a week.

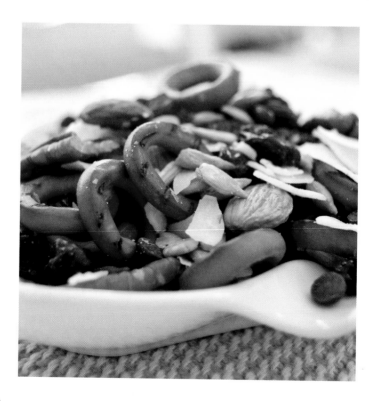

Baking / Desserts / Snacks

Rilee's Mish Mash Mix

This nut-free trail mix is a lifesaver on busy days when we need a grab-and-go snack. I control the sweetness level and the fact that it's free of gluten and nuts, so I feel good letting my children nibble when they want. And it's yummy so I can sneak handfuls while they're at school.

¼	**C (40 g) raw pumpkin seeds**
¼	**C (40 g) raw sunflower seed kernels**
¼	**C (40 g) roasted salted sunflower seed kernels**
¼	**C (22 g) organic unsweetened coconut flakes**
¼	**C (40 g) organic dried cherries**
¼	**C (40 g) organic raisins**
¼	**C (35 g) gluten-free pretzels**
1	**Tbsp mini chocolate chips**

1. Mix all ingredients in a large zip-top bag to combine.
2. Store in an airtight container for up to a week.

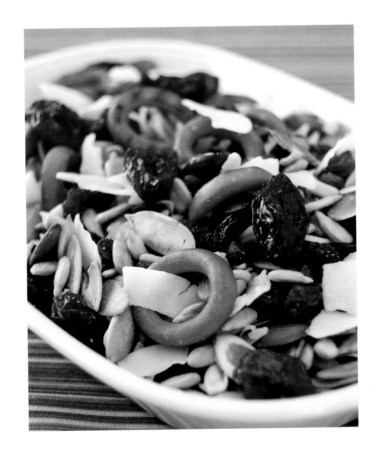

Toasted Pumpkin Seeds

Great by themselves, sprinkled on salads, or tossed on butternut squash soup (p. 198), these spiced pumpkin seeds deliver great taste and nutrition. Pumpkin seeds possess anti-inflammatory properties and are high in phospho-rous, magnesium, iron, and zinc, making this a great go-to snack for the whole family!

1	**Tbsp coconut oil**
⅔	**C (100 g) shelled, raw green pumpkin seeds (pepitas)**
½	**tsp sea salt**
¼	**tsp pumpkin pie spice**
¼	**tsp chili powder**

1. Heat oil over medium-high heat.
2. Add pumpkin seeds and cook, stirring often, until golden brown, about 4 minutes.
3. Transfer seeds to a small bowl and toss with salt and spices.

Option:

~Try toasted pecans or walnuts instead of pumpkin seeds for a change.

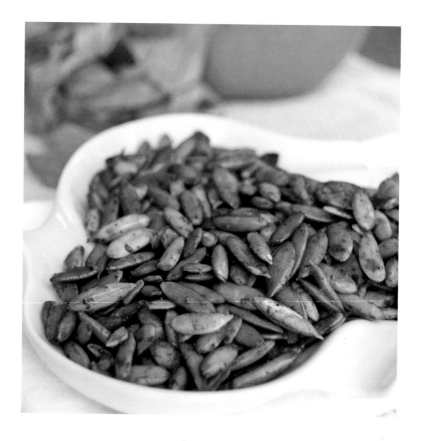

Coco Loco Bananas

We call these "loco" because they look a little crazy on the plate. But boy do they taste great! Sometimes the ugly, messy snacks are the ones the kids love best.

2	**Tbsp almond butter**
1	**Tbsp raw organic honey**
2	**organic bananas, cut in half and then sliced lengthwise down the middle**
2	**tsp organic cocoa powder**
¼	**C (22 g) toasted unsweetened organic coconut flakes**

1. Mix almond butter and honey until blended.
2. Roll banana in cocoa powder.
3. Spread some of the almond butter mixture over the cut side of each banana.
4. Sprinkle toasted coconut over tops.
5. If needed, freeze for 10 minutes until everything sets.
6. Devour!

Options:

~My kids love a little extra honey drizzled on top

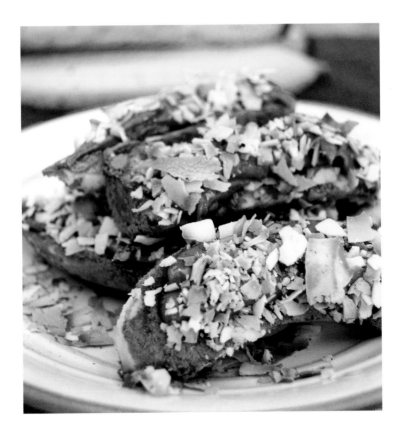

Chocolate Fondue

We make this fondue every New Year's Eve. The kids look forward to it all year long because they know there will be a tray of fresh fruits just waiting to be dunked into this delicious chocolate pool. It's one of those treats that seem bad for you, but isn't really too bad as far as indulgences go. With fresh fruit, dark chocolate (antioxidants!), and coconut milk high in medium-chain fatty acids, you don't have to beat yourself up for indulging in this yum-merific dessert on a special night.

1	C (240 mL) lite canned coconut milk
9	oz (about 250 g) GF DF chocolate chips (we use Enjoy Life)
3	oz (about 84 g) 85% GF DF dark chocolate (Trader Joe's has a couple of options)
1½	tsp pure vanilla extract
½	tsp pure almond extract
~	Lots of fresh fruits for dipping: pitted cherries, strawberries, orange slices, kiwi slices, cubed apples, cubed pineapple, sliced bananas, etc. If you're feeling particularly naughty, you can dunk Homemade 'Shmallows (p. 364) and Graham Crackers (p. 302) too!

1. Heat coconut milk over medium heat in a saucepan.
2. When bubbles form around the edges, add chocolate chips, dark chocolate, vanilla, and almond extracts. Remove from heat and whisk until smooth.
3. Transfer to a fondue pot and keep on low.
4. Dunk and have fun!

Tip:

~Freeze leftover fondue in a jar with a tight-fitting lid. When needed, let thaw in the fridge and then reheat in the microwave until warm. Stir.

Option:

~I like to surprise the kids for school lunch sometimes. I heat ½ C fondue and another ⅓ C coconut milk. Heat and whisk until combined. Refrigerate in a small container and put in the lunchbox with fruit and GF pretzels. Makes a great dip!

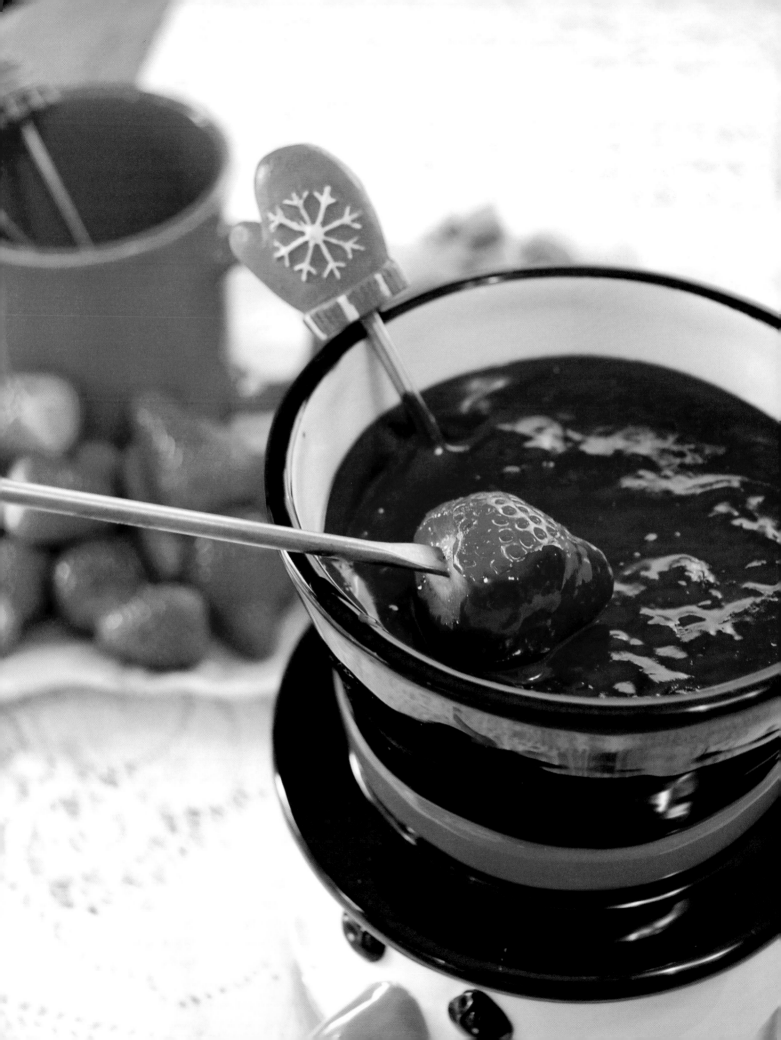

Coconut Whipped Cream

Whipped cream can be difficult to let go when dairy becomes a dietary enemy. I mean, there's just nothing that complements short cake or pumpkin pie quite like a dollop of creamy goodness. Well, now you can have that creamy finish on any dessert, and I promise, it quite rivals the real thing.

1	can (about 450 mL) full-fat coconut milk, chilled
1	tsp pure vanilla extract
2	Tbsp coconut nectar
1	tsp coconut flour
¼	tsp xanthan gum

1. Place a stainless steel bowl and hand-mixer beaters in the freezer for about 30 minutes prior.
2. In the cold bowl, add coconut milk and beat with hand mixer (and cold beaters) for 1 minute.
3. Add in vanilla, nectar, flour, and xanthan gum.
4. Beat 2 minutes.
5. Cover and freeze 30 minutes.
6. Remove from freezer and blend again with hand mixer for about 30 seconds.
7. Serve immediately.
8. Store leftovers in a jar with a tight-fitting lid for up to 3 days.

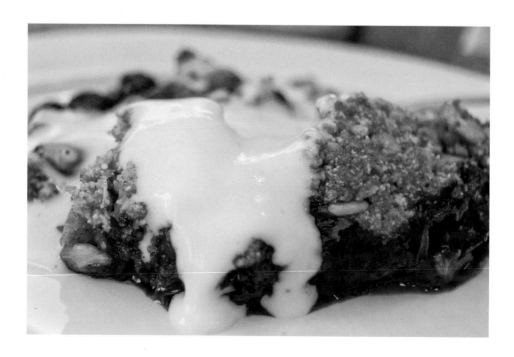

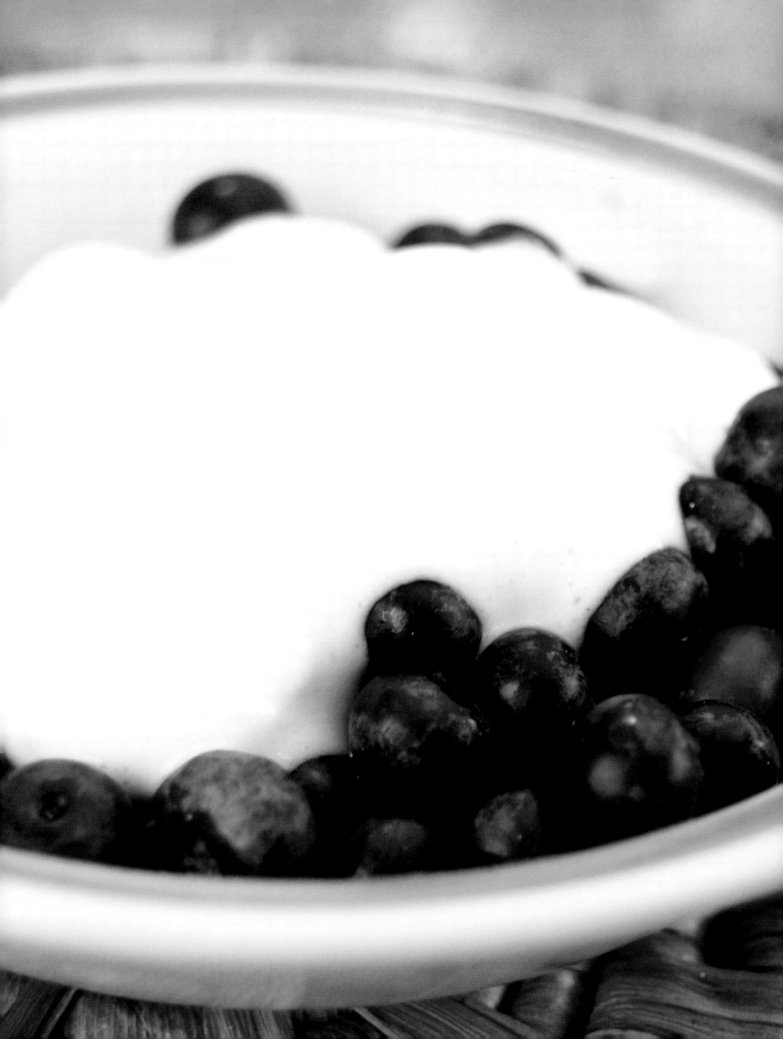

Sugar Cookie Icing

If you've ever wondered how to make that perfect sugar cookie icing that spreads perfectly and dries a little bit hard and shiny without cracking, then look no further! Perfect for Sugar Cookies (p. 294), this frosting is subtle in flavor but gorgeous on any cookie. I like to use natural food colorings such as beet juice for light and dark pink, turmeric mixed with a tiny amount of water for yellow, and of course, blueberry juice for blueish purple.

2	C (200 g) organic powdered sugar
2–3	Tbsp nondairy milk
1	Tbsp golden syrup (I used Lyle's brand)
1	Tbsp nondairy butter, very soft
½	tsp pure vanilla extract
¼	tsp pure almond extract

1. In a medium bowl, whisk together all ingredients until it is smooth and glossy. Start with 2 Tbsp of milk and only add more if needed. Icing should be medium thickness, not too thin and runny, but thin enough to be squeezed out of piping bags.

2. Separate the frosting into 3 bowls. Leave 1 bowl white. Add beet juice to one for pink. Add turmeric mixed with a few drops water for the yellow.

3. Scoop each into a piping bag, or zip-top bag with the corner cut off, and squeeze onto cookies.

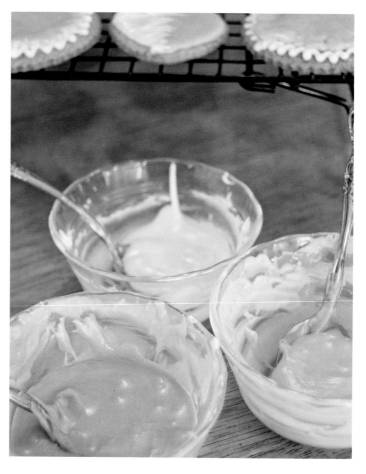

Baking / Desserts / Snacks

Maple Glaze

Sweet maple flavor really accents various baked items nicely. For starters, try it on cinnamon rolls, Apple Cinnamon Scones (p. 76), and Sweet Potato Spice Cookies (p. 282). Then let your imagination run wild!

2	**C (200 g) organic powdered sugar**
1	**tsp softened nondairy butter**
1	**tsp maple extract**
2–3	**Tbsp nondairy milk**

1. In a medium bowl, whisk together powdered sugar, butter, maple, and 1 Tbsp of milk. If it's too dry, add another Tbsp of milk, until desired consistency. Whisk until smooth.
2. Use a fork to drizzle icing over cookies, scones, etcetera.

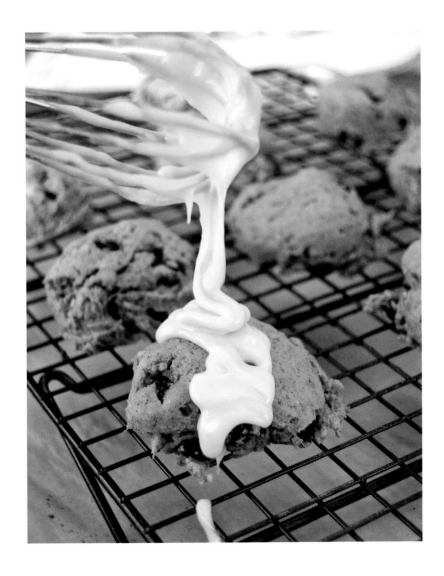

Sandwich Bread

I know there are a lot of flours in this recipe, but please do not give up on it before you try it! When you take the gluten and eggs out of bread, which is pretty much the entire make up of the bread, you must add things back in to provide taste, texture, and moisture. This combination has turned out, without fail, beautiful loaf after loaf of bread for my family. The pea flour is added because of its high protein content. If you do not want to buy another flour, replace it with almond meal (I use pea flour because my daughter has a nut intolerance). And potato flour (not starch!) is added because it gives any loaf of gluten-free yeast bread that texture we love so much. Give it a try, I will bet that you'll love it as much as we do!

Yeast Mixture:

1	C (240 mL) warm water
¼	C (60 mL) raw organic honey
1	Tbsp dry active yeast

Dry Ingredients:

1	C (120 g) sorghum flour
¼	C (30 g) amaranth flour
¼	C (30 g) coconut flour
¾	C (90 g) teff flour
2	tsp potato flour
2	tsp pea flour (or almond meal)
1¼	C (150 g) potato starch
1½	C (150 g) tapioca starch
1½	Tbsp xanthan gum

Wet Ingredients:

¼	C (30 g) flax meal mixed with ¾ C (180 ml) hot water
½	C (120 mL) unsweetened organic applesauce
⅔	C (160 mL) coconut oil, melted
2	tsp raw apple cider vinegar
1	tsp molasses (optional, but I love the flavor and color it gives the bread)
¼–¾	C (60–180 mL) warm water (add a little at a time until dough is the right consistency)

1. Whisk together dry ingredients, set aside.
2. Preheat oven to its lowest setting, or on "warm," about 150°–170°.
3. Heat water for the yeast mixture in the microwave for about 2 minutes, or until temperature is around 100°–110°. Add honey and yeast, mix gently to combine. Set aside in a warm place, like on top of the stove or in the microwave, to proof and become frothy, for 5 minutes.
4. Grease 1 loaf pan and 1 mini loaf pan.
5. In a stand mixer fit with the paddle attachment, mix dry ingredients, yeast mixture, and wet ingredients, reserving some of the warm water. Blend on high for 2 minutes to fully incorporate. Dough should be the consistency of wet bread dough. Almost like a thick muffin batter. It will not be like regular bread dough that is dry and can be handled. If it's too thick, add a little more water and blend again. Be careful though, a thick batter will rise well, if there is too much water and the batter is runny, it will collapse after baking.
6. Pour batter into the large loaf pan, about ¾ up the sides. Fill the mini loaf pan with remaining dough, also about ¾ up the sides. If needed, smooth tops of loaves with a wet spoon.
7. Place loaf pans in the oven. Let them rise for about 30–45 minutes, or until dough is higher than the sides of the pans.
8. Raise oven temperature to 425°. Bake for 15 minutes.
9. Lower temperature to 350° and bake an additional 15 minutes for the mini loaf and an additional 40–45 minutes for the regular loaf. Tops should be browned and the loaves will sound hollow when you tap lightly on the tops. If they become too brown during baking, cover loosely with a piece of foil as they finish.
10. Cool loaves for 10 minutes in the pans, then remove loaves from pans and cool completely on a wire rack before slicing.

Tips:

~See freezing directions at the front of the book to freeze the remaining slices of bread . . . if there are any!

Makes 1 large loaf and 1 mini loaf

Baking / Desserts / Snacks

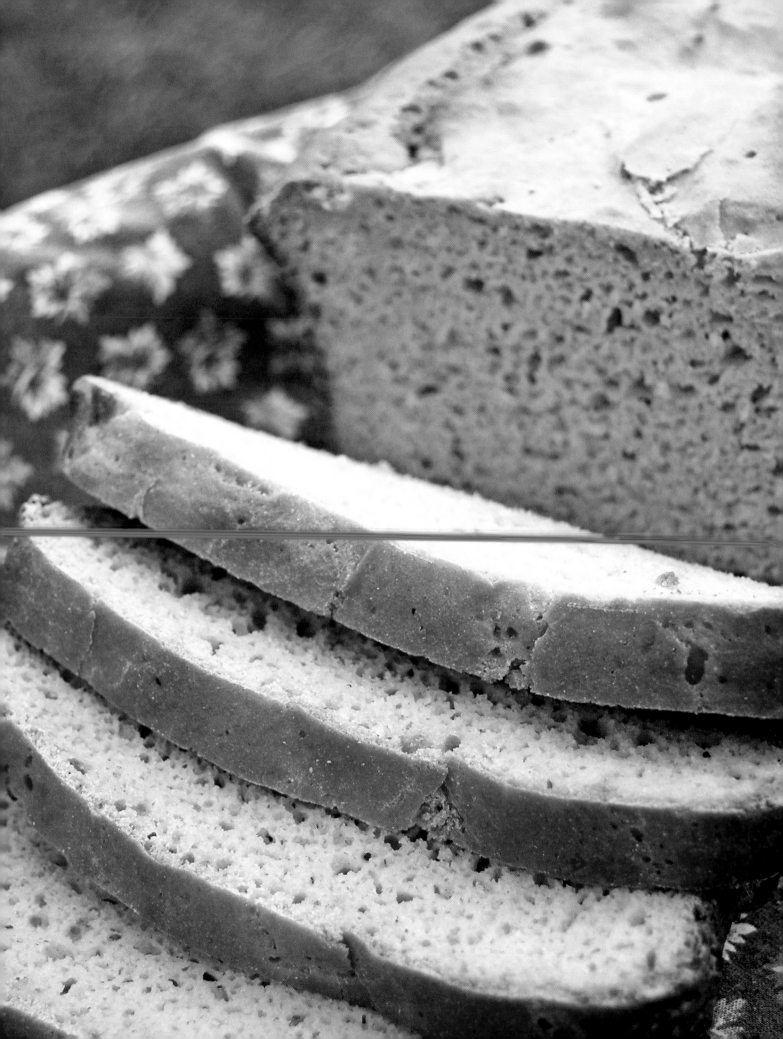

No-Yeast Quick Rolls

Next to good sandwich bread, this recipe for quick and easy rolls will be filed under "I can't live without it" in your recipe card files. Taking just a few minutes to whip up and less than 30 minutes to bake, these soft yet crusty rolls are the perfect side to any weeknight meal. And yes, they are so easy to make you won't mind mixing a quick batch, even on a Monday. They are great on their own, or use with sandwiches, soups, and even as hamburger buns! And don't worry if you have leftovers (not likely, but occasionally it happens)—just crunch up stale rolls into bread crumbs to use as a coating on fish or chicken. Or dice into cubes, toast, and freeze to use in stuffing at Thanksgiving. Delicious and versatile!

Dry Ingredients:

½	C (60 g) sorghum flour
¼	C (30 g) millet flour
½	C (60 g) teff flour
½	C (60 g) potato starch
½	C (60 g) tapioca starch
1½	tsp xanthan gum
½	tsp sea salt
¼	tsp granulated garlic
¼	tsp granulated onion
2	tsp baking powder

Wet Ingredients:

1	Tbsp flax meal mixed with ¼ C (60 mL) hot water
2	Tbsp raw organic honey
2	Tbsp organic unsweetened applesauce
½	C (120 mL) coconut oil, melted
1	tsp raw apple cider vinegar
½	C (120 mL) warm water

Topping:

~ Olive oil

~ Sea salt

Options:

~ Sesame seeds, poppy seeds, herbs

1. Mix hot water and flax meal in a small bowl and set aside.
2. In a large mixing bowl, whisk together dry ingredients. If you're feeling crazy, you can add about 2 tsp dried Italian seasoning to this for some tasty herbed rolls! But if this makes you nervous, we can slow down a bit and save that creativity for later. Let's take a deep breath and move on to the next step.
3. Add wet ingredients (flax meal, honey, applesauce, oil, vinegar, and water). Mix for 1 minute on medium speed until well blended.
4. Drop dough by spoonfuls onto parchment-lined baking sheet. Dough balls should be about 2½ inches in diameter.
5. Drizzle olive oil over tops of rolls, then sprinkle with coarse sea salt. If you're still feeling a little on the wild side, you can also sprinkle poppy seeds or sesame seeds on top for variety.
6. Bake at 350° for about 25 minutes, or until slightly golden on top, and the tops spring back when you push on them.

Makes 8

Baking / Desserts / Snacks

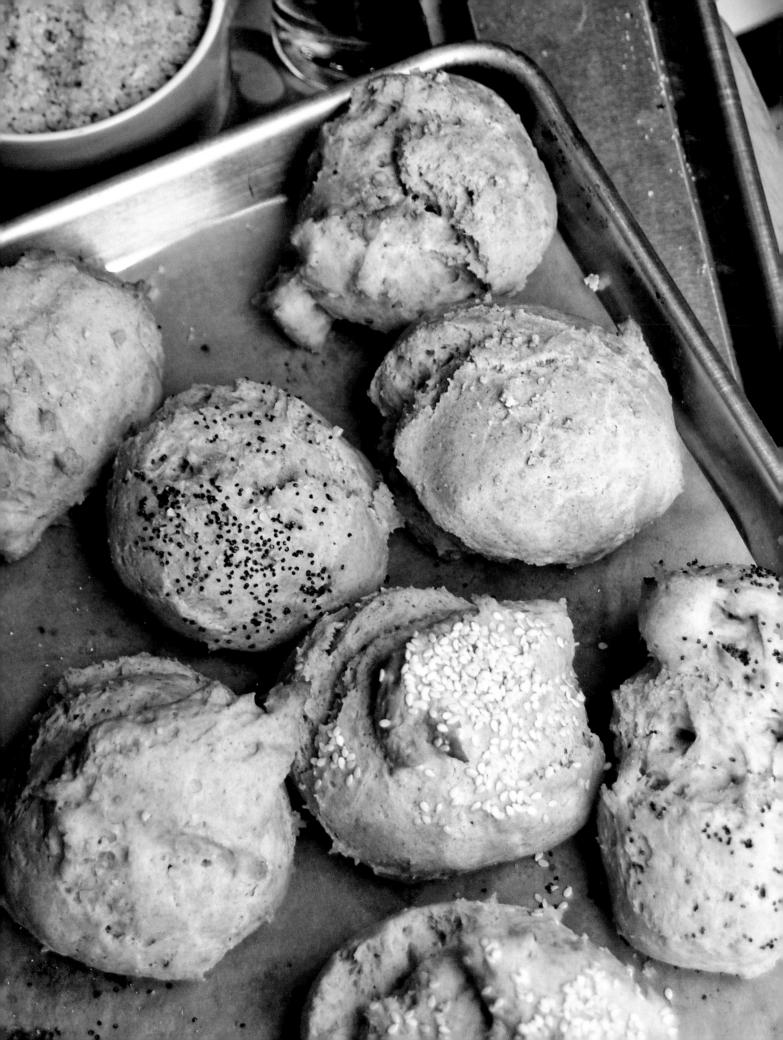

Breadsticks

Missing soft, chewy breadsticks? Look no further! Perfect for dipping in homemade spaghetti sauce (p. 248) or as a side to any dinner, these breadsticks will leave you feeling like you've had the real thing. Recipe can easily be doubled for extras!

Yeast Mixture:

¾ C (180 mL) warm water
2 tsp active dry yeast
1 Tbsp raw organic honey

Dry Ingredients:

⅓ C (40 g) sorghum flour
⅓ C (40 g) amaranth flour
¾ C (90 g) potato starch
½ C (60 g) tapioca starch
¾ tsp sea salt
2 tsp xanthan gum
½ tsp granulated garlic
2 tsp Italian seasoning

Wet Ingredients:

1 Tbsp olive oil
2 tsp raw apple cider vinegar

Add Ons:

~ Olive oil
~ Sea salt
~ Freshly ground pepper
~ Nondairy cheese (Daiya)
~ Organic palm shortening for greasing baking sheet, such as Spectrum vegetable shortening
~ Brown rice flour for dusting your pan

1. Whisk together dry ingredients, set aside.
2. Preheat oven to its lowest setting or on warm (about 150°).
3. Heat water for the yeast mixture in the microwave for about 1 minute, or until temperature is around 100°–110°. Add honey and yeast, mix gently to combine. Set aside in a warm place, like on top of the stove or in the microwave, to proof and become frothy, for 5 minutes.
4. In a stand mixer fit with the paddle attachment, mix dry ingredients, yeast mixture, and wet ingredients until fully incorporated. Blend on high for 30 seconds. Dough should be the consistency of wet bread dough, very thick but sticky.
5. Divide into 6 balls.
6. Grease a baking sheet. Sprinkle it lightly with rice flour. Place dough balls on pan and dust dough lightly with rice flour.
7. Using light quick fingers, shape and roll dough into sticks. Use additional rice flour if needed, being careful not to use too much, which will make the dough grainy. This may take some practice so don't worry! After a time or two, you will get a feel for the dough and know how to work with it.
8. Brush tops with olive oil. Sprinkle with sea salt, pepper, and cheese.
9. Place pan in warm oven and let the breadsticks rise for 20 minutes.
10. Turn heat up to 425° and bake for 25 minutes, or until browned and cooked through.
11. Cool for a 5 minutes on a cooling rack and serve.

Makes 6 large breadsticks

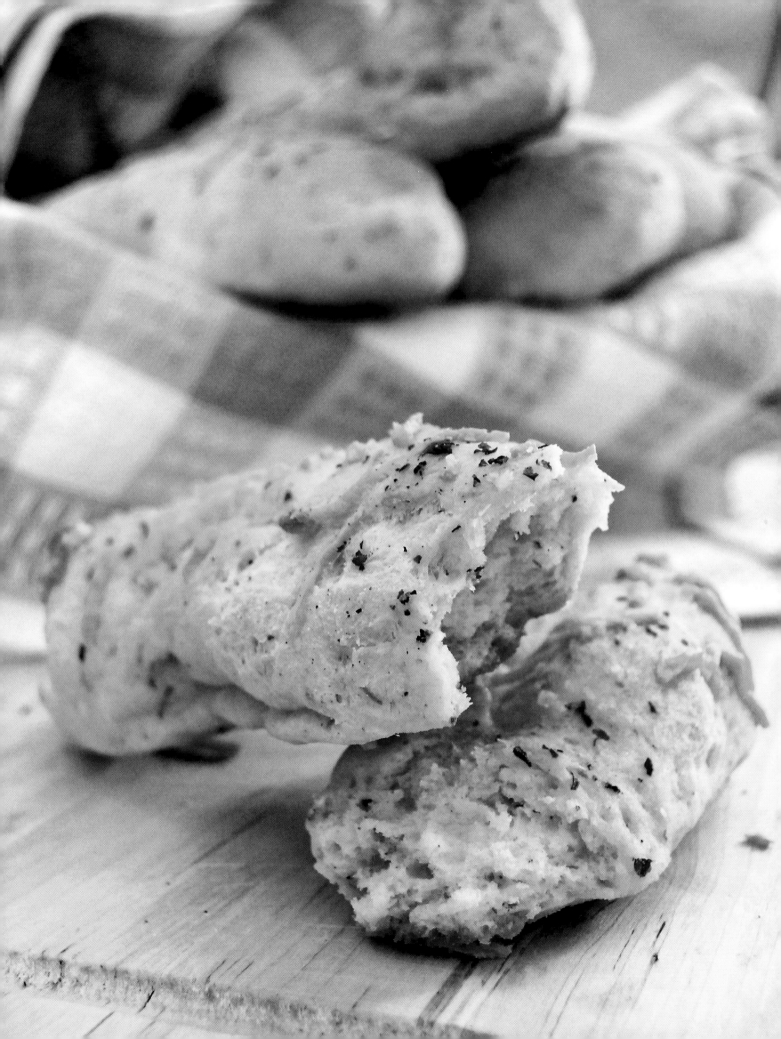

Quick Bread Crumbs/Cubes

One of the biggest hurdles in the gluten-free kitchen is adapting old recipes to our new lifestyle. And the recurring thorn in my side was always bread crumbs for recipes. For a while I actually baked a whole loaf of fresh bread only to let it dry out so I could make crumbs and cubes for various dishes. Well no more! This quick recipe and time-saving method allows you to whip up bread crumbs any time you need them with just a little effort. And if you happen to be in the zone and make these ahead of time, the crumbs or cubes freeze perfectly for later use as well.

Dry Ingredients:

½	C (60 g) sorghum flour
½	C (60 g) teff flour
½	C (60 g) potato starch
½	C (60 g) tapioca starch
2	tsp xanthan gum
½	tsp sea salt
2	tsp baking powder
¼	tsp granulated garlic
¼	tsp granulated onion

Wet Ingredients:

1	Tbsp raw organic honey
3	Tbsp unsweetened organic apple-sauce
½	C (120 mL) coconut oil, melted
1	tsp organic raw apple cider vinegar
½	C (120 mL) warm water

1. Whisk together dry ingredients, set aside.
2. In a stand mixer, blend together honey, applesauce, oil, and vinegar until combined.
3. Slowly add dry ingredients alternately with the warm water. If dough is too dry, add additional water, a teaspoon at a time, until dough comes together.
4. On a baking sheet covered with parchment paper, spread dough evenly across the pan.
5. Bake in a 350° oven for 20–25 minutes or until baked through and top starts to brown.
6. Remove from oven, cool completely.
7. If using for bread crumbs, crumble and break bread into crumbs, spread on another baking sheet and toast until browned.
8. If using for bread cubes for a stuffing or dressing, cut bread into bite-sized cubes, spread on a baking sheet and toast until lightly browned (or if you have time, let the bread cubes sit on a baking sheet in your cold oven for a day or so to dry out).

Baking / Desserts / Snacks

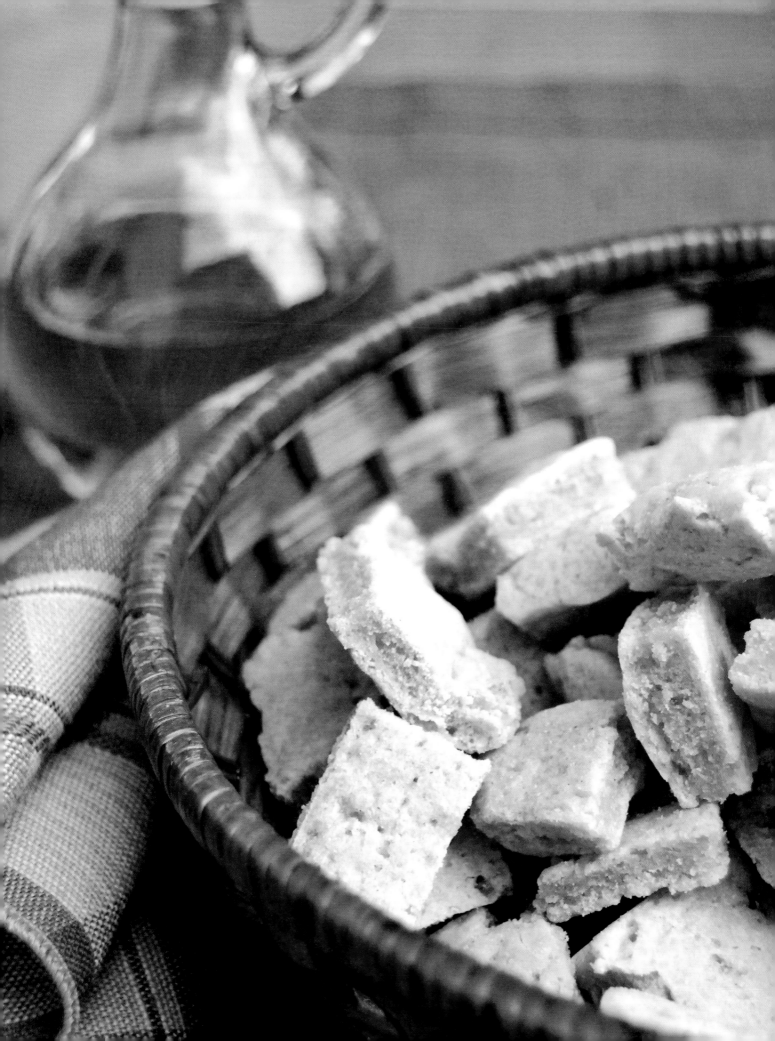

Kalamata Mini French Bread

You will never miss gluten-filled bread with this handy recipe around. Delicious kalamata olives pair nicely with olive oil and sea salt to create a crusty, true-to-form French bread that is the perfect side to any meal. And you can easily double the recipe for extra!

Yeast Mixture:

¾	C (180 mL) warm water
2	tsp active dry yeast
1	Tbsp raw organic honey

Dry Ingredients:

½	C (60 g) sorghum flour
¼	C (30 g) amaranth flour
¾	C (90 g) potato starch
½	C (60 g) tapioca starch
¾	tsp sea salt
2	tsp xanthan gum

Wet Ingredients:

1	Tbsp olive oil
2	tsp raw apple cider vinegar

Add Ins:

¾	C (110 g) chopped kalamata olives
1	tsp chopped fresh rosemary

Add Ons:

- ~ Olive oil
- ~ Sea salt
- ~ Organic palm shortening for greasing your pan, such as Spectrum vegetable shortening.
- ~ Brown rice flour for dusting your pan

1. Whisk together dry ingredients, set aside.
2. Preheat oven to its lowest setting or on warm (about 150°).
3. Heat water for the yeast mixture in the microwave for about 1 minute, or until temperature is around 100°–110°. Add honey and yeast, mix gently to combine. Set aside in a warm place, like on top of the stove or in the microwave, to proof and become frothy, for 5 minutes.
4. In a stand mixer, fit with the paddle attachment, mix dry ingredients, yeast mixture, and wet ingredients until fully incorporated. Blend on high for 30 seconds. Dough should be the consistency of wet bread dough, very thick but sticky.
5. Divide into 2 balls.
6. Grease a baking sheet. Sprinkle it lightly with rice flour. Place dough balls on pan and dust dough lightly with rice flour.
7. Using light quick fingers, shape and roll dough into mini loaves of French bread. Use additional rice flour if needed, being careful not to use too much, which will make the dough grainy.
8. Brush tops with olive oil. Sprinkle with sea salt.
9. Place pan in warm oven and let the loaves rise 25–30 minutes.
10. Turn heat up to 425 and bake for 35 minutes, or until browned and loaves sound hollow when you tap on them.
11. Cool and slice. Delicious as is or dipped in olive oil!

Makes 2 mini loaves

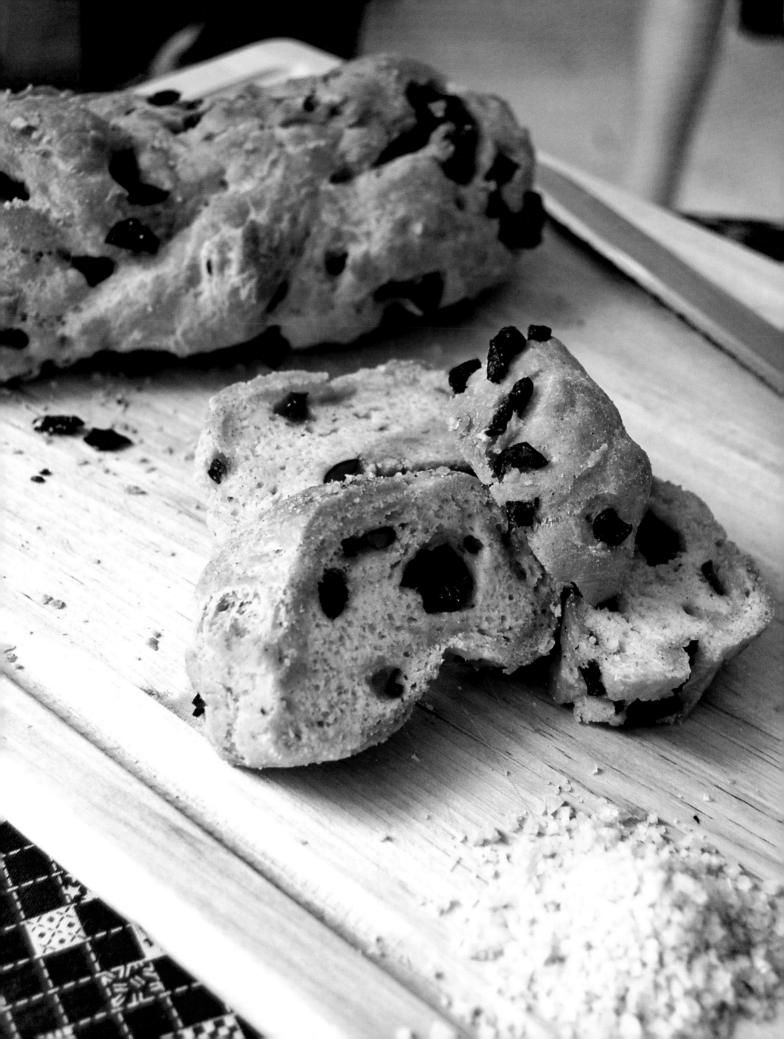

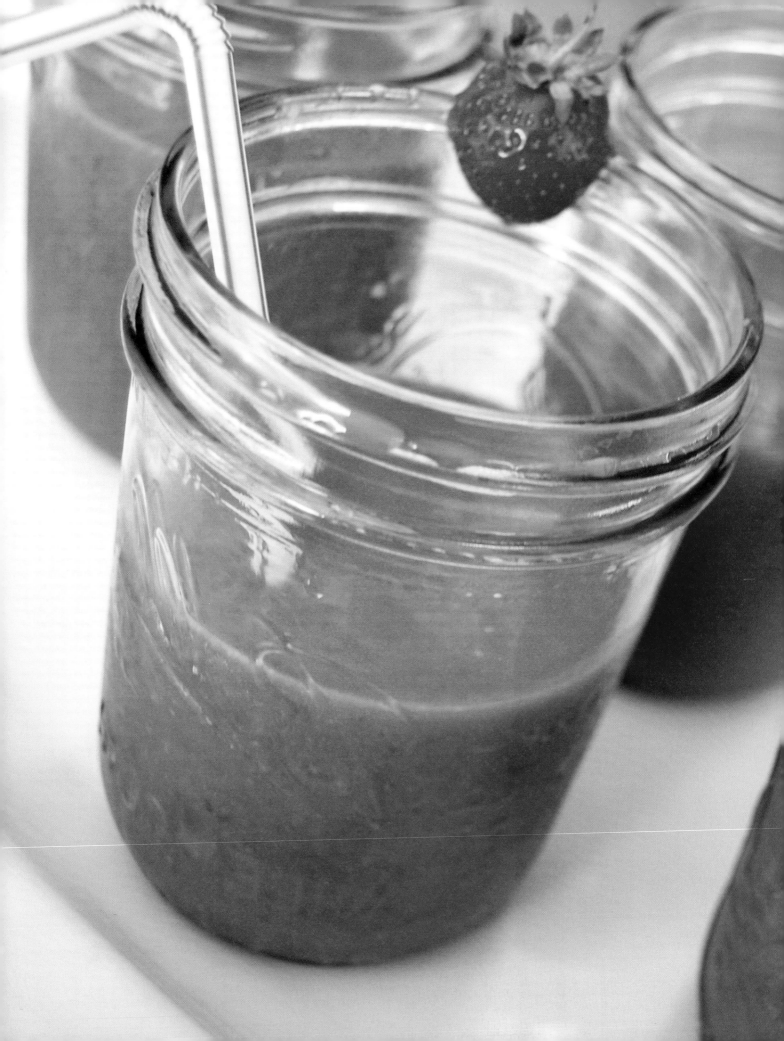

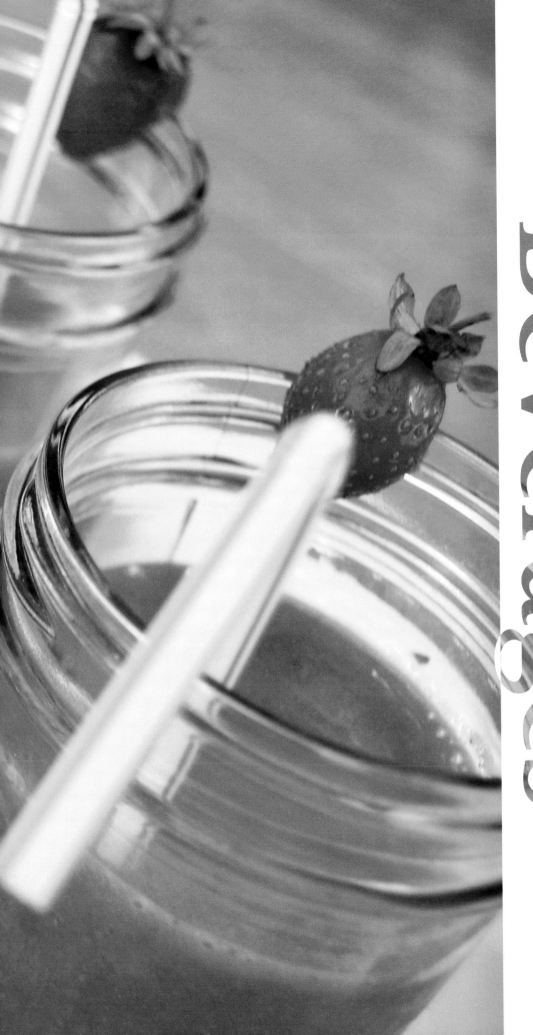

Beverages

Cool as a Cucumber Blueberry Smoothie

The combination of fresh cucumbers and fragrant blueberries is like a summer breeze in a glass! I always like sneaking a veggie or two into smoothies when the kids aren't looking, and this combination worked extremely well. Makes great popsicles too!

1	organic cucumber, peeled, seeded, and sliced
¾	C (180 mL) nondairy milk, such as light coconut milk
2	C (300g) frozen organic blueberries
1	Tbsp raw organic honey
2	tsp pure vanilla extract
1	C (240 mL) water

1. Place all ingredients in a blender and blend until smooth. If too thick, add additional water as needed to thin.

Makes four 6-oz glasses plus more for freezing

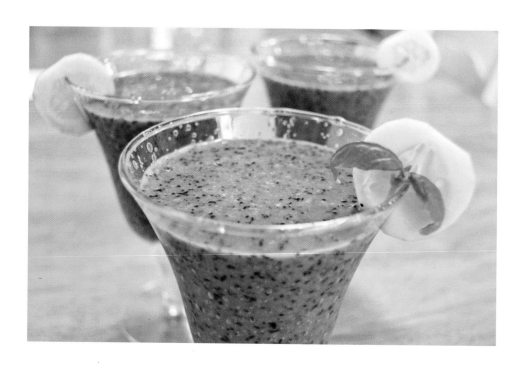

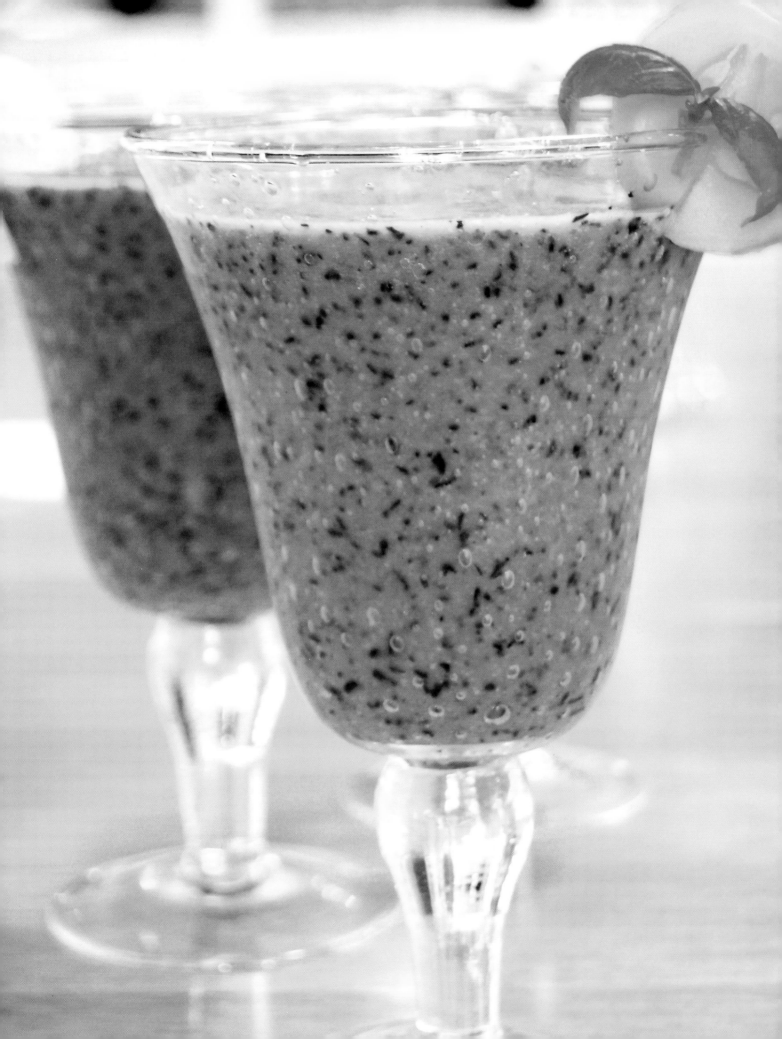

Strawberry Nectarine Smoothie

A bright, sweet, summer combination of juicy, ripe nectarines and sweet, red strawberries. And no matter what those smoothie places say, nature did just fine, so there's no need to add any extra sugar.

¾	C (180 mL) canned lite coconut milk
1	C (240 mL) water
2	tsp pure vanilla extract
2	C (300 g) frozen organic strawberries
1	organic nectarine, sliced
2	tsp coconut nectar or raw organic honey (optional—especially if the strawberries are really sweet)

1. Add all ingredients to a blender. Blend until smooth and creamy. If too thick, add a little more water until desired consistency. If too thin, add a few more frozen strawberries and blend until incorporated.

Tip:

~*Freeze leftover smoothies in popsicle molds for great after-school snacks you don't have to worry about!*

Makes six 6 oz glasses plus a little extra for freezing

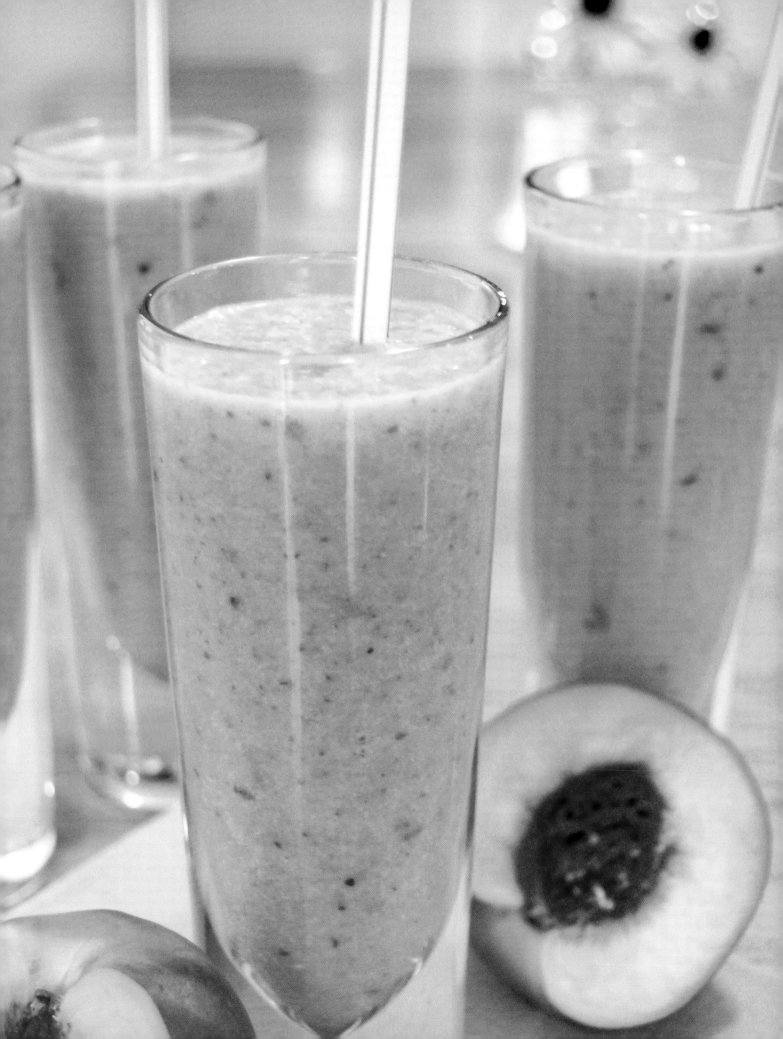

Strawberry Smoothie

Variety with smoothies is great to have, but sometimes it's hard to beat a classic like straight-up strawberry. Nothing else in here to overshadow that amazing red berry's flavor!

¾	C (180 mL) canned lite coconut milk
1	C (240 mL) water
2	tsp pure vanilla extract
2	C (300 g) frozen organic strawberries
2	tsp coconut nectar or raw honey (optional—especially if the strawberries are really sweet)

1. Add all ingredients to a blender. Blend until smooth and creamy. If too thick, add a little more water until desired consistency. If too thin, add a few more frozen strawberries and blend until incorporated.

Tip:

~Freeze leftover smoothies in Popsicle molds for great after-school snacks you don't have to worry about!

Makes six 6 oz glasses plus a little extra for freezing

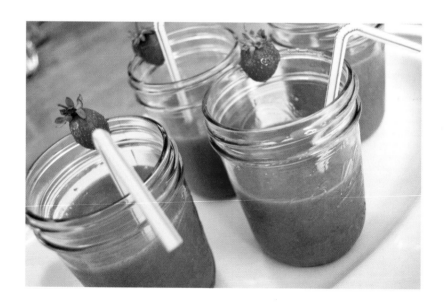

Beverages

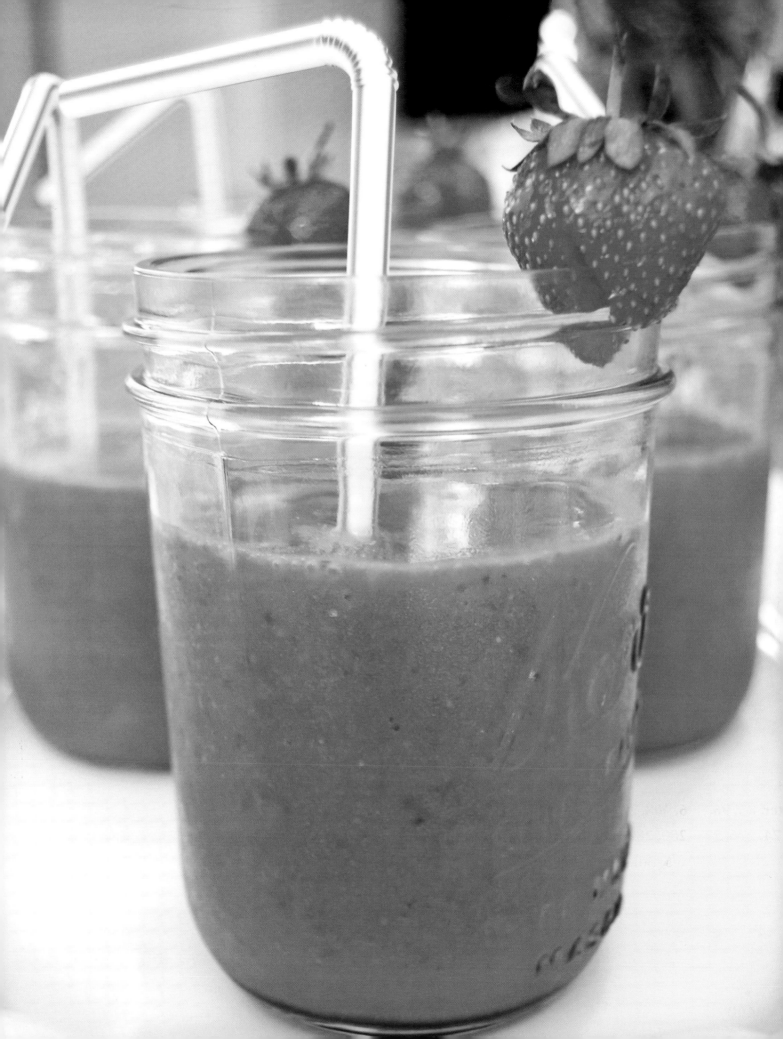

Orange Manius

If you've ever been to a mall, pretty much anywhere in America, then you've probably had one of those delicious, creamy, orange blended drinks that a certain chain produces. Well, now you can have that exact flavor at home, with no added sugar and who knows what else! These also make amazing frozen Popsicles, if there are any leftovers!

2	C (475 mL) organic orange juice
½	C (120 mL) nondairy milk (such as lite coconut milk)
2	Tbsp raw organic honey
1	Tbsp pure vanilla extract
~	Ice cubes (as many or few as you like)

1. Add all ingredients to the blender and blend until smooth. Add additional ice cubes as necessary to obtain desired thickness.

Makes six 6 oz glasses plus a little extra for freezing

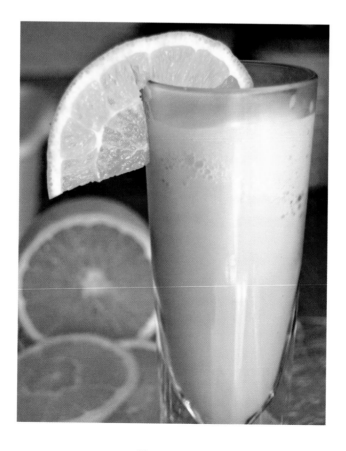

Rhubarb Lemonade Spritzer

This sweet (but not overly sweet) and refreshing drink hits the spot on an August afternoon. I love the distinct flavor rhubarb gives it, and it's nice having a different way to use my rhubarb, rather than the standard pie. Rhubarb is very hearty, easy to grow, and fairly forgiving, making it a perfect plant for my garden!

6	C water
⅓	C (80 mL) coconut nectar
¼	C (60 mL) raw organic honey
¼	C (50 g) organic evaporated cane juice
6	C (900 g) coarsely chopped fresh rhubarb
~	Zest of 1 large lemon
~	Juice of 1 large lemon
~	Sparkling water

1. In a saucepan, bring water, coconut nectar, honey, and cane juice to a boil.
2. Add rhubarb. Return to a boil and simmer over low heat for 5 minutes.
3. Add lemon zest and stir in gently.
4. Strain mixture into a bowl, allowing pulp to drain for 10 minutes without pressing.
5. Pour liquid into a pitcher and add lemon juice. Refrigerate at least 1 hour. This can be made several days in advance.
6. To serve, mix one portion syrup with an equal portion of unflavored sparkling water.

Makes six 6 oz glasses

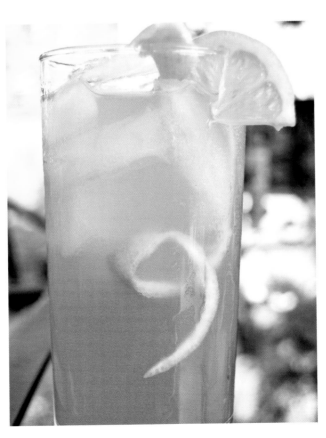

Pink Lemonade

I love lemonade in the summer, but could never get over the huge amount of sugar it took to offset those potent lemons. Then I started playing with different sweeteners. I started with straight honey, but wasn't happy because that was all you could taste. The combo of coconut nectar and honey really add the sweetness necessary without an overpowering flavor of either. Feel free to reduce the coconut nectar to ¼ C if your pucker can handle it!

⅓ C (80 mL) coconut nectar

¼ C (60 mL) raw organic honey

1 C (240 mL) water

1 C (240 mL) fresh squeezed lemon juice

3–4 C (700–950 mL) cold water

1–2 tsp beet juice (I like to boil beets, strain the liquid and cool. Store in a sealed container in the freezer until needed. Defrost enough to get a few teaspoons out and refreeze.)

1. In a medium saucepan heat nectar, honey, and 1 C water until honey has dissolved. Let cool for 10 minutes.
2. In a pitcher, combine lemon juice, 3 C cold water, and nectar/honey mixture. Taste. If too strong, add additional C of cold water.
3. Add beet juice and stir, until desired color is achieved.
4. Refrigerate until cold and serve over ice.

Tip:

~*When purchasing lemons, make sure to pick them up before buying. Heavier lemons yield more juice than the lighter ones. You can really feel the difference!*

Makes 1 large pitcher

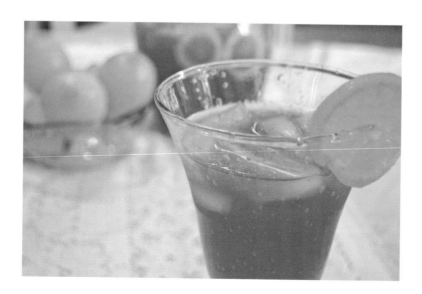

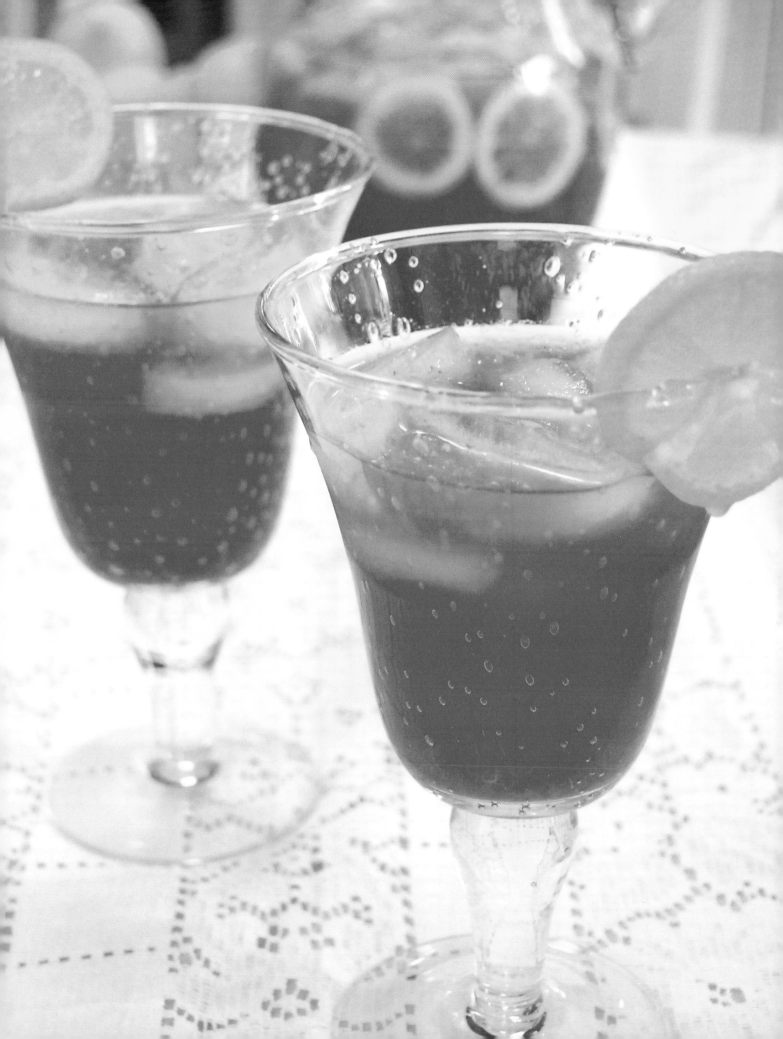

Watermelon Juice

Watermelon is so naturally sweet, it makes a fantastic summer drink. And once again, it also makes an even better Popsicle, so make a full batch so you can freeze any leftovers!

1	small organic seedless watermelon, rind removed, cubed, and chilled
1	lime wedge
2	Tbsp honey

1. Fill a blender almost to the top with watermelon cubes.
2. Squeeze lime wedge over watermelon.
3. Pour honey over watermelon.
4. Blend on high until fully pureed. Serve immediately or freeze in Popsicle molds.

Makes four 6 oz glasses plus a little extra for freezing

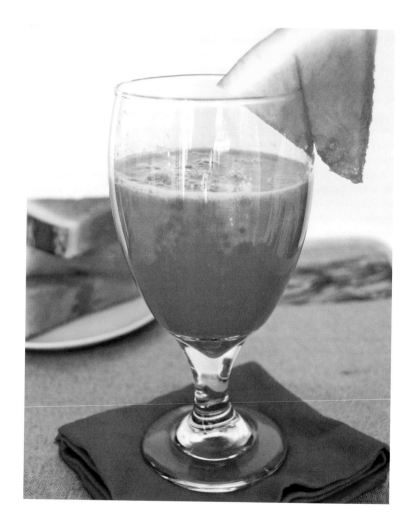

Beverages

Quick Pumpkin Latte

Sometimes, especially in the fall months, I want a little extra something in my coffee, without the added cost and sugar that typically comes with those corner coffee houses. And I especially don't want to spend fifteen minutes in the morning steaming "milk" to make a latte at home. This little concoction works wonders to satisfy that craving, yet I can make it a cup at a time in just a few minutes, right in the comfort of my bathrobe.

1	C (240 mL) of your favorite brewed coffee
¼	tsp pure vanilla extract
~	Pinch of pumpkin pie spice
2	tsp canned pumpkin (pumpkin puree)
~	Nondairy milk to taste
~	Coconut nectar to taste (or sweetener of your choice)

1. Brew coffee and pour into a coffee cup. Add vanilla, pumpkin pie spice, and canned pumpkin.
2. Add milk and coconut nectar to your taste.
3. Enjoy a fall morning!

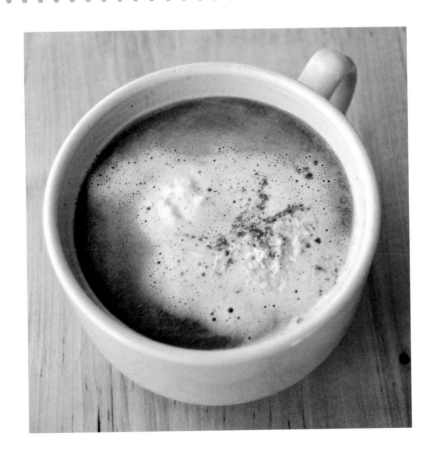

The Healthy Gluten-Free Life

Hot Cocoa

My kids love hot cocoa. All winter long that's the number one request each morning. We love the blend of milks for this recipe because it gives a creamy rich taste without one milk overpowering the rest on flavor. I like the simplicity of adding chocolate chips, but feel free to add cocoa powder and sweetener of your choice if you prefer!

1	can (about 400 mL) lite coconut milk
2	C (475 ML) rice milk
1	C (240 mL) almond milk
1	vanilla bean, sliced and insides scooped out into the milk
1	tsp pure vanilla extract
5	oz (140 g) GF DF chocolate chips (Enjoy Life)

1. Heat the milks, inside of vanilla bean, and vanilla bean pod in a saucepan over medium heat.
2. When mixture starts to bubble around the edges, add chocolate chips and vanilla extract. Whisk until chocolate is melted and is well combined.
3. Remove vanilla bean pod.
4. Serve with soft, pillowy homemade 'Shmallows (p. 364).

Options:

~Great mixed in your coffee.

~Freeze leftovers to reheat later.

~Garnish with a sprinkle of cinnamon and cinnamon sticks.

~Add ½ tsp pure peppermint extract and garnish with GF candy canes or peppermint sticks for yummy peppermint patties!

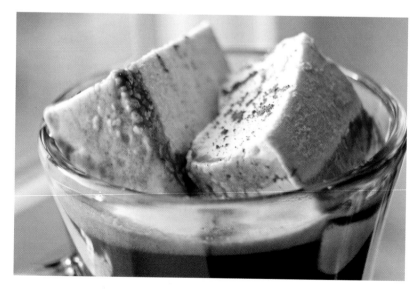

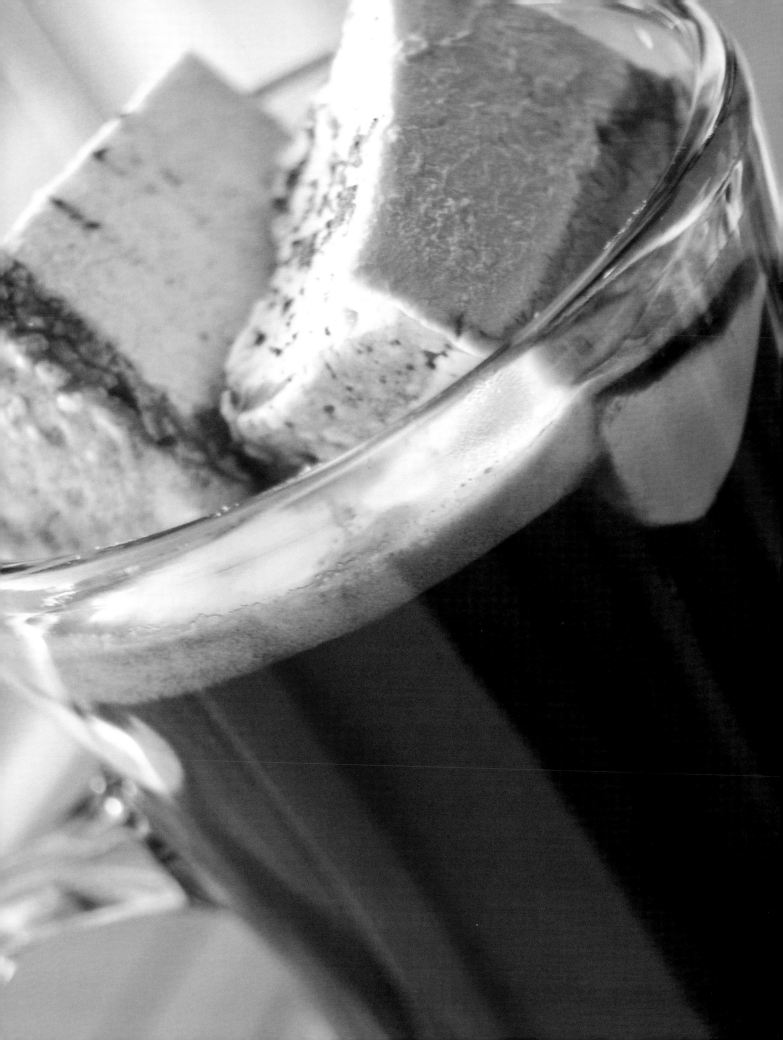

Pumpkin Martini

The first time we made these martinis at Thanksgiving everyone responded the same way, "Pumpkin in a martini?" It didn't sound great, but we gave it a go anyway, and we are so glad we did! They were a hit and we've made them every year since. The combination of orange, pumpkin, and cinnamon make a really unique and delicious pre-meal drink.

~	Ice
1	oz (30 mL) GF vodka, chilled
1	oz (30 mL) GF vanilla liqueur
1½	oz (45 mL) organic orange juice
1	Tbsp organic pumpkin puree (canned pumpkin)
~	Pinch of cinnamon
~	Pinch of nutmeg

1. Fill a cocktail shaker with ice.
2. Add the vodka, vanilla liqueur, orange juice, pumpkin puree, and a pinch of cinnamon.
3. Shake well and strain into a cocktail or martini glass.
4. Garnish with a pinch of nutmeg.

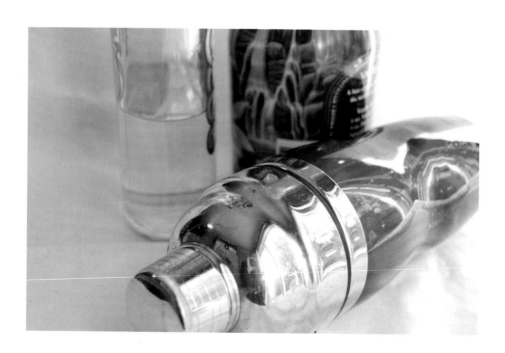

Beverages

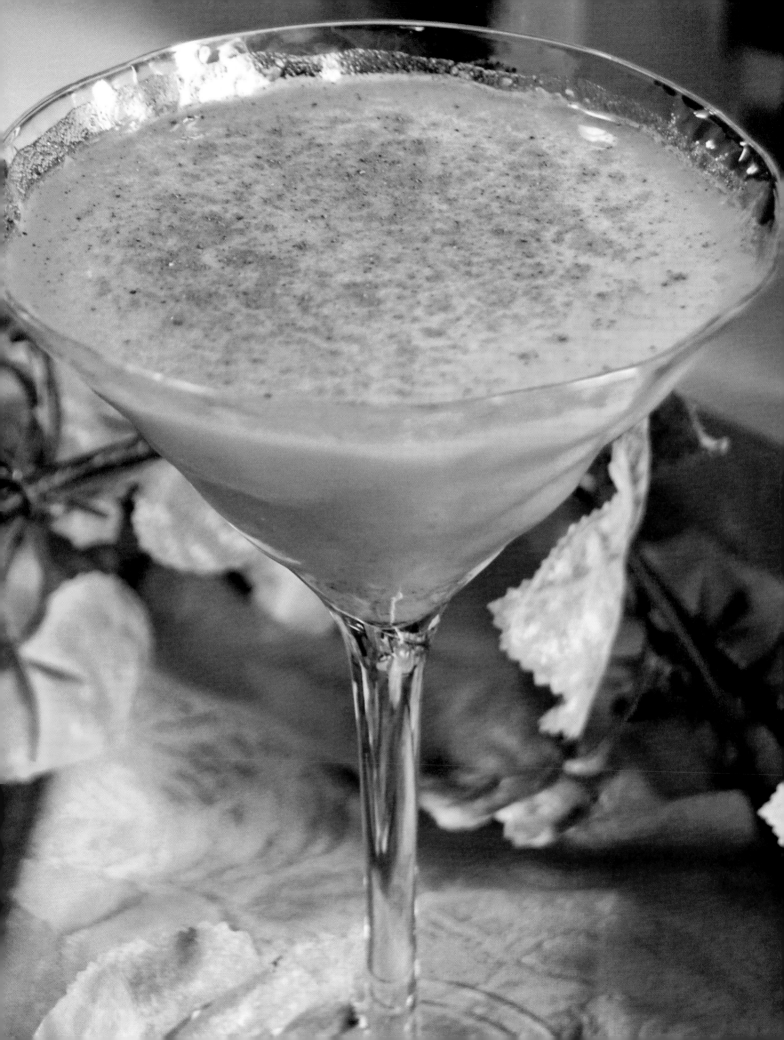

School Lunches

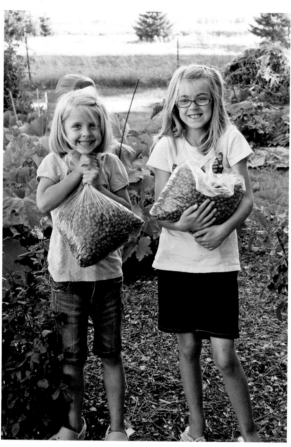

When it comes to school lunches, most parents stand, staring at the fridge at 7 AM trying to figure out what to shove into that tiny box. We don't usually put a lot of thought into school lunches because, let's face it, life is busy and dinner is enough to think about during the week. That's when the prepackaged food-like items get purchased—in a moment of exhausted weakness at the supermarket. But when you have kids with food intolerances, this isn't an option. That's a good thing! I'm not sure Lunchables and Twinkies should be options, nor am I certain they are technically food.

So now we know we need real food, but how many things can we make that are sim-ple and quick? The options are endless . . . but you don't need them to be.

I'm not sure how we parents got into the habit of believing our kids needed a huge variety for their lunches. Kids are pretty habitual creatures, and trust me, they don't mind eating the same thing over and over if it's something they like. My advice is to find those few things they love that are healthy and acceptable, and let 'em have at it all week. Kids do not need a menu of choices each and every day for lunch.

At my house, we keep a list on the fridge of seven or eight lunches that my kids like, and that's what we rotate through. Changing a veggie or fruit in their lunches keeps things interesting enough. You don't need to cook a gourmet meal each morning. And if you need proof, ask your kids what they want for lunch and I can guarantee they will list the same four or so items.

There are a few accessories that will help with the lunchtime conundrum. First, buy a wide-mouth food bottle (a.k.a. Thermos). The school year is through the winter, in most parts of the country, and it's oh so easy to fill that thing with soups and leftovers. Also, let your kids pick out a cool lunch carrier. We have moved way beyond the metal and plastic lunchboxes of our youth, so get online and check out the array of cool lunch carriers out there. Here are a couple of my favorites:

Laptop Lunches:	http://www.laptoplunches.com
LunchBots:	http://lunchbots.com
PackIt:	http://www.packit.com
Thermos:	http://www.thermos.com/product_catalog.aspx?CatCode=FOOD

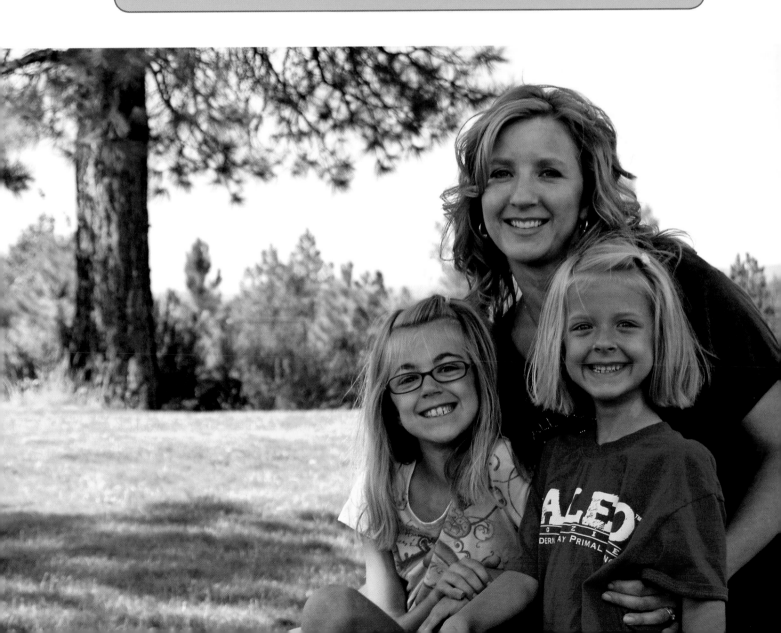

To help you along, here is a week's worth of school lunches that we use all year long:

Monday: Ham Roll Ups (GF Ham rolled around lettuce, carrot sticks and non-dairy cheese. Or use any sliced veggies they love!), sliced cucumbers, small organic apple.

Tuesday: Chicken GF Noodle Soup (p. 132), ½ slice Pumpkin Bread (p. 314).

Wednesday: Hot Dogs (Applegate Farms organic grass-fed hot dogs. Cook hot dogs in the morning and place in a warmed wide-mouth food jar. Stays hot until lunchtime!), with ketchup for dipping, carrot sticks, and tangerine.

Thursday: Citrus Chicken Pasta Salad (p. 142), small chocolate chip cookie (p. 274).

Friday: PB & F (p. 96) on an English Muffin (p. 88) or Sandwich Bread (p. 384), sliced peppers, a piece or two of organic beef jerky.

And when it comes to your child's school, you need to be a fairly loud voice regarding your concerns and expectations for your child's care. No one will protect your child or be as aware of their needs as you will. Schools are extremely understaffed and overworked. Teachers and administrators need education before they can possibly understand the extent to which food allergies affect our kids. Don't be afraid to speak up and speak up often. Be there at every party and function. Be your child's advocate at school! If they know you are present constantly, they will be more likely to pay attention to your needs. It's easy to forget a child's needs when they are feeding 400, so be noisy about it!

Ingredient Index

Almond Butter, 296, 310, 362, 377

Almond Meal, 150, 164, 276, 280, 288, 310, 318, 348, 384

Almonds, 48, 104, 116, 280, 296, 368, 374

Amaranth Flour, 192, 274, 278, 284, 302, 304, 384, 388, 392

Apples, 50, 60, 62, 76, 234, 358, 378

Artichokes, 128, 216

Avocado, 56, 174, 176, 196, 266

Bacon, 78, 140, 176, 206, 236, 244

Bananas, 82, 316, 347, 354, 359, 377-378

Beef, Ground, 70, 84, 150, 156, 162, 164

Beef, Hot Dogs, 190, 194

Beef, Short Ribs, 152

Beef, Steaks, 154, 160, 262

Beef Flank Steak, 148, 158

Black Beans, 196, 238

Black Olives, 184

Blueberries, 54, 58, 68, 92, 396

Broccoli, 236

Brown Rice, 206, 222

Brown Rice Flour, 58, 60, 62, 72, 74, 76, 80, 82, 88, 90, 92, 94, 182, 192, 218, 224, 280, 286, 294, 300, 302, 304, 314, 318, 320, 328, 330, 336, 340, 348, 350, 356, 388, 392

Brussels Sprouts, 220

Butternut Squash, 198

Cabbage, 104, 204, 228

Capers, 128, 186

Carrots, 62, 104, 116, 118, 132, 152, 172, 230, 234, 240, 268

Cauliflower, 214

Celery, 132, 138, 142, 144, 152, 184, 234, 268

"Cheese", 78, 174, 178, 196, 244, 388

"Cream Cheese", 170, 314

Cherries, 312, 344, 347, 375, 378

Chicken, 100, 102, 104, 106, 108, 110, 112, 114, 116, 118, 120, 122, 124, 126, 128, 130, 132, 134, 136, 138, 140, 142, 144, 188, 206, 268

Chocolate Chips, 274, 278, 280, 284, 296, 298, 306, 309-310, 332, 336, 344, 359-360, 362, 366, 368, 374-375, 378, 408

Chocolate Sandwich Cookies, 334, 342

Cocoa Powder, 280, 284, 304, 306, 310, 324, 326, 330, 336, 377

Coconut, 62, 82, 106, 276, 278, 288, 290, 296, 309-310, 312, 320, 359, 374-375, 377

Coconut Aminos, 102, 104, 112, 116, 120, 134, 136, 158, 160, 180, 206, 212, 228, 238

Coconut Butter, 310

Coconut Flour, 106, 162, 164, 234, 276, 290, 310, 380, 384

Coconut Milk, 72, 74, 76, 80, 86, 162,

198, 218, 244, 320, 332, 342, 344, 346, 352, 354, 378, 380, 396, 398, 400, 402, 408

Coconut Nectar, 92, 94, 252, 342, 344, 346, 348, 380, 398, 400, 403-404, 407

Coffee, 336, 338, 407

Corn Meal, 190

Corn Tortillas, 174, 196

Cranberries, 94, 136, 252, 286, 312, 318, 374

Cucumbers, 116, 184, 226, 396

Dark Chocolate, 306, 359, 378

Dates, 310, 312

Golden Syrup, 364, 382

Grapes, 138

Green Beans, 212

Green Onions, 102, 104, 114, 116, 138, 142, 170, 180, 198, 206, 244

Halibut, 182

Jam or Jelly, 74, 80, 108

Kalamata Olives, 392

Kale, 144

Leek, 198, 234

Mango, 166

Marshmallows, 308

Masa Harina, 232

Millet Flour, 58, 316, 322, 324, 328, 386

Molasses, 384

Mushrooms, 110, 116, 162, 170, 234, 242

Nectarine, 398

Nondairy Butter, 82, 96, 126, 208, 244, 270-271, 274, 276, 278, 280, 282, 284, 286, 288, 292, 294, 300, 306, 308-310, 322, 324, 326, 328, 330, 336, 338-339, 340, 350, 354, 382-383

Palm Shortening, 80, 192, 359, 362, 366, 368, 388, 392

Pasta, 132, 142, 178, 184

Pea Flour, 356, 384

Peaches, 96, 350

Peanut Butter, 96, 292, 298, 308, 366

Peas, 104, 206, 230

Pecans, 54, 60, 76, 82, 234, 278, 282, 306, 348, 354, 370, 374,

Pineapple, 166, 174, 347, 378

Pinto Beans, 238

Pistachios, 220

Pomegranate Seeds, 220

Popcorn, 372

Poppy Seeds, 255, 340, 386

Pork, Ground, 84, 164

Pork, Ham, 64, 206

Pork, Italian Sausage, 150, 170, 234

Pork Chops, 166, 174

Pork Roast, 168, 172

Pork Tenderloin, 264

Potato Chips, 126

Potato Flour, 384

Potatoes, 56, 172, 198, 244

Pretzels, GF, 296, 374-375

Pumpkin Seeds, 198, 290, 309, 312, 375-376

Pumpkin, canned, 82

Quinoa, 48, 50, 52, 54, 282

Radishes, 116, 184

Raisins, 52, 62, 90, 236, 282, 290, 296, 309, 312, 372, 374-375

Rhubarb, 403

Salmon, 180, 186

Sesame Seeds, 102, 104, 116, 154, 180, 206, 309, 386

Shrimp, 178, 184, 188, 206

Sorghum Flour, 58, 60, 66, 72, 74, 76, 80, 82, 86, 88, 90, 92, 94, 188, 192, 210,

224, 274, 278, 280, 282, 284, 286, 292, 294, 300, 302, 306, 314, 316, 318, 320, 322, 324, 328, 330, 336, 340, 350, 352, 384, 386, 388, 390, 392

Sparkling Water, 403

Spinach, 64, 78, 146

Strawberries, 48, 96, 271, 347, 378, 398, 400

Sugar Snap Peas, 104

Sunbutter, 96, 296, 298, 309, 362

Sunflower Seeds, 52, 290, 296, 312, 374

Sweet Potatoes, 64, 118, 210, 282

Teff Flour, 58, 60, 62, 66, 72, 74, 76, 82, 86, 88, 90, 92, 94, 210, 224, 274, 278, 284, 292, 294, 306, 314, 316, 318, 320, 322, 324, 328, 330, 336, 340, 350, 352, 356, 384, 386, 390

Tomato Paste, 134, 150, 156, 160, 172, 248, 251

Tomato Sauce, 134, 150, 156, 160, 248, 251

Tomatoes, 78, 174, 176, 178, 184, 196, 202, 222, 248

Turkey, Ground, 116, 146

Unflavored Gelatin, 364

Vanilla Ice Cream, 334, 360

Vanilla Liqueur, 410

Vodka, 410

Walnuts, 50, 62, 74, 122, 138, 142, 286, 316, 318

Water Chestnuts, 236

Watermelon, 406

Yeast, 88, 90, 92, 94, 192, 384, 388, 392

Zucchini, 56, 208, 242

Recipe Index

BREAKFASTS

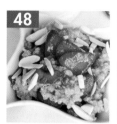
48 Vanilla Honey Quinoa with Strawberries & Almonds

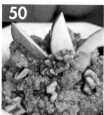
50 Apple Cinnamon Quinoa

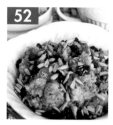
52 Brown Sugar & Cinnamon Quinoa

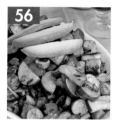
54 Maple Pecan Quinoa with Blueberries

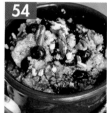
56 Sausage Veggie Hash

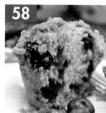
58 Blueberry Crumb Muffins

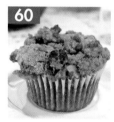
60 Apple Crisp Muffins

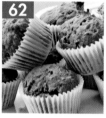
62 Morning Glory Muffins

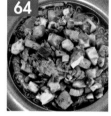
64 Hammin' it up Morning Scramble

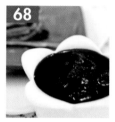
66 Pancakes

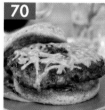
68 A Better Blueberry Syrup

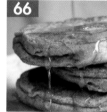
70 Quick Breakfast Sausage

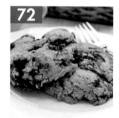
72 Teff Scones

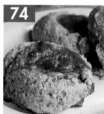
74 Strawberry Walnut Scones

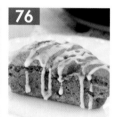
76 Apple Cinnamon Scones

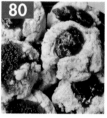
78 Breakfast Stack

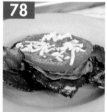
80 Jellied Biscuits

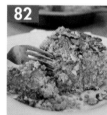
82 Banana Crumb Coffee Cake

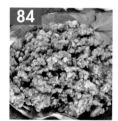
84 Homemade Chorizo

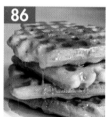
86 Waffles

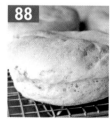
88 Famous Celiac Maniac English Muffins

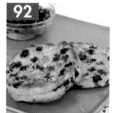
90 Cinnamon Raisin English Muffins

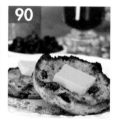
92 Blueberry English Muffins

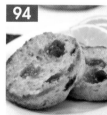
94 Cranberry Orange English Muffins

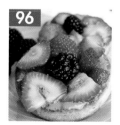
96 Breakfast PB & F

ENTRÉES

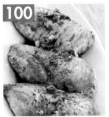
100
Balsamic Chicken

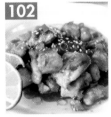
102
Ginger Lime Chicken Bites

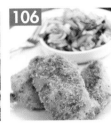
104
Oriental Chicken Salad

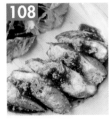
106
Coconut Chicken Strips

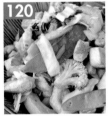
108
Raspberry Glazed Chicken

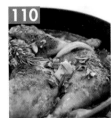
110
Skillet Rosemary Chicken

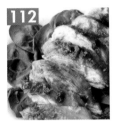
112
Citrus Ginger Chicken

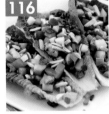
114
Grilled Lime Chicken

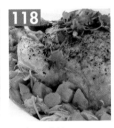
116
P.F. Chicken Lettuce Cups (as in, Pretty Fantastic!)

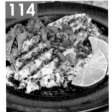
118
Crock Pot Chicken

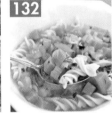
120
Sweet and Sour Chicken Stir Fry

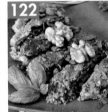
122
Walnut Basil Chicken

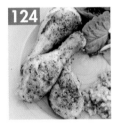
124
Baked Chicken Legs

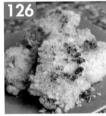
126
Chippy Chicken Thighs

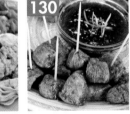
128
Lemon Artichoke Chicken Piccata

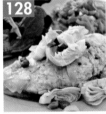
130
Garlic Rosemary Chicken Bites

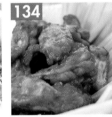
132
Classic Chicken Noodle Soup

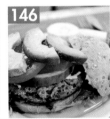
134
Chicken Wings

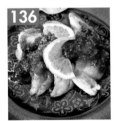
136
Cranberry Chicken Fingers

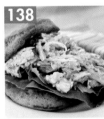
138
My Favorite Chicken Salad

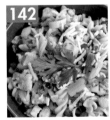
140
Bacon Wrapped Chicken Bites

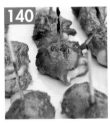
142
Citrus Chicken Pasta Salad

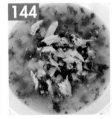
144
Rosemary Kale Chicken Soup

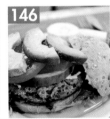
146
Favorite Turkey Burgers

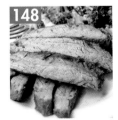
148
Flank Steak Rub

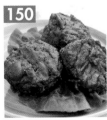
150
Mini Meatloaves

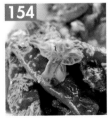
152
Holy Cow! Short Ribs

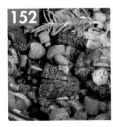
154
Grilled Marinated Tri-Tip

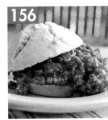
156
Sloppy Joes

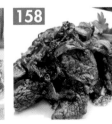
158
Quick Burgundy Beef w/Caramelized Onions

The Healthy Gluten-Free Life

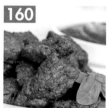
160 Steak Bites

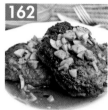
162 Salisbury Steak w/Mushroom Gravy

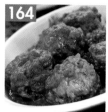
164 Italian Meatballs

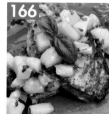
166 Pork Chops w/Pineapple Mango Salsa

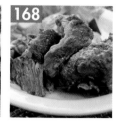
168 Dutch Oven Pork Roast

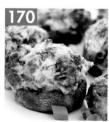
170 Stuffed Mushrooms

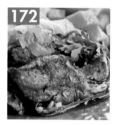
172 Garlicky Crock Pot Pork Roast

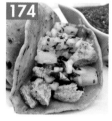
174 Pork Tacos w/Pineapple Salsa

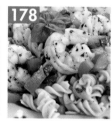
176 BLAT's To Go (Bacon, Lettuce, Avocado & Tomato)

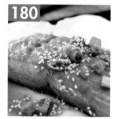
178 Shrimp Basil Pasta

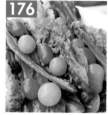
180 Ginger Salmon

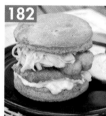
182 Filet O' GF Fish Sandwiches

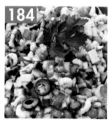
184 Bay Shrimp Veggie Salad

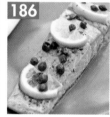
186 Baked Lemon Caper Salmon

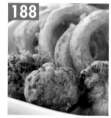
188 Batter Mix

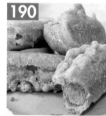
190 Corn Dogs

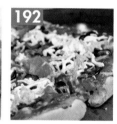
192 Pizza Crust

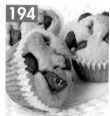
194 Corn Dog Cupcakes

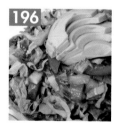
196 Black Bean Tostadas

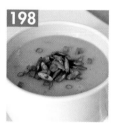
198 Butternut Squash Soup

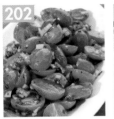
Cherry Tomato Salad

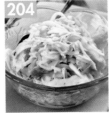
Simple Slaw

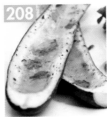
Fried Rice

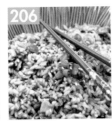
Zucchini Boats

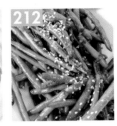
Sweet Potato Biscuits

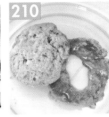
Garlicky Green Beans

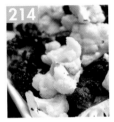
Roasted Cauliflower

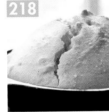
Artichokes
with Garlic Dill Mayo

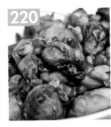
Cornbread

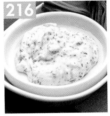
Pan-Roasted Brussels
Sprouts

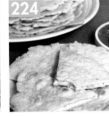
Spanish Rice

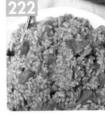
Flour Tortillas

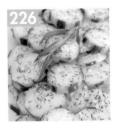
Cucumber Salad

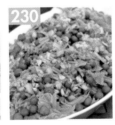
Sweet and Sour Cabbage

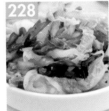
Easy Peasy Carrot Salad

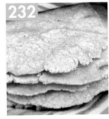
Corn Tortillas

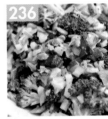
Sausage Veggie Stuffing

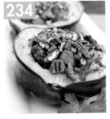
Broccoli Salad

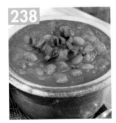
Easy Beans

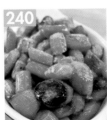
Honey Glazed Carrots

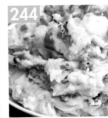
Zucchini with Mushrooms

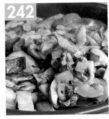
Famous Mashed Potatoes

SAUCES/RUBS/DRESSINGS/MISC.

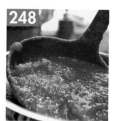
248 Spaghetti (and Pizza) Sauce

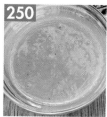
250 Honey Mustard Dipping Sauce

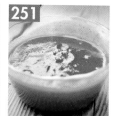
251 BBQ Sauce

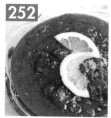
252 Sugar-Free Cranberry Sauce

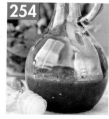
254 Balsamic Vinaigrette

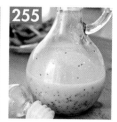
255 Poppy Seed Dressing

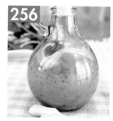
256 Garlic Vinaigrette

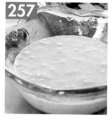
257 Cranberry Vinaigrette

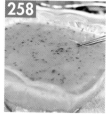
258 Italian Vinaigrette

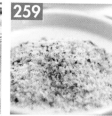
259 Salad Seasoning

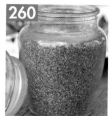
260 Taco Seasoning

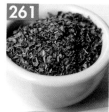
261 Italian Seasoning

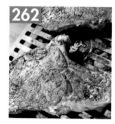
262 Steak Rub

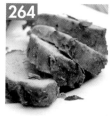
264 Pork Tenderloin Rub

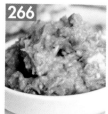
266 Speedy Guacamole

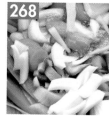
268 Shortcut Chicken Stock

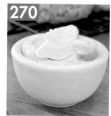
270 Honey Butter

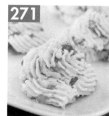
271 Strawberry Honey Butter
A Christmas morning treat!

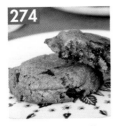
274 As Needed Chocolate Chip Cookies

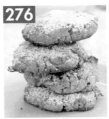
276 Grain-Free Lemon Cookies

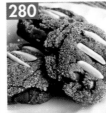
278 High Desert Cookies

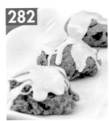
280 Chocolate Almond Cookies

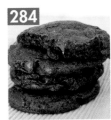
282 Sweet Potato Spice Cookie

284 Double Trouble Chocolate Chip Cookies

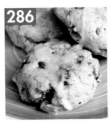
286 Cranberry Walnut Cookies

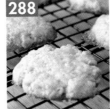
288 Almond Orange Coconut Cookies

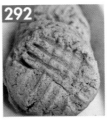
290 No'Oatmeal Raisin Cookies

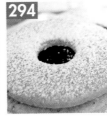
292 Peanut Butter Cookies

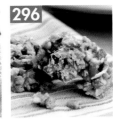
294 Sugar Cookies

296 No Bake Cookies

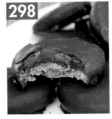
298 Sunbutter Patty Tagalongs

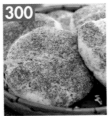
300 Snickerdoodles

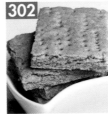
302 Graham Crackers

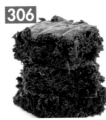
304 Chocolate Graham Crackers

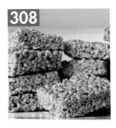
306 Fudgy Brownies

308 Cocoa Rice Crisp Squares

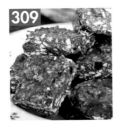
309 Chunky Cocoa Crisp Snack Bars

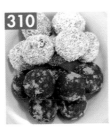
310 Almond Butter Nut Balls

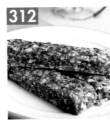
312 Macadamia Bars

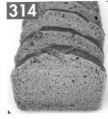
314 Pumpkin Bread

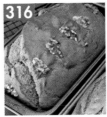
316 Banana Bread

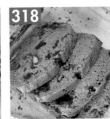
318 Cranberry Walnut Bread

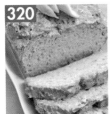
320 Orange Olive Oil Bread

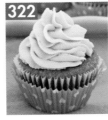
322 Vanilla Cupcakes

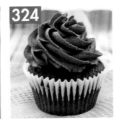
324 Chocolate Cupcakes

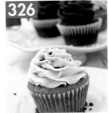
326 Vanilla / Chocolate Buttercream Frosting

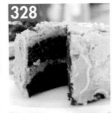
328 Easy-Bake Oven Mix Vanilla Cake

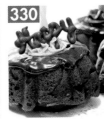
330 Birthday Bundts

BAKING/DESSERTS/SNACKS

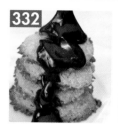
332 Chocolate Ganache

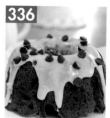
334 Flower Pot Cakes

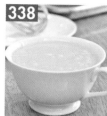
336 Java Chip Bundt

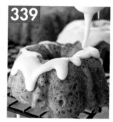
338 Mocha Java Glaze

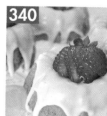
339 Lemon Icing

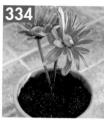
340 Lemon Poppy Seed Bundt

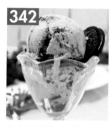
342 Cookies 'n' Cream Coconut Milk Ice Cream

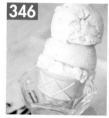
344 Chocolate Cherry Almond Ice Cream

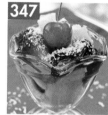
346 Vanilla Ice Cream

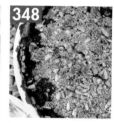
347 Frozen Banana Splits

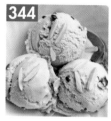
348 Berry Crisp

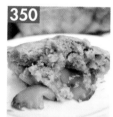
350 Peach Cobbler

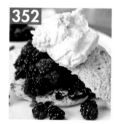
352 Shortcakes

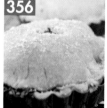
354 Pecan Praline Bananas

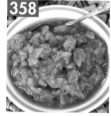
356 Pie Crust

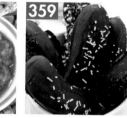
358 Pie Apples (a.k.a. Cooked Apples)

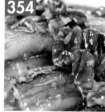
359 Frozen Chocolate Dipped Bananas

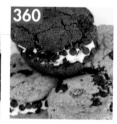
360 Ice Cream Sandwiches

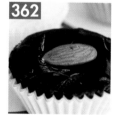
362 Butter Cups

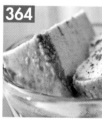
364 Homemade 'Shmallows

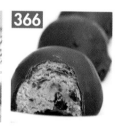
366 Cookie Doh Bites I'm sorry.

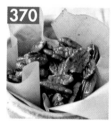
368 Nut Clusters

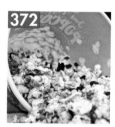
370 Spiced Maple Pecans

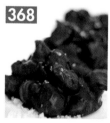
372 Cinnamon Sugar Popcorn

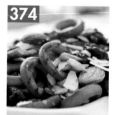
374 Makenna's Mix

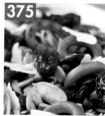
375 Rilee's Mish Mash Mix

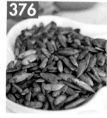
376 Toasted Pumpkin Seeds

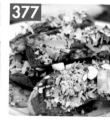
377 Coco Loco Bananas

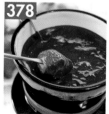
378 Chocolate Fondue

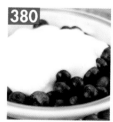
380 Coconut Whipped Cream

BAKING/DESSERTS/SNACKS

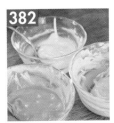
382 Sugar Cookie Icing

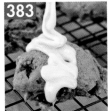
383 Maple Glaze

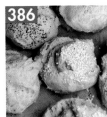
384 Sandwich Bread

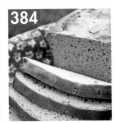
386 No-Yeast Quick Rolls

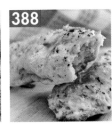
388 Breadsticks

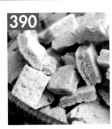
390 Quick Bread Crumbs/Cubes

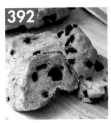
392 Kalamata Mini French Bread

BEVERAGES

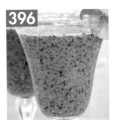
396 Cool as a Cucumber Blueberry Smoothie

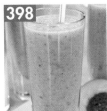
398 Strawberry Nectarine Smoothie

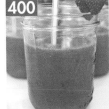
400 Strawberry Smoothie

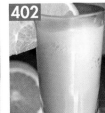
402 Orange Manius

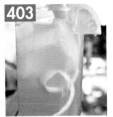
403 Rhubarb Lemonade Spritzer

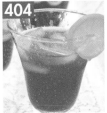
404 Pink Lemonade

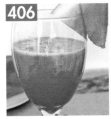
406 Watermelon Juice

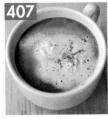
407 Quick Pumpkin Latte

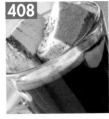
408 Hot Cocoa

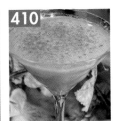
410 Pumpkin Martini

Resource Index

Azure Standard	http://www.azurestandard.com	Extracts, honey, yeast, maple syrup, sea salt, cocoa powder, canned pumpkin, coconut oil, sucanat, baking powder, baking soda, Spectrum organic palm shortening, gallon glass storage jars
Costco	http://www.costco.com	Organic applesauce, McCormick Spices, organic evaporated cane juice, organic raisins, organic almond butter
Bob's Red Mill	http://www.bobsredmill.com	Sorghum, brown rice, amaranth, potato starch, tapioca starch, arrowroot, coconut flour, almond meal, millet, pea flour, golden flaxseeds, xanthan gum
Earth Balance	http://www.azurestandard.com	Soy free "butter" or vegan buttery sticks
Lodge Cast Iron	http://lodgemfg.com	Cast iron cookware
US Wellness Meats	http://www.grasslandbeef.com	Grass-fed, pastured meats
Really Raw Honey	http://www.reallyrawhoney.com/	Raw, unprocessed honey
Teff Co	http://www.teffco.com	Maskal Ivory Teff Flour
Whole Foods	http://www.wholefoodsmarket.com	Quinoa flour, organic brown sugar, organic powdered sugar, red wine vinegar, balsamic vinegar, poppy seeds, sesame seeds, Spectrum organic palm shortening, olive oil, coconut oil

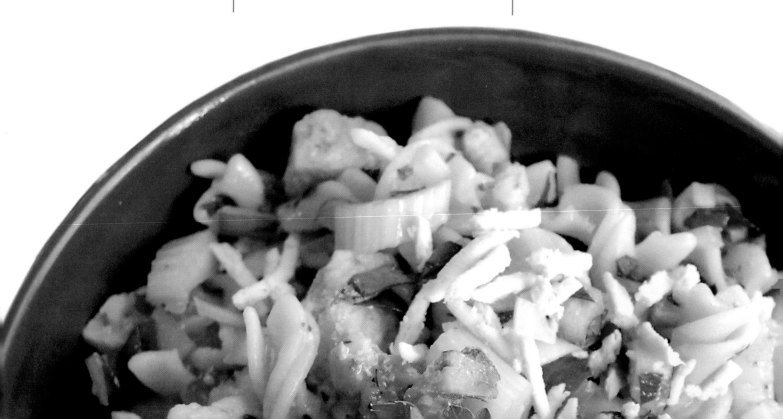

Trader Joes	http://www.traderjoes.com	Canned coconut milk, chocolate chips, dark chocolate, olive oil, nuts, seeds, organic fruits and veggies, sun butter
Coconut Secret	http://www.coconutsecret.com	Coconut aminos, coconut nectar, coconut crystals, coconut flour
Bragg	http://www.bragg.com	Liquid aminos, apple cider vinegar
Daiya	http://www.daiyafoods.com	Non dairy, casein free cheeses
Authentic Foods	http://authenticfoods.com	Xanthan Gum
Wright's Natural Hickory Seasoning Liquid Smoke	http://www.bgfoods.com/wrights/	
Let's do organic	http://edwardandsons.com/ldo_shop_coconut.html	Coconut flakes, shredded coconut, coconut butter, Sprinkelz (jimmies), ice cream cones
Enjoy life	http://www.enjoylifefoods.com	Mini chocolate chips
McCormick	http://www.mccormick.com/	Spices, but not spice blends, as they do not guarantee their blends are free of gluten. The straight spices are gluten-free.
Turtle Mountain/So Delicious	http://www.turtlemountain.com	Coconut milk: beverages, kefir, ice cream, yogurt
Glutino	http://www.glutino.com/our-products/snacks/cookies/chocolate-vanilla-creme-cookies	Chocolate vanilla sandwich cookies
Wilderness Family Naturals	http://www.wildernessfamilynaturals.com	Coconut oil and coconut products
Tropical Traditions	http://www.tropicaltraditions.com	Coconut oil, organic unrefined red palm oil
Eat Wild	http://eatwild.com	
Weston A. Price Foundation	http://www.westonaprice.org	
Local Farmer's Markets	http://www.localharvest.org	
Local CSA (community supported agriculture)	http://www.localharvest.org/csa	
Your local GIG group	http://www.gluten.net	
The Healthy Gluten-Free Life	www.thehealthyglutenfreelife.com	
Help Finding a CSA	www.nal.usda.gov/afsic/pubs/csa/csa.shtml	
Help Finding a CSA	www.eatwellguide.org	

Research Index

(1) Jefferson, W. N., E. Padilla-Banks, and R. R. Newbold. (2007). Disruption of the developing female reproductive system by phytoestrogens: Genistein as an example. *Molecular Nutrition and Food Research*, 51(7): 832–844. doi:10.1002/mnfr.200600258

(2) Jefferson, W.N., D. Doerge, E. Padilla-Banks, K. A. Woodling, G. E. Kissling, and R, Newbold. (2009). Oral exposure to Genistin, the glycosylated form of Genistein, during neonatal life adversely affects the female reproductive system. *Environmental Health Perspectives*, 117, 12, 1883–1889. doi:10.1289/ehp.0900923.S1

(3) Chavarro, J. E., T. L. Toth, S. M. Sadio, and R. Hauser. (2008). Soy food and isoflavone intake in relation to semen quality parameters among men from an infertility clinic. *Human Reproduction*, 23(11): 2584–2590. doi:10.1093/humrep/den243

(4) Van Duursen, M. B. M., and S. M. Nijmeijer. (2011). Genistein induces breast cancer-associated aromatase and stimulates estrogen-dependent tumor cell growth in *in vitro* breast cancer model. *Toxicology*, 289(2–3): 67–73. doi:10.1016/j.tox.2011.07.005

(5) Arentz-Hansen, H., and B. Fleckenstein. (2004). The molecular basis for oat intolerance in celiac disease patients. *PLoS Medicine*, 1, 1, 6. doi:10.1371/journal.pmed.0010023

(6) This concept, known as glycemic load, was first popularized in 1997 by Dr. Walter Willett and associates at the Harvard School of Public Health.

(7) Lim, Jung; Michele Mietus-Snyder, Annie Valente, Jean-Marc Schwarz, and Robert H. Lustig (May 2010). The role of fructose in the pathogenesis of naFlD and the metabolic syndrome. *Nature Reviews Gastroenterology & Hepatology* 7(5): 251–264. doi:10.1038/nrgastro.2010.41. http://www.nature.com/nrgastro/journal/v7/n5/full/nrgastro.2010.41.html.

(8) Stanhope, K. L. (2009). Consuming fructose-sweetened, not glucose-sweetened, beverages increases visceral adiposity and lipids and decreases insulin sensitivity in overweight/obese humans. *Journal of Clinical Investigation*, 5(119): 1322–1334. doi:10.1172/JCI37385.

(9) Kretowicz, M. (2011). The impact of fructose on renal function and blood pressure. *International Journal of Nephrology*. doi:10.4061/2011/315879

(10) Ouyang, X. (2008). Fructose consumption as a risk factor for non-alcoholic fatty liver disease. *Journal of Hepatology*, 48(6): 993–999.

(11) http://www.naturesblessings.com.ph/cocosugar.htm

(12) http://www.canolacouncil.org/facts_gmo.aspx

About the Author

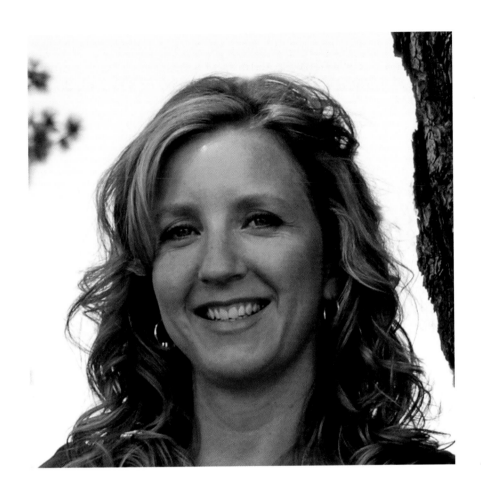

Tammy Credicott is a part-time blogger, full time entrepreneur, the wife of a Celiac (affectionately called The Maniac), and mom to two girls with gluten, dairy, and egg intolerances.

Tammy lives in Bend, Oregon, where she created the successful gluten-free, dairy-free, egg-free wholesale bakery, *The Celiac Maniac*. A self-taught home cook extraordinaire and *Food Network* junkie, she has transformed her family's health with the creation of simple, healthy, allergy-friendly recipes that fit their busy lifestyle. And in her spare time, Tammy likes to help her husband, The Maniac, with recipes and photography for his newly published *Paleo Magazine*, a publication dedicated to a naturally gluten-free lifestyle based on ancestral health science.

Visit **www.thehealthyglutenfreelife.com.**

Recipe Notes

Recipe Notes

Recipe Notes